Defending Standardized Testing

Defending Standardized Testing

edited by

Richard P. Phelps

LAWRENCE ERLBAUM ASSOCIATES, PUBLISHERS
2005   Mahwah, New Jersey   London

Lawrence Erlbaum Associates, Inc., Publishers
10 Industrial Avenue
Mahwah, New Jersey 07430
www.erlbaum.com

Cover design by Kathryn Houghtaling Lacey

Library of Congress Cataloging-in-Publication Data

Defending standardized testing / edited by Richard P. Phelps.
        p. cm.
    Includes bibliographical references and index.
ISBN 0-8058-4911-4 (cloth : alk. paper)
ISBN 0-8058-4912-2 (pbk. : alk. paper)
1. Achievement tests—United States. 2. Education—Standards—United
    States.   3. Educational accountability—United States.   I. Phelps,
    Richard P.
LB3060.3.D44   2004
371.26'2—dc22
                                                            2004053779
                                                            CIP

Books published by Lawrence Erlbaum Associates are printed on acid-free paper, and their bindings are chosen for strength and durability.

Printed in the United States of America
10 9 8 7 6 5 4 3 2 1

Contents

Foreword   vii

Introduction and Overview   xi

1   Persistently Positive: Forty Years of Public Opinion   1
on Standardized Testing
Richard P. Phelps

2   High-Stakes Testing: Contexts, Characteristics,   23
Critiques, and Consequences
Gregory J. Cizek

3   The Rich, Robust Research Literature on Testing's   55
Achievement Benefits
Richard P. Phelps

4   Some Misconceptions About Large-Scale Educational   91
Assessments
Dean Goodman and Ronald K. Hambleton

5   The Most Frequently *Unasked* Questions About Testing   111
Stephen G. Sireci

6 Must High Stakes Mean Low Quality? Some Testing   123
Program Implementation Issues
George K. Cunningham

7 Whose Rules? The Relation Between the "Rules"   147
and "Law" of Testing
Chad W. Buckendahl and Robert Hunt

8 Teaching For the Test: How and Why Test Preparation   159
is Appropriate
Linda Crocker

9 Doesn't Everybody Know That 70% is Passing?   175
Barbara S. Plake

10 The Testing Industry, Ethnic Minorities,   187
and Individuals With Disabilities
Kurt F. Geisinger

11 A School Accountability Case Study: California API   205
Awards and the *Orange County Register* Margin
of Error Folly
David Rogosa

12 Leave No Standardized Test Behind   227
Mary Lyn Bourque

Appendix A: Polls and Surveys That Have Included   255
Items About Standardized Testing: 1954 to Present

Appendix B: Some Studies Revealing Testing   281
Achievement Benefits, by Methodology Type

Author Index   331

Subject Index   337

Foreword:
The Rest of the Story

John Fremer

Founder, Caveon Test Security, Washington Crossing, PA

If you rely on the media for information about standardized testing, then this book offers a much-needed "rest of the story." All too frequently, a press report begins with a set of factual statements about a testing program, followed by overwhelmingly negative comments about the test, the use under discussion, and the overall value of standardized testing. The sources most often cited are individuals or groups that are fundamentally opposed to all the major applications of high-stakes testing in school and society.

Why is it that so much commentary about testing comes from its critics rather than its supporters? I believe part of the reason to be that those who develop tests or conduct testing research focus primarily on their own tests or research and not on presenting a case for testing in the media. Some of the largest companies in the field do employ communications staff charged with building and maintaining a positive view of their employer. These individuals, however, are viewed (with good reason) as spokespersons for the testing companies, and not as independent observers of the testing scene. The professors who conduct research on testing and train future generations of testing professionals might be viewed as able commentators, but they are not well known to reporters, and it is no one's job to circulate lists of these professors so their voices can be heard. To bring some balance into the public discussion of testing, we need some means for the public to find the words of those who truly understand testing, but who have no axe to grind. This describes well the volunteer mission accepted by Richard Phelps for the past several years, and the raison d'être of Defending Standardized Testing.

Phelps has challenged an extraordinarily distinguished group of senior testing professionals to make the case for testing. The result, however, is not the kind of one-sided presentation in which the critics of testing most often engage. This book's contributors recognize that test making is difficult and that testing programs can have flaws, just like everything else humanity produces. *Defending Standardized Testing's* authors, however, make a very strong case for the beneficial value of well-developed tests.

Basically, testing is a systematic means of collecting information. Analyzing thoughtfully what kind of information might be helpful, and then obtaining it, helps one to make a better decision. This is just as true where standardized tests are used as it is in other venues. The person who carefully researches competing products and reads informed reviews of product effectiveness increases the probability of a wise purchase. The employer who creates an internship program where prospective employees perform tasks similar to those of regular employees will make more informed hiring decisions than one who relies on "gut instinct" to choose new hires.

As someone who has been collecting criticisms of testing for more than 40 years, I appreciate this book's seminal contribution to the story of testing. I hope readers become a bit more skeptical of the extravagant negative comments often presented in the press as "proven facts," rather than highly slanted perspective. Readers have an opportunity here to review thoughtful analyses derived from a scholarly, not an adversarial, perspective.

Testing critics, unfortunately, tend to rely on the rhetorical style of the legal and political professions. One presents only those snippets of information that favor's one's own case, leaving to the other side the job of presenting its best case. This style can work in the courtroom when both sides are represented by counsel of equal skill and commitment. Whether it works effectively in the political arena is, perhaps, more debatable.

Presenting a complete analysis is the rhetorical method of responsible academics and researchers. One presents all salient points on an issue, acknowledging merit in opposing positions. It is even possible to show respect for those with whom one disagrees, recognizing that one's own perspective could change over time with the acquisition of new information and more experience.

In closing, I must acknowledge that I have spent more than 40 years working in the mainstream of standardized testing. I have worked for the largest non-profit testing company, Educational Testing Service, and the largest commercial test publisher, now known as Harcourt Educational Measurement. I now am co-founder and executive of a company devoted exclusively to enhancing the security of high-stakes tests, Caveon Test

Security. I chose to work in the testing field immediately after completing my doctoral studies in educational psychology because I thought that standardized testing made the largest contribution to society of any of the fields I had studied. I have had that view confirmed many times, and I greatly appreciate the value of testing that is well conceived and well implemented.

To argue against good testing at the highest conceptual level, one needs to dismiss the idea that relevant information can lead to better decisions. This is a fundamentally weak position, no matter how often or how stridently it is stated.

Introduction

There is, perhaps, no issue more visible among current education reforms than standardized testing. Most reform efforts of the past couple of decades have attempted to raise academic standards and, often, testing is considered an essential component of the effort, necessary to prompt attainment of and gauge the extent to which standards are followed or attained. Some critics, however, view the push for standards and testing as precisely what ails American education. In this latter view, current calls for increased standards and testing are actually considered harmful. Those who assume such a perspective would diminish—or even extinguish—the presence of high-stakes educational achievement testing.

Through a broader lens, testing disputes can be seen as a clash of philosophical positions. One position advocates competition, rewards merit or accomplishment, embraces individual responsibilities and acknowledges individual differences. The other position discourages competition, rewards effort and process, embraces collective responsibilities, and strives for equity. Accordingly, adherents to the latter position view testing generally as an impediment to reform, an antiquated technology that reflects an antiquated view of teaching, learning, and social organization, perpetuates inequality, and serves the ends of cultural, political and educational oppression.

Likewise, opposition over standardized testing can be seen as a clash of interests. One position advocates measurement of the performance of public organizations, public disclosure of information, and the implementation of programs the public clearly wants. The other position asserts that measurement and disclosure unleash forces that pervert natural instructional processes and unnecessarily produce adversarial relationships between teacher and student, school and parent, and educators and the public.

Most of those with expertise in educational testing acknowledge its benefits in private conversation and sometimes in technical journals. But, we believe that those benefits have been insufficiently articulated in public discussions of testing. The success of the American educational system is not well served by the absence of an articulate defense of testing from the public square.

Meanwhile, the testing profession continues to advance the state of the art, improving tests' accuracy, dependability, and utility. Never before has obtaining such an abundance of accurate, rich, and useful information about student learning been possible.

WHERE WE COME IN

It has been our observation that many testing experts (a.k.a., psychometricians) tend to stick close to their trade, writing technically proficient research articles and instructional manuals. Goodness knows there is a need for such work, particularly in these testing times. Moreover, those testing experts most fond of their trade tend to practice it directly, working in test development at private firms or in test administration at government agencies. In either line of work, these testing proponents ordinarily are prohibited from expressing any opinions about testing policy. As contractors to governments, test development firms or individual consultants have no legitimate role in promoting public policies and would be foolish to do so (lest they alienate some faction in the political process for whom they may, one day, wish to work). As unelected public servants, state or local testing directors are obliged to execute the assessment policy of their elected superiors and guard their public statements, for fear of a lawsuit if they were to say the wrong thing. This tends to leave the more political discussions of testing policy to testing opponents, some of whom have testing expertise and some of whom have not.

Indeed, anyone interested in learning about standardized testing who reads the education policy literature first, may well see no reason to bother reading the more technical psychometric literature. Much education policy research condemns the use of any type of standardized testing the least bit controversial (e.g., with high-stakes, externally controlled, aptitude tests). Furthermore, after reading primers of the testing critics, the technical tomes of the psychometricians may well seem imposing.

As a result, a large number of articles and books have been written over the past decade on testing policy and the worth, or lack thereof, of standardized testing. Few of them have been written by measurement specialists who support the use of external, high-stakes standardized testing, the kind that is most controversial.

In an effort to fill this void, we have written *Defending Standardized Testing*, with the intention to:

1. document the public support for testing and the realized benefits of testing;
2. explain and refute some of the common criticisms of testing;
3. acknowledge the genuine limitations, and suggest improvements to testing practices;
4. provide guidance for structuring and administering large-scale testing programs in light of current public preferences and the federal No Child Left Behind Act requirements; and
5. present a vigorous defense of testing and practical vision for its promise and future.

WHY THIS BOOK?

To our knowledge, no book like this has ever before been written. Not only is there a need for this book to fill a void in education policy debates but, just as importantly, to explain the debate to nonspecialists interested in education reform. Accurate, factual, and current information about testing can be difficult to acquire for many reasons. For reasons of self-interest or adherence to an ideological position, some education researchers portray testing in an inaccurate manner. Journalists tend to report on testing in terms that lean toward the sensational and emphasize any untoward consequences of testing. Such reporting may be due to naiveté, expediency, ideological sympathy, convenience, the negative nature of news, or simply because well-reasoned counterpoints are unarticulated by those testing experts with whom they speak.

In being critical of the advocacy of those who would abandon testing, we admittedly assume a risk of being labeled advocates as well, albeit advocates *for* testing. We must admit that, to some extent, we are guilty as charged. There is no getting around it: *Defending Standardized Testing* is an "advocacy" book. What we advocate, however, is a balanced approach to the role of testing. Moreover, we believe—and we think that this belief is a foundational principle in healthy democratic republics—that the availability of well-reasoned positions capturing *both* perspectives on any issue is necessary for informed decision making.

So, this is both a "how to" and a "why to" book.

This is also an extremely well-informed book. Every author is both an accomplished researcher and practitioner. All of us hold PhDs. All of us have published extensively in technical journals. All of us have accumulated abundant experience working directly for government testing agencies or under contract to them. All of us are well-known nationally in education research circles.

As the more intrepid reader will discover, we do not agree on all points, and some of the current debates raging within the community of testing experts are represented in our book. Even what many outsiders might regard as the most confusing (or most bemusing) current debate in standardized-testing policy—that over item format—creeps into the book. One author firmly believes that only the demonstrably most reliable test item format—machine-scorable multiple choice—merits a legitimate place in high-stakes accountability systems. Other authors advocate the greater use of other item formats.

Although we do disagree on some points that most outside observers likely would perceive to be minor, we do agree on the major points. All of us, for example, advocate the use of standardized testing, even in high-stakes accountability systems, and believe that standardized tests represent a beneficial and, in certain circumstances, superior technology, one clearly better than all available alternatives.

ORGANIZATION AND OVERVIEW

Our book consists of twelve chapters. The first half comprises the "why to" section, the second half the "how to."

Only a few years ago, some education leaders and journalists frequently touted a "the public backlash" against standardized testing, as if it were a fact. Whatever happened to that backlash, Richard Phelps asks? The short answer is that there never was one. In "Persistently Positive: Forty Years of Public Opinion on Standardized Testing" (chap. 1), he digs through hundreds of surveys and polls from the 1960s to the present and summarizes not only the public's preferences on the topic but that of education providers as well.

The public does have some reservations about high-stakes testing when it is employed in certain extraordinary ways, but the underlying support for the systematic use of standardized testing for all its most common purposes has remained steadfast and strong for at least four decades. There does appear to be some diminution in support in recent years, particularly among teachers. Among education's consumers, however, most polls still show testing supporters outnumbering detractors by threefold or greater.

Many critiques of high-stakes testing for pupils in K–12 education have identified actual or potential negative consequences of typical mandated tests. However, there is actually scant evidence regarding a few of the asserted negative consequences, and no evidence of many of the others. More

importantly, in the literature on high-stakes testing, the positive consequences are routinely unaddressed.

In "High-Stakes Testing: Contexts, Characteristics, Critiques, and
Consequences" (chap. 2), Gregory Cizek documents some current controversies regarding the effects of high-stakes external testing, and compiles a
list of some of these positive consequences, their rationales, and the supporting evidence. Cizek argues that both positive and negative consequences should be recognized and weighed when crafting assessment
policy or evaluating the results of testing and accountability systems.

Peruse the press coverage and the more prominent education journals
over the past decade and one can easily find statements like "Despite the
long history of assessment-based accountability, hard evidence about its effects is surprisingly sparse, and the little evidence that is available is not encouraging." Unfortunately, many folk who do not know any better
sometimes believe such proclamations. So, Richard Phelps has exhumed
some of the research literature in "The Rich, Robust Research Literature on
Standardized Testing's Achievement Benefits" (chap. 3).

Standardized tests can produce at least three benefits: improved diagnosis (of student's strengths and weaknesses); improved prediction and selection (for college, scholarships, or employment) and; most controversial,
improved achievement. That is, do students in school systems with testing
programs learn more than their counterparts in school systems without?
An abundance of evidence demonstrates that they do.

Citing examples from their considerable experience in test program
implementation and evaluation in Massachusetts, Maryland, Virginia,
and Kentucky, with the National Assessment of Educational Progress,
and elsewhere, Dean Goodman and Ron Hambleton outline the most
prominent "Misconceptions About Large Scale Educational Assessments" (chap. 4). They specifically counter allegations that large-scale assessments: are too expensive and time consuming, are full of flaws and
biased against minorities, do not assess what is taught, over time are non-
equivalent, set standards too high, and often use only a single test to decide high school graduation.

"The Most Frequently Unasked Questions About Testing" (chap. 5)
helps make the transition from the "why to" focus to the "how to" focus of
the book. In his chapter, Stephen Sireci uses this framework to illustrate and
dispel myths about standardized testing. The five unasked questions are:
(1) What is a standardized test?; (2) What is reliability?; (3) What is validity?; (4) How are passing scores set on tests?; (5) Where can I get more
information about a test?

As Sireci illustrates, standardized tests are actually designed to promote fairness and to reconcile the important goals of reliability and validity. The chapter explains how, illustrates proper and improper methods

for setting passing scores, and tells people where to go for more information about a test.

Forty-eight out of 50 states have established high-stakes testing programs, which are being used to determine whether students have mastered state standards. Although much of the surrounding controversy focuses on whether such programs should be implemented at all, the technical qualities of the assessments are often not examined closely enough. In "Must High-Stakes Mean Low Quality?" (chap. 6) George Cunningham describes some better and worse ways of implementing a statewide, high-stakes assessment.

In some cases, problems arise because different groups, with different values and goals and very different ideas about tests, may be separately involved in the legal mandate, the assessment system design, its implementation, or the reporting of test results. Even when all interests are aligned, the task of setting up statewide, high-stakes tests is technically quite challenging. But, usually, all the separate stakeholder interests are not aligned, and the clash of goals and interests can lead to challenges.

Legal challenges to standardized educational testing are well-established and generally fall into two broad areas: statutory (e.g., Title VI and Title VII of the Civil Rights Act of 1964) and constitutional (e.g., Fourteenth Amendment of the United States Constitution). In "Whose Rules? The Relation Between the "Rules" and "Law" of Testing" (chap. 7), Chad Buckendahl and Robert Hunt discuss some of the legal challenges that educational testing programs have defended over the past 30 years.

The *Standards for Educational and Psychological Testing* (of the AERA, APA, & NCME, 1999) and other requirements for testing programs are then discussed as they represent the agreed-upon professional guidelines of the testing community. Most of the chapter focuses on how the psychometric elements of the testing programs were defended in two landmark challenges to standardized, educational testing, *Debra P. v. Turlington* and *GI Forum v. Texas Education Agency*. The chapter concludes with general recommendations for defending high-stakes testing programs in the future.

In "Teaching For the Test: How and Why Test Preparation is Appropriate" (chap. 8) Linda Crocker addresses the myth that all teaching to the test is necessarily immoral and instructionally unproductive. She reviews appropriate practices that teachers can use with published test specifications to ensure that their own curricula and instructional coverage are meeting students' instructional needs. She also describes how teachers can develop student test-taking and problem-solving skills that generalize to a variety of future performance situations that students may face. Finally, she also contrasts appropriate and inappropriate standardized test preparation practices.

Standardized tests are used for many purposes. In high-stakes settings, often these tests are used to make critically important decisions. Such decisions include which students are eligible for high school graduation, which applicants pass a licensure test, and who, among the qualified applicants, will receive scholarships or other awards or prizes. To make these decisions, typically one or more score values are identified from the test-score distribution as the "cutscore" or "passing score." As the evocative chapter title from Barbara Plake suggests, to most members of the public, the methods used for determining these score values are a mystery. After all, "Doesn't Everybody Know That 70% is Passing?" (chap. 9).

Plake addresses the issues concerning using arbitrary and capricious passing scores (e.g., the 70% rule) and presents methods that are available to set valid and defensible passing scores. Her chapter focuses both on the methods and on the best practices for determining recommended passing scores. She also covers issues related to policy decisions, such as who has the final responsibility for setting passing scores and how often these passing scores should be revisited. Her most important message is that there is a well-established set of procedures for standard setting.

Whereas standardized tests do not "standardize minds" as some testing critics assert, in many cases, they do assume that the student test takers have an equal ability and opportunity to learn the subject matter tested. That may not always be the case, particularly with disabled students and limited-English proficient students. Indeed, some of these students may be uniquely challenged to take a test. In "The Testing Industry, Ethnic Minorities and Individuals with Disabilities" (chap. 10), Kurt Geisinger reviews the issues and argues that, while the tests or the test administrations may need to be different, the education of disabled and LEP students will benefit from the use of standardized testing. Geisinger provides an historical lesson in how the testing industry, and society as a whole, have quickly responded to the challenges.

In "A School Accountability Case Study: California API Awards and the *Orange County Register* Margin of Error Folly" (chap. 11) the statistician David Rogosa dissects one of the more technical statistical conundrums in the current debate over accountability systems. Some testing opponents argue that some accountability systems (e.g., California, North Carolina, and NCLB) are naive to rely on measurements of year-to-year changes in test scores, as those changes are too statistically "volatile" (i.e., erratic). Such is the nature of test scores, the students who produce them, the tests (that change from year to year), and test administrations, which can never be exactly the same.

A tempting argument, perhaps, but misinformed. Rogosa illustrates the flaws in the empirical basis for the argument, and ascribes the "volatility" claims to some fairly simple misinterpretations of some fairly simple statistics.

Standardized testing plays a key role in the federal No Child Left Behind Education (NCLB) Act. In "Leave No Standardized Test Behind" (chap. 12), Mary Lyn Bourque itemizes both the testing requirements and how each of them affects the structure and character of U.S. public education—the impact on curriculum, professional development, and classroom and instructional decisions. First, she lays out the historical background, summarizing 1990s era reform ideas, and reminds the reader that two earlier presidents (Bush and Clinton) proposed national testing programs, too. Second, Bourque describes the context of the legislative deliberations leading to NCLB. Third, she specifies the principle requirements, including annual testing and adequate yearly progress. Fourth, she evaluates the early impact of NCLB on the major components of school reforms already in progress, such as curriculum and instruction, and professional development. Fifth, she assesses the progress of states in preparing for and meeting NCLB requirements. Finally, she anticipates the legacy of NCLB.

We wrote this book with the intention of reaching a wide audience, and so have endeavored to minimize the use of technical jargon. Some use of technical terms, however, was unavoidable.

1

Persistently Positive: Forty Years of Public Opinion on Standardized Testing

Richard P. Phelps
Third Education Group

Public-opinion polls make good news copy, but are much maligned as a source of data for research, and for rather compelling reasons. For example:

- Polling is episodic. Pollsters poll when a topic is topical, and not when it is not. This leaves researchers without baselines, time series, or benchmarks for making comparisons.
- Often, polls are written quickly as stories emerge in the news and before they sink, leaving little time to pretest and edit items. Too often, the result is poorly written questions and a too frequent use of terms with ambiguous or varied meanings, which produce ambiguous results.
- Pollsters are often unfamiliar with a topic and, as a result, may pose questions based on naïve or inaccurate assumptions.
- Pollsters often work for hire, and the preference of clients for certain results can be satisfied all too easily.
- Neither the government nor anyone else regulates the quality of polls or pollsters. Anyone can hang out a shingle and call themselves a polling expert.

1

Just as there exist a variety of pollsters, polls themselves vary widely in quality. On even the most fundamental aspect of polling—the sampling—one finds great disparity. The typical political poll taken during an election campaign consists of no more than single telephone call attempts to a representative random sample over a single weekend, garnering a response rate of 20% of that sample or less. It is common with such "quick-and-dirty" polls for its methodology report, if one is written, to wax eloquent on the high quality of the sample selection, and neglect completely to mention the pathetically low response rate, which degrades the representativeness of the sample. As the political pundit Ariana Huffington once quipped, the lonely or unemployed—those most dependably at home and with time on their hands to talk to pollsters—are over-represented in poll results and are, consequently, making public policy decisions for the rest of us (Huffington, 2003a, 2003b).

Moreover, response rates have been declining precipitously for more than a decade, most likely due to public revulsion toward telemarketing. As one of the nation's leading pollsters remarked recently, "response rates are getting so low, they're starting to get scary." A half-century ago, when many polls were still conducted door-to-door and face-to-face, response rate percentages in the high nineties were ordinary. Today, pollsters feel lucky when they exceed 50.[1]

This begs the question: If public-opinion poll data are so untrustworthy, where can one find a better gauge of the public's preferences? Perhaps in elections and referenda? Unfortunately, at least in the United States, elections and referenda have serious response-rate problems, too. They attract only a small, usually unrepresentative, minority of the electorate to the polls, to choose among sharply constrained, limited choices, which were themselves made by small, exclusive elites within political parties or interest groups. Moreover, election outcomes are subject to multiple manipulations that can pervert the electorate's true wishes, including gerrymandering, asymmetric financing, unfair candidate marketing (particularly just prior to election day), and bad weather.

Despite their flaws, opinion polls and surveys may represent the best available alternative for divining the public's wishes in our democracy, arguably even better than the very expensive, highly controlled and monitored official elections.

Besides, not all polls are "quick and dirty." High-quality polls take the time and make the effort to reach the more difficult-to-reach folk in order to make their samples truly representative in result as well as in design. More patient pollsters typically allocate 2 weeks of time for telephone calling and for repeated attempts to reach the busier, the seldom-at-home, and the re-

---

[1]Ironically, new anti-telemarketing regulations could help pollsters as pollsters, charities, and other nonsales-oriented organizations are held exempt.

calcitrant. Any more, the better polls also supplement a standard sample questionnaire with small focus groups of key subgroups that delve more deeply and expansively into a topic.

Even the "quick-and-dirty" polls can provide useful insights, however, when reinforced by other polls and surveys conducted concurrently or by multiple efforts on the part of one pollster. Political polls in high-profile elections, for example, are seldom taken in isolation but, rather, form patterns of responses retrieved in series and batches. Particularly when conducted by experienced political pollsters with sufficient knowledge to appropriately adjust results to compensate for response group biases, the patterns can tell a trustworthy story.

Having said that, experience and insight with election polls do not necessarily translate all that well to education issue polls. Some pollsters have developed an expertise with the subtleties of public opinion on education issues, but more have not.

Still, despite their flaws, public-opinion polls on education issues in general and standardized testing in particular remain important as unique representations of the public's preferences (Phelps, 1998). Moreover, they provide a counterweight to the numerous program evaluations and surveys conducted by education professors and education interest groups that, overwhelmingly, solicit the attitudes and opinions only of other educators—teachers and administrators.

Table 1.1 displays my count of the numbers of studies, both polls and surveys, which posed questions about standardized testing, classified by type of respondent group—education providers (i.e., teachers, administrators, education professors) and education consumers (i.e., the public, parents, students, policymakers). There is some double counting of studies, as some surveyed multiple groups of respondents.

TABLE 1.1
Respondent Groups in Public-Opinion Polls and Research Surveys

	Number of Testing Studies: 1965–2002	
	Respondent Group	
	Education providers: administrators, board members, teachers, education professors	**Education consumers**: public, parents, students, employers, politicians, higher education
Public opinion polls	13 (5%)	232 (95%)
Research studies (evaluations, surveys)	56 (73%)	21 (27%)

Source. See Appendix A.

The relevant point here is not that public-opinion polls have outnumbered research studies. Many of the polls counted in this tabulation posed only one or two questions on standardized testing, whereas the research studies, on average, posed more. It is not the relevant point that the opinions of education consumers have been solicited more often than those of education providers as, there too, the studies of consumer opinion tend to have posed fewer questions on testing than those of education provider opinion.

In Table 1.1 it is the row percentages to which I wish to draw attention. Most testing research studies are conducted by education professors, and, generally, they solicit the opinion of their fellow education providers. Moreover, their research tends to be school bound. Even in the majority of their research studies that did solicit the opinion of education consumers, those consumers were students, in school. Only two testing program evaluations or research studies from the past several decades solicited the views of the general public or employers. Only five solicited the views of parents.

If it were not for public opinion polls, virtually all the empirical data on the public's testing policy preferences would come from education providers. And their self-interest in the issue can differ dramatically from that of education consumers.

PLACING THE TOPIC OF STANDARDIZED TESTING IN CONTEXT

Granted, standardized tests are rarely the first thing on the mind of most poll respondents, even when they are thinking about education. What is? It is sad to say—order and discipline, and not academics.

Certainly, education professors focus on academic issues—issues that to most of the public sometimes seem rather arcane. Public Agenda's late-1990s poll, *Different Drummers*, exposed the large dimensions of the vast rift that separates the education issue priorities of parents and education professors (Farkus, 1997). Order and discipline top the priority list for the public and parents. They rest near the bottom, for the majority at least, of education professors. Either the education professors in the Public Agenda poll did not take complaints about discipline seriously, did not consider discipline important, or thought, as a reasonable interpretation of the poll results would suggest, that problems of order and discipline were the fault of incompetent teachers (i.e., the teachers they trained).

One of the few education poll items with enough persistence to produce a trend line over the years is the Phi Delta Kappa (PDK) Gallup Poll's "the biggest problem" in education. The PDK-Gallup poll iterates with religious certainty—exactly once a year since the 1970s. It would be too much to ask for "the biggest problem" item to be, in all its important aspects, exactly the same every year. The question posed has not changed much over the years, but the coding and classification of the open-ended responses has.

Nonetheless, "the biggest problem" series is the longest and most dependable in the history of education polls. Figure 1.1 summarizes the series. The many and varied responses are collapsed into a number of categories we can work with, with proper adjustments made in the interest of historical continuity, when possible, for the everchanging categorization methods of the PDK-Gallup folk. In the end, four categories survived the winnowing process: (1) discipline, respect, fighting; (2) funding, low pay, poor facilities; (3) drugs, drink; and (4) poor curriculum, education quality, administration.

Needless to say, the fourth category—the one where testing and accountability would be placed—garners the least interest over the years. Except for the 1980s, when drugs and drink looked to take over first place for good, order and discipline have always been on top, and by some substantial margin.

As the *Phi Delta Kappan* put it:

Over the past 10 years, drug abuse ranked first among local school problems seven times and once tied with lack of proper financial support. From 1969

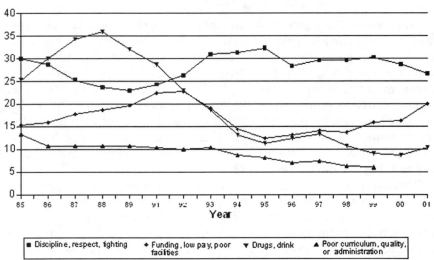

**Percent of adults thinking it is among
the biggest problems of local schools, by year**

| ■ Discipline, respect, fighting | ◆ Funding, low pay, poor facilities | ▼ Drugs, drink | ▲ Poor curriculum, quality, or administration |

FIG. 1.1.   Percent of adults thinking it is among the biggest problems of local schools, by year. (*Note.* In order to smooth natural volatility, data were converted to a 3-year moving average.) *Source*: Elam (1995).

to 1985, every poll but one ranked lack of discipline as the top problem. It is interesting that problems related to such critical matters as curriculum, quality of the teaching staff, and the academic performance of students never make it to the top of the list. (Elam, Rose, & Gallup, 1996, p. 49)

IF DISCIPLINE IS THE SCHOOLS' BIGGEST PROBLEM, WHAT DO WE DO ABOUT IT?

To respond to this question, let us step back a bit. In a PDK-Gallup poll in which issues of "discipline, respect, fighting" were cited more than twice as often as any other "education problems," the same respondents were also asked: How often do you think each problem occurs in [your] public schools? A list of potential problems was delivered.

Here are the responses, listed in their rank order of popularity, along with the percent responding "most of the time" or "fairly often" (in the parenthesis) (Elam, 1995).

(1) Schoolwork and homework assignments not completed (64%)
(2) Behavior that disrupts class (60%)
(3) Skipping classes (56%)
(6) Use of drugs at school (53%)
(8) Sloppy or inappropriate dress (47%)
(9) Cheating on tests (46%)

Apparently, the concept of "discipline" includes *academic* behaviors, such as completing homework, showing up to class, and doing one's own work or, more generally, behaviors such as responsibility, diligence, organization, and self-reliance. Alternatively, a large majority of parents and the public might believe a greater emphasis on academic achievement in the schools likely to reduce the order and discipline problem. In that, they would agree with the research literature, in which the correlation between an academic focus on the one hand, and order and discipline on the other, seem to very strong, indeed. Give the students something meaningful to do, and they are more likely to behave.

This hypothesis is reinforced when the public is asked directly, not what the problems are, but how to fix them. Granted, a large proportion of the respondents mentioned discipline and character issues, 50% and 39%, respectively, but more mentioned academic and quality control issues, such as "more attention to basic skills" (51%), "raise academic standards" (27%), and "emphasize career education" (38%).

In general, education standards and quality issues seem to rise more prominently in respondents' minds when:

Question: Which ... would do most to improve the quality of public education overall?	
Proposed Action	Percent citing
... more attention to basic skills	51
... raise academic standards	27
... increase amount of homework	14
... emphasize career education	38
Quality control issues TOTAL	130
... enforce stricter discipline	50
... emphasize moral development	39
Discipline and character issues TOTAL	89
... raise teachers' salaries	14
Funding issues TOTAL	14

FIG. 1.2.   *Source*: Elam, 1998.

- responses are selected from a list (thus, not drawn strictly from respondent's near term memory of episodic and negative news reports);
- all of public education, not just the local schools, are considered; and
- the focus of the question is on how to improve the schools, not what the problems are.

It may be simple common sense that brings topics like order, discipline, and drugs to mind when the public is asked about school problems. After all, those problems do exist in some schools and, after all, they are not supposed to. Schools, at least in the public's mind, are supposed to be places where students learn academic subject matter. Given that, imposing order and discipline, and ridding the schools of drink and drugs, could certainly help matters, but, in and of themselves, they make students no more learned.

TRENDS IN POLL ITEMS ON STANDARDIZED TESTING

I ran computer searches through poll item data bases, including the Roper Center's and Polling the Nations, to retrieve hundreds of items on testing, dating back to the 1960s. I also collected any I could by other means, such as Web searches, library searches, and requesting similar information from organizations that have, at some time in the past, conducted polls or surveys on education issues.

I won't pretend that I have captured all the relevant poll items, but I would imagine that I have come pretty close, at least for those to be found in U.S. national polls. In Fig. 1.3 I chart their numbers by year.

This tabulation includes only public-opinion poll items and not survey items from program evaluations (which would make a much flatter pattern over time). Thus, this graph represents the frequency with which the topic of standardized testing reached the level of public awareness necessary for pollsters to wish to pay attention to it.

At some risk of speculation, let me try to interpret some of the trend represented in the graph. One notices right away that the popularity of poll questions on testing seems to have increased over time. But, the rise has been irregular. The late 1960s and early 1970s had few relevant items and most of them referred to IQ testing, rather than district- or state-level achievement tests. The late 1970s and early 1980s show some pickup in interest coinciding with *the minimum competency era*, a period when most U.S. states and many school districts installed basic-skills high school graduation test requirements. Another blip in interest, in 1984, coincides with the release of the controversial *A Nation at Risk* report, with its call for higher standards and stiffer accountability in education.

1991 marks the arrival of the first of three major national testing proposals by three consecutive presidents. President George H. W. Bush's American Achievement Tests proposal was followed in 1997 by President Bill Clinton's

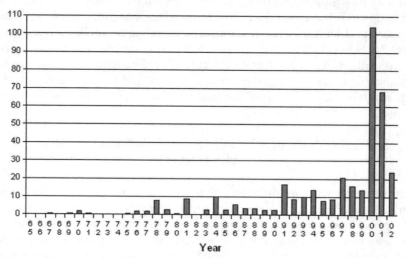

FIG. 1.3.   Items on standardized testing in national polls, by year.
Source: Appendix A.

Voluntary National Tests proposal and, in 2000, by presidential candidate George W. Bush's national accountability scheme, to eventually be entitled the *No Child Left Behind Act*. Each proposal seems to have induced a spike in the number of questions posed on the topic standardized testing, such as one might expect from any issue given intense presidential attention.

This pattern of public interest reflects an inherent irony in testing policy in particular, as in education policy in general. The U.S. Constitution makes no mention of education, so, any public action on education is reserved to the discretion of our country's original founding entities, the states. Legally, education is a state matter, but the direction of its public debate is often determined nationally.

It seems apparent that pollsters pay more attention to testing when a national testing proposal is under consideration. Granted, a number of statewide polls on education have included items on standardized testing, but, even they more frequently ask about national, rather than state, testing programs.

As for the presidential testing proposals, the public response has been overwhelmingly positive. The measure presented in Table 1.2 and throughout the rest of the chapter distills a poll item response down to one number. *Percentage point differential* (pp dif) is the percentage responding favorably to a question, minus the percentage responding unfavorably. Other, neutral responses—don't know, no opinion, no answer—are disregarded.

SEMANTIC SENSITIVITY ANALYSIS

Some common criticisms of poll data for social science research use were made at the outset. A general problematic feature of poll items is their inconsistency. Pollsters tend to live in the moment, and reasonably so given that, usually, they are paid to provide very current information as it flowers, information whose value tends to wilt quickly. Sometimes pollsters re-

TABLE 1.2
Number and Results of Polls on Presidential Testing Proposals

	Number of Polls	Mean pp dif
George H. W. Bush's American Achievement Tests (1990–1992)	6	+52
Bill Clinton's Voluntary National Tests (1997–1999)	6	+48
George W. Bush's No Child Left Behind (2000–2002)	14	+57

Source. Multiple polls (1990–2002).

peat questions at different points in time and publish the results as then-and-now comparisons, which can be very informative.

Unfortunately, it is probably more common for a pollster to deny any relevance to old items and write new ones from scratch even when old ones might do. The result for a researcher trying to patch together a time series of public opinion is a set of questions on the exact same topic, but worded slightly differently. In most cases, slightly different wordings make items non comparable; it does not take much of a difference in a question to move a response a few percentage points.

It can be delightfully edifying when pollsters make small alterations intentionally, that is, change just one characteristic of a question to see how different the response is. If the altered question is posed to the same respondent group as the original question, one can calculate how much weight the single altered characteristic bears in the public mind.

With this semantic sensitivity analysis, studying poll items can seem rather analytical, even scientific. Gratefully, there exist many instances of pollsters asking a set of questions while altering a single characteristic, allowing us to conduct semantic sensitivity analyses, and on some key topics. I describe some below. Again, percentage-point differential (pp dif) is the percentage responding favorably minus the percentage responding unfavorably (percentages for no opinion, don't know, and no answer are ignored).

Surprisingly, the public, by 23 percentage points preferred *requiring* school districts to administer standardized tests over leaving the matter optional, and, among the choices for test content, the basic skills were most popular (see Table 1.3).

There is a wide swing in preferences for standardized test use from the most popular, most benign use of student academic diagnosis—a use virtually everyone supports—to various accountability purposes (see Table 1.4). The percentage point differential declines from +79 for diagnosis to +39 for ranking schools and +28 for grade promotion testing. Mind you, +28 still

TABLE 1.3
What Should Tests Measure? Should They be Required?

Do You Favor or Oppose Requiring Standardized National Tests to Measure ... ?

	pp dif
... the academic achievement of students	+60
... knowledge in 5 core subjects	+80
... problem-solving skills	+74
... ability to write a clear composition	+75
... making these tests optional for school districts?	+37

Source. Elam, 1995.

TABLE 1.4
How Should Tests be Used?

Do You Think Tests Should be Used to ... ?	pp dif
... identify area in which students need help.	+76
... rank the local public schools.	+39
... determine if a student advances to the next grade	+28
... determine the level of funding school receives	−18
... determine how much teachers should be paid	−14

Source. Rose, et al. (1997).

represents a strong majority; a +28 dif could be produced by a response split of 58% in favor, 30% opposed, and 12% neutral.

Even among accountability options, there remains a wide swing in preferences. The +28 for grade promotion testing falls to −18 for linking school funding to test scores.

The proportion of the public in favor of graduation exams is huge, has been for decades, and remains so today (see Table 1.5). Among those testing opponents who are willing to concede this fact, some are fond of arguing that opinion will change when parents' own children are in the school system.

In fact, parents are often stronger supporters of high-stakes testing than nonparents. Low-income parents are often stronger supporters of high-stakes testing than higher income parents. In the poll results displayed below, parentage reduced the positive differential, but only by 4 percentage points even if the child failed the exam once. Graduation exams' popularity is reduced further when parents are told their children will not graduate. But, even then, the pp dif is +68, which means that fewer than 16% of parents objected to graduation exams even if they knew their own child would not graduate.

TABLE 1.5
Steadfast in Support of Graduation Exams

Should Students be Required to Pass Tests to Graduate?	+90
... if your child failed the first time?	+86
... if your child did not receive a diploma?	+68
... if 20% of low income students did not receive a diploma?	+55

Source. Market Opinion Research (1985).

Indeed, graduation exams lose more support when respondents are told large numbers of low-income students—other parents' children—will not graduate.

There seems to be much more support—+27 pp differential more—for an indirect, than for a direct, federal government role (see Table 1.6). In this, and on most other issues, the No Child Left Behind Act, with its federal initiation of broad parameters but state discretion over details, seems crafted to perfectly fit public preferences.

In one of these semantic sensitivity analyses, we witnessed parents willing to cut poor children who failed tests more slack than they would their own children (see Table 1.7). Just about everyone seems to believe that schools in poor neighborhoods, and the poor children who attend them, are academically disadvantaged.

There exists enormous reluctance to punish those perceived to be disadvantaged, yet few seem willing to let poor students and schools completely off the hook. Proposals to help make up for disadvantages garner very strong public support. They include more funding for schools in poor neighborhoods; subsidies for tutors, after-school, Saturday, and summer school programs; multiple chances to pass exams with tutoring help as long as is needed; and so on.

As any accountant, economist, or labor union negotiator might say, the difference between giving money and taking it away is merely perception and semantics. It all depends on the starting point and the level of expectations, but, perception can be important, and the lesson for any politician in

TABLE 1.6
What Should be the Federal Role in a National Testing Program?

Federal Government Should …	*pp dif*
… support a national testing program (PDK '87)	+57
… create national standardized tests (Newsweek '98)	+30

TABLE 1.7
What to Do With Poor, and Consistently Poor, Performing Schools?

What Should be Done With Schools Serving Low-Income Communities That Score Consistently Poorly in Reading and Math Tests … ?	
… provide additional funds to help raise standards	+70
… replace the principal	−10
… close the school	−71

Source. Louis Harris (2001).

these poll numbers is that rewards programs are far more popular than punishment programs (see Table 1.8).

HAS THERE EVER BEEN A PUBLIC "TESTING BACKLASH?"

The short answer is … no. Many prominent educators and many journalists, in the years 2000 and 2001, described "grass roots movements" forming, crowds of placard-waving students and parents taking to the streets, and majority opinion turning against "this new breed of tests" (i.e., state mandated high-stakes tests). It was wishful thinking by testing opponents that fed on itself. So many said there was a backlash, those who listened assumed there must be, as did those who listened to them, and those who listened to them. Unfortunately, too much education research is disseminated this way.

Public support for high-stakes testing is consistent and long standing, and majority opinion has never flipped from support to opposition, as the word *backlash* would imply. Poll items on the high-stakes testing issue date back to 1958 for graduation tests and to 1978 for grade-level promotion tests.

These are large positive differentials for either type of high-stakes test (see Table 1.9). A 45 percentage point differential could be produced by a split of 72.5% favorable, 27.5% unfavorable, or 70% favorable, 25% unfavorable, 5% neutral. That's a popular landslide. Interestingly, the two differentials are approximately the same—between 45 and 50.

Public, parental, and even student support for high-stakes standardized testing remains "rock solid" today, to use Public Agenda's words, despite a several-year flood of negative media coverage.

Support for high-stakes testing among education providers is not quite as strong, but it is still very strong (see Table 1.10).

Nonetheless, prolonged and intense opposition to a testing proposal seems capable of pealing away some support. Figure 1.4 shows the regression in public support, over the course of 7 months, for the testing requirements in President George W. Bush's No Child Left Behind bill during the

TABLE 1.8
Carrots Preferred to Sticks

Do You Favor or Oppose … ?	
… giving less federal money to states where schools fail to improve	−24
… using federal money to reward states where results improve	+27

Result is similar for "districts" or "schools," in place of "states." *Source.* Louis Harris (2001).

TABLE 1.9
Summary of Public Opinion on High-Stakes Requirements
(Among Education Consumers [i.e., public, parents, students, employers, etc.])

	Number of Polls	Mean pp Dif
Support for high school graduation test requirement	33	+47.3
Support for grade-level promotion test requirement	23	+45.3

Source. Multiple polls and surveys (1958–2003).

TABLE 1.10
Summary of Public Opinion on High-Stakes Requirements
(Among Education Providers [i.e., teachers, administrators, board members, etc.])

	Number of polls	Mean pp dif
Support for high school graduation test requirement	26	+34.3
Support for grade-level promotion test requirement	5	+38.4

Source. Multiple polls and surveys (1978–2003).

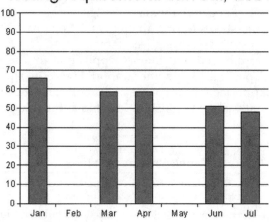

Positive differential in favor of NCLB testing requirement: Jan-Jul, 2001

FIG. 1.4.   Positive differential in favor of NCLB testing requirement: Jan–Jul, 2001.

14

period it was debated in the Congress. The same item was posed to the public five times, in both CBS and AP polls. The positive differential in favor of the plan declined steadily from 65 to 48 percentage points.

Still, 48 percentage points represents a very large buffer of support; less than one quarter of the public was opposed and, of course, the bill passed into law later that year.

There exists one group—teachers—with which support for testing has declined over the years. Teachers in the 1970s and 1980s were overwhelmingly supportive of standardized testing and, in particular, high-stakes testing. Then, the high stakes were intended only for the students. Now, many states have raised the stakes for teachers as well and, not surprisingly, that has eroded support.

Any more, polls may or may not find majority teacher support for high-stakes tests, depending on the context. For example, the American Federation of Teachers' Albert Shanker Institute found a noticeable decline in teacher support for "standards, testing and accountability" from 1999 (73% strongly or somewhat in favor) to 2001 (55%; Business Roundtable, 2003).

Another indicator implies some diminution in public support for high-stakes standardized tests, although hardly anything that could reasonably be considered a "backlash." It is the increase in the number of respondents asserting there may be too much testing now, or too much emphasis on testing. Figure 1.5 displays the percentage point differential by year, from 1997 to 2002, of responses to an identical item posed (by 8 pp) in the PDK-Gallup Poll four times during that period. The differential started out positive in

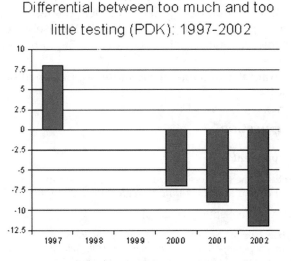

FIG. 1.5. Differential between too much and too little testing (PDK): 1997–2002.

1997 (in this case positive means more respondents thought there was "too little testing" than thought there was "too much testing"). By 2002, the differential was –12.

THEN, HOW MUCH TESTING SHOULD THERE BE?

Most poll items on this topic ask if there should be more or less testing, which (naively) assumes the respondent knows how much there is currently. The results for such items can be virtually meaningless.

Two recent polls, however, asked how much large-scale standardized testing respondents thought there should be, with no assumption made or suggested regarding the current amount. In the first (AAP/Franz, 2000), respondents were given a choice of one or two tests per year: 49% chose one and 50% chose two. In the second (NEA/Tarrance, 2001), their choice was annual testing or no, with 69% responding yes, and 27% asserting that annual testing was excessive.

Combining information from both polls, we can conclude that more than two-thirds of the public favors a testing frequency of once-per-year, at least. Some of the two-thirds want more.

HOW TO MANIPULATE POLL RESULTS

Sometimes, poll questions are written poorly, and it is unintentional. Other times, poll questions seem to be written with a deliberate intention of skewing the results. Unfortunately, that intention can be all too easily realized.

Even if an organization has hired one of the more responsible pollsters, and they write responsible questions, the results themselves can usually be manipulated toward one's preferences before they are reported to the public.

Below are examples of some of the more popular methods for biasing items and results.

Biasing the Question

Lead the respondent:

Q. "Do you think the teachers in your school focus so much on preparing for standardized tests that *real learning* is neglected … ?" [italics added]

(Public Agenda, September, 2000)

[*The suggestion here, of course, is that preparation for standardized test must be "false" learning or, perhaps, not learning at all, and who would want their child wasting any amount of time in "false learning" or no learning?*]

Q. "Student success at meeting the standards would be determined by so-phisticated assessments, including written essays, rather than multiple-choice tests."

(AFT, Peter D. Hart, 1994)

[*Who wouldn't pick the "more sophisticated" option? By the way, how did the venerable old essay tests, which have been around for millennia and are written by ordinary teachers every day, become "more sophisticated" than multiple-choice tests, which are only several decades old and designed by PhDs?*]

Q. "Do you have any particular concerns or opinions about any of these standardized tests?"

(National Science Foundation, Boston College, 1992)

[*This is the only question in a long interview about the effects of mandated testing to which a teacher could have responded with an opinion supportive of tests. The responses to this single question formed the set from which the researchers compiled the results declared for teacher support for or rejection of testing in general. The question, however, specifically requests negative information—"concerns." Everyone has concerns; no one believes that standardized tests are perfect.*]

Pose a false choice:

Q. "In your opinion, which is the best way to measure student academic achievement—by means of test scores, or by classroom work and homework?"

(PDK-Gallup, 2002)

Q. "In your opinion, should the primary use of achievement tests be to determine how much students have learned or to determine the kind of instruction they need in the future?"

(PDK-Gallup, 2001)

[*In fact, no one ever faces these choices. There is no school in the U.S. where tests have replaced class or home work. Tests are supplements to the other activities, not replacements. Moreover, test scores and class and home work are quite different, used in different ways and for different purposes, and are not directly comparable. Surprisingly, a large minority of respondents to this item chose test scores. Besides, tests can easily be used, singly or in combination, both to determine how much students have learned or the kind of instruction they need.*]

Constrain the choice:

Q. "The state-mandated test motivates previously unmotivated students to learn?"

(Boston College NBETPP, 2003)

[*Why ask only about "previously unmotivated students," why not ask about all students? Is it, perhaps, because that will reduce the likelihood of a negative response? Abundant evidence from polls, surveys, and controlled experiments shows that student achievement is higher where there are testing programs, everything else held equal (see chap. 3, this volume).*]

Assert a false assumption:

Q. "It's wrong to use the results of just one test to decide whether a student gets promoted or graduates. Would you say you agree or disagree with this view?"

(Public Agenda 2000; Public Agenda/*Education Week*, 2000)

Q. "A student's progress for one school year can be accurately summarized by a single standardized test." [agree, disagree]

(AASA, Luntz/Laszlo, 2000)

Q. "Do you think it is fair or unfair to use a single standardized test to determine what a student knows or has achieved?"

(CNN, *USA Today*, 2001)

Q. "Do you favor or oppose using a single standardized test in the public schools in your community to determine whether a student should be promoted from grade to grade? ... should receive a high school diploma?"

(PDK-Gallup, 2001)

[*There is no state in the country making graduation decisions solely based on one test, or even based on multiple tests, but many respondents will not know that. Most graduation exams are set at a junior-high level of difficulty and students are given many opportunities over a several year period to pass. Moreover, no where are standardized tests the only graduation requirement; there are attendance, course distribution, course accumulation, course completion, public service, and other requirements, all of which must be met or passed satisfactorily before a student receives a diploma. Even the author would oppose using a single test to determine a diploma; ironically, a strong majority of respondents in the PDK-Gallup poll supported using a single standardized test for grade promotion and graduation decisions.*]

Pose only negative questions (re: stress, pressure, adverse outcomes, political conspiracy).

[Examples: Boston College, 1990, 2003; AASA-Luntz/Lazlo; PDK-Gallup, 2002, 2003; Corbett & Wilson, 1987]

Learn over time which questions wordings get the responses one favors, which do not, and continue to use the former.

[Example: the past several years of PDK-Gallup polls.]

Biasing the Poll Results

Add the Neutral Percentage to the Choice One Favors.

A poll item's neutral responses (e.g., don't know, no opinion, no response) usually count for little in the reporting of results, as in the calculation of the percentage point differential, used in this and other studies, where they are simply ignored. Some more enterprising reporters, however, manage to use the neutral percentage in ways that benefit their point of view.

Association for Supervision and Curriculum Development (ASCD)-Sylvan Learning Centers-Harris Interactive Poll 2000. From the ASCD press release ...

"Approximately half [of the poll respondents] disagree or are undecided about whether these tests should determine graduation."

[*actual results:* "agree" 51%, "disagree" 38%, "neither" 11%]

"Nearly half find inconsistencies between their children's standardized test results and their report cards."

[*actual results:* "consistent" 40%, "not consistent" 16%, "in some areas but not others" 44%]

"Half [of parents] are unsure of or do not know what the state standardized tests measure."

[*actual results:* "yes" 50%, "no" 23%, "not sure" 27%]

[In the summary report written by the polling firm—Harris Interactive—the same information is presented thus: "Half of the respondents say that they know what their state's educational assessments measure. The other half are split fairly evenly between not knowing and not being sure" (p. 9).]

Emphasize the Results One Favors and Ignore the Others.

[Good examples—the ASCD and AASA press releases of 2000, in which virtually all the results supportive of testing were ignored. In the case of the AASA, one entire poll, of the two they commissioned, was ignored.]

Code Responses or Define Terms in a Manner That Skews Results.

(Boston College-National Science Foundation survey of math and science teachers-1991) In a 1990 study by researchers at Boston College, math and science teachers were asked to render their opinions regarding the effect of mandated testing on their programs. The study authors recorded the comments made by the respondents, classified them as positive or negative, counted them, and then calculated the percentages positive and negative.

According to the tabulations, 83% of math teachers and 67% of science teachers cited negative effects, whereas only 47% of math teachers and 28% of science teachers cited positive effects (West & Viator, 1992b).

These results contrasted dramatically with those from other teacher surveys of the era. But, the contrary conclusions may have a lot to do with the rather convoluted design of the Boston College study. First, respondents were chosen selectively. There were all in urban, "high-minority" public school districts, and high school teachers in the sample were limited to those with classes of "average and below average" students (West & Viator, 1992b).

Second, the specific interview question that elicited opinions on the effects of mandated tests was biased toward negative answers. The question was: "Do you have any particular concerns or opinions about any of these standardized tests?" (West & Viator, 1992a, p. 6).

Third, the Boston College researchers classified as "negative" responses that others might classify as neutral or positive. For example, if a teacher

said that her students "didn't test well," it was interpreted by the researchers as a "major source of invalidity" and a "negative" comment, even
though students can test poorly for dozens of reasons, including not studying or not paying attention in class (West & Viator, 1992a). The researchers
pretty much classified any effect a mandated test had on altering a teacher's
instructional program as negative. Any high-stakes mandated test will alter
a teacher's instructional program; many would argue that is exactly what it
is supposed to do.

The Boston College/NSF study also decided to add to the usual definitions of
"higher order thinking" the aspect of "communicating," which was interpreted to mean, in the context of a test, writing out a response. As a student
does not "communicate" when completing a multiple-choice test item, the
Boston College study declared that all multiple-choice tests "tap only lower-
order thinking."

The Decline in Quality of the Phi Delta Kappan Polls

For decades, the most reliable source of polling on any education issue was
the Phi Delta Kappa organization. It has contracted with the Gallup Organization annually to pose a couple of dozen questions to representative samples of U.S. adults and parents (in its "Poll of attitudes toward the public
schools," as it is now called). Not only has the alliance been steady and dependable, some years during the 1960s, 1970s, and 1980s, they were the
only ones asking about education issues.

The polls conducted by the partnership from the 1960s into the early
1990s, I would surmise, were largely written by the Gallup Organization.
The poll items had the clean, crisp (some would say bland) character of
those written by experts.

By the mid- to late-1990s, I would further surmise, something changed.
Some of the old standard questions, including several of those that elicited
strong support for standardized testing over the years, disappeared, never
to be used again. In their place, new questions appeared that, I would argue, were less professional and more leading, presumptive, or ambiguous
(see, e.g., the aforementioned sections "Pose a false choice" and "Assert a
false assumption"). All items are now proposed and screened by a committee of Phi Delta Kappa members and invitees. (For additional insight, see a
devastating critique of the 35th Annual PDK Poll (2003), by Schneiders,
with additional comments by Bowers.)

From the mid-1980s to the year 2000, the *Phi Delta Kappan* magazine also
administered a teacher survey entirely of its own design and administration.
Five surveys in all were conducted by mail. Their response rates were very
low, around 20% but, responsibly, PDK did report the response rate. Results
of the *PDK Teacher Polls* were fairly interesting in that they seemed on virtually all issues to be diametrically opposite those of other teacher polls.

Part of the explanation could be the low response rate. But, a larger part of the explanation could be that only PDK members were polled. A brief glance through the tables of contents of a few *Phi Delta Kappan* magazines would show anyone well enough that the organization harbors a particular point of view, and few with differing points of view would feel much like they belonged and, so, probably do not. Moreover, I would argue that many of the poll questions were transparently biased, designed to achieve predetermined results.

The poor quality of the *PDK Teacher Polls* was discussed even within PDK and, to its credit, the organization decided on its own to discontinue the series. It is unknown, at least to this correspondent, if the decline in quality of the annual *Phi Delta Kappan*-Gallup poll of public attitudes is also being discussed in the boardroom in Bloomington.

CONCLUSION

Public support for widespread and consequential use of standardized testing is overwhelming, and has been since pollsters first posed questions about tests. Over several decades, the scale of the large magnitude of public support has barely budged. Indeed, the public would like to see standardized tests administered: more often (more than once a year), and for all the purposes for which they are now administered, as well as some for some others (e.g., regular, periodic recertification tests for teachers and administrators).

Was there ever a "public backlash against testing," as so many education insiders (and journalists) claimed? Not really. Trend data show that public opinion can be moved some by a persistent onslaught of negative insinuation. But, a change from a barely perceptible minority to a tiny minority opposed to testing can hardly be validly described as a "widespread," "grassroots," "groundswell," of "concerned parents and students." The "backlash" was, to borrow a phrase from a couple of prominent testing opponents, a "manufactured crisis."

Certainly, many parents will "game the system" if they see that standards are not being enforced, or that they are being enforced arbitrarily. Most parents put their children first. But, decades of surveys reveal that a very large majority of parents want standards to matter and want them to be enforced uniformly. Indeed, one finds larger majorities in favor of standards enforcement among parents than among the general public. That difference persists even when the parents are reminded of the possibility that their own children might be held back a grade or denied graduation.

ACKNOWLEDGMENTS

The author thanks the Educational Testing Service, whose research fellowship support freed up the time necessary to begin this study and, in particular, the advice and support of Richard Coley, Carla Cooper, Linda DeLauro, and Drew Gitomer. The able assistance of the staff of ETS's Brigham Library and of Terris Raiford, on a summer fellowship at ETS, also were crucial to the completion of this work.

REFERENCES

[*Note.* All polls mentioned are listed in Appendix A, where they are arranged in reverse chronological order.]

Bowers, W. (2003). Personal correspondence, December 29.

Business Roundtable. (2003, March). *What parents, students and teachers think about standards, tests, accountability ... and more.* New York: Author.

Elam, S. M. (1978). *A decade of Gallup Polls of attitudes toward education: 1969–1978.* Bloomington, IN: Phi Delta Kappa, p. 263.

Elam, S. M. (1995). *How America views its schools: The PDK/Gallup Polls, 1969–1994.* Bloomington, IN: Phi Delta Kappa, p. 44.

Elam, S. M., Rose, L. C., & Gallup, A. M. (1996, September). The 28th annual Phi Delta Kappa/Gallup Poll of the Public's Attitudes Toward the Public Schools. *Phi Delta Kappan, 78*(1), 49.

Farkus, S., Johnson, J., & Duffett, A. (1997). *Different drummers: How teachers of teachers view public education.* New York: Public Agenda.

Franz, J. D. (2000, June). *Association of American Publishers: Survey of Parents: Final report.* Sacramento, CA: J. D. Franz Research.

Harris, L. (2001, March). The Harris Poll [retrieved from Polling the Nations database, April 16, 2003].

Huffington, A. (2003a, May 8). The 77 percent solution. *Working for change.*

Huffington, A. (2003b, May 19). Just say 'No' to pollsters. *Business Week Online.*

National Endowment for the Arts/The Tarrance Group. (2001, February 7). [Retrieved from Polling the Nations database, April 16, 2003].

Phelps, R. P. (1998, Fall). The demand for standardized student testing. *Educational measurement: Issues and practice, 17*(3), 5–23.

Rose, L., Gallup, C., Alec, M., & Elam, S. M. (1997, June). Attitudes toward the public schools. *Phi Delta Kappan,* 41–56.

Schneiders, G. (2003). The 35th Annual Phi Delta Kappa/Gallup Poll: SDS Comments. Schneiders, Della, Volpe, & Schulman.

West, M. M., & Viator, K. A. (1992a). *The influence of testing on teaching math and science in grades 4–12: Appendix D: Testing and teaching in six urban sites.* Chestnut Hill, MA: Boston College.

West, M. M., & Viator, K. A. (1992b). *Teachers' and administrators' views of mandated testing programs.* Chestnut Hill, MA: Boston College.

2

High-Stakes Testing: Contexts, Characteristics, Critiques, and Consequences

Gregory J. Cizek
University of North Carolina at Chapel Hill

Qualitative research conducted on standardized tests has demonstrated conclusively the value of these instruments. In a major book, *Improving Schools by Standardized Tests*, in which the research results were collected and reported, teachers unequivocally and enthusiastically praised the such tests. Consider the following perceptions drawn from a sample of teachers (identified in the study by their initials).

E.M.W.: *"My appreciation of having had the privilege of introducing standardized tests in my school cannot be too strongly emphasized .... No school can accurately determine the progress of its pupils, either as a group or individually, without using these tests"* (p. 126).

V.L.W.: *"I now consider standardized tests the only fair means of measuring a pupil's ability and progress .... The saving of time and energy from the old method of examinations and, above all, the fact that they showed up in every study the weak points of each pupil was truly remarkable"* (p. 127).

L.E.M.: *"I think that standardized tests are the greatest boon that has ever been invented for the benefit of teachers, especially for those who are interested in* *and conscientiously working to obtain the best possible results with each child" (p. 128).*

The teachers not only expressed their strong support for standardized tests, but also commented on their students' perceptions.

A.N.H.: *"To me, another proof that these tests are helpful is the fact that they create a marked degree of enthusiasm on the part of the pupils. They look forward eagerly to the testing time, each one eager to do his or her best. I believe that the enthusiasm thus aroused is a stepping-stone to better work and, therefore, to better results" (p. 129).*

G.E.S.: *"They are a great benefit to children. I find that a child who takes the standardized tests two or three times a year does much better work, and also does it much more quickly. The children enjoy them .... Instead of dreading an 'examination' as they used to do, they are simply overjoyed at the prospect of taking a 'test' (p. 133).*

In the same study, the students were interviewed. The students' own comments corroborated their teachers' observations about the value and positive effects of standardized testing.

Student 1: *"I think the tests have helped me in many ways. They have helped me to work both faster and better, and I have more interest in getting ahead in my studies" (p. 135).*

Student 2: *"I think the standardized tests are the best kind to have. They tell us where we pupils belong and what we have to work up on. They tell us what we are weak in .... I like them very much. I don't know of anything better that we could have" (p. 137).*

Student 3: *"I think the standardized tests are a good thing. They show you where you stand in your studies and whether you are keeping up in your grade or not. They help you work with greater speed and accuracy" (p. 139).*

Student 4: *"I am always glad when we have the tests. I try to do better each time they come around ... and I think they help us a lot. I hope we have some more very soon" (p. 142).*

THE CURRENT CONTEXT

The preceding endorsements by teachers and students alike are real, although the book from which they are sampled was authored by Samuel Brooks in 1922. It is safe to say that students' and teachers' perceptions about testing have changed somewhat since that time, when objective testing was first being introduced. The consequences—both intended and unintended—of this new form of testing were widely recognized and effusively praised as uniformly positive.

From a vantage point nearly 80 years later, it is clear to many specialists in educational testing, education reformers, and increasingly for the American public generally, there are concerns about the unintended consequences of testing.

Perhaps *concerns* is too polite a term to characterize the malevolent outcomes cited and apocalyptic predictions proffered by critics of high-stakes tests. Opponents of such tests assail mandated, high-stakes testing as abusive of individual school children, misinformative for policy makers, harmful for those who practice in the field of education, and detrimental to real progress in education reform.

Who hasn't heard the criticisms of high-stakes tests? The shop-worn complaints include assertions that they:

- increase teacher frustration and burnout,
- make young children cry and/or vomit,
- increase student drop-out rates,
- reduce classroom instructional time,
- measure only lower order ("drill and kill") content,
- militate against academic excellence,
- narrow the curriculum,
- widen the achievement gap,
- reproduce social inequalities,
- promote cheating, and
- are biased.

These apprehensions largely lack support in the scholarly testing journals. Particularly, it is perhaps because they lack foundation that it is distressing to see the extent to which they have worked their way into what many commentators, critics, and even well-meaning parents and educators "know" about testing. Unfortunately, the critics "know what ain't so."[1] Before describing the fundamental errors of the critics, some background on high-stakes testing and reactions to testing are presented.

HIGH-STAKES TESTING DEFINED

It is perhaps important to first be clear about the kind of testing we are considering. To be precise, it is not all testing that is at issue, or even all standardized testing—only so-called "high-stakes" testing. That is, concerns center on tests to which positive or negative *consequences* are attached. Examples of such consequences include promotion/retention decisions for students, salaries or bonuses for educators, and state recognition of high-performing (or state take-over of low-performing) schools.

---

[1]This phrase is borrowed from one of the shrillest of the critics (see Bracey, 1989).

Of course, there have always been high-stakes tests. Testing historians have traced high-stakes testing to civil service examinations of 200 B.C., military selection dating to 2000 B.C., and Biblical accounts of the Gilead guards. Mehrens and Cizek (2001) related the story of the minimum competency exam, told in the book of Judges, that took place when the Gilead Guards challenged the fugitives from the tribe of Ephraim who tried to cross the Jordan river.

> 'Are you a member of the tribe of Ephraim?' they asked. If the man replied that he was not, then they demanded, 'Say Shibboleth.' But if he couldn't pronounce the H and said Sibboleth instead of Shibboleth he was dragged away and killed. So forty-two thousand people of Ephraim died there. (Judges 12:5-6, *The Living Bible*)

CRITIQUES OF HIGH-STAKES TESTING

To observe that high-stakes tests have a long history is not to say that the issues surrounding high-stakes tests have remained unchanged. For example, the scriptural account just related lacks the characteristics of some currently popular reactions to high-stakes tests. Nothing is mentioned regarding which verbal skills should be tested, how to measure them, how "minimally proficient" performance should be defined, whether paper–pencil testing might have been cheaper and more reliable than performance assessment, whether there was any adverse impact against the people of Ephraim, or what remediation should be provided for those judged to be below the standard. Maybe the Gilead Guards should have abandoned their test altogether because the Ephraimites didn't have the opportunity to learn to pronounce *shibboleth* correctly, because the burden of so many oral examinations was a top-down mandate, or because listening to all those Ephraimites try to say *shibboleth* reduced the valuable instructional time available for teaching young members of the tribe of Gilead the real-life skills of sword fighting and tent making (Mehrens & Cizek, 2001).

TESTING ON THE RISE

Whether educator, parent, student, or testing specialist involved in K–12 education, the central role of testing in American schools is unmistakable. If high-stakes testing had been a recognizable force in the education arena prior to the introduction of Public Law 107-110, the prominence of—and resistance to—testing has only increased with the passage of that law, better known by its colloquial title, the No Child Left Behind (NCLB) Act of 2001. Among its most visible features is the requirement that all states establish rigorous assessments for Grades 3 through 8 in reading, mathematics, and science. As a testing specialist, it is with a sense of awe that I approach this dramatic expansion of large-scale testing: Urgent requests for assistance with technical testing problems and the desperate need to train, recruit, and retain a vastly greater number of testing personnel have induced some of my measurement colleagues jokingly to refer to the law as "No psychometrician left behind."

WE HAVE SEEN THE ENEMY AND IT IS TESTING

Although it is certain that high-stakes testing has been around for centuries, it is perhaps the recent increases and consequential nature of current testing that has fueled critiques of testing. The critiques range from homegrown to pseudo-scientific. For example, on the homegrown side, the vernacular of most teachers includes anecdotes describing the despair experienced by earnest students who were denied a diploma as a result of a high-stakes test, illustrations of how testing has narrowed the curriculum, first-hand accounts of frustration and anxiety brought about by testing, and sad tales of bright, young pupils sobbing, vomiting, and surrendering in the throes of test anxiety.

Such anecdotes have become the grist of a mill widely referred to as the *testing backlash*. This movement is characterized by sentiments about the effects, expense, extent, and content of student testing that cannot be ignored. Interestingly, the strong disaffection for testing driving the backlash most commonly originates from within the education profession. Indeed, an impartial reader of much published opinion in the education field could easily conclude that testing is the most dire threat facing the postmodern world.

This side of the testing backlash often takes the form of commentary or data analysis in periodicals produced for educators, educational researchers, and policy makers. For example, in just one recent issue of the widely read magazine for educators *Phi Delta Kappan*, commentator Alfie Kohn (2001) urged teachers to "make the fight against standardized tests our top priority ... until we have chased this monster from our schools" (p. 349). Another article in the same issue described high-stakes testing as "the evil twin" of an authentic standards movement (Thompson, 2001, p. 358). A third article praised 22 educators and parents for their efforts to derail, resist, or sabotage testing (Ohanian, 2001). Without sparing the hyperbole, consistent critic Gerald Bracey (2002) summed up the critics' perspective: "High standards and high-stakes testing are infernal machines of social destruction" (p. 32). If nothing else, published commentary concerning high-stakes testing has been remarkable for its uniformity. The conclusion: High-stakes tests are uniformly bad.

The titles of some of these articles leave little room to misinterpret the authors' perspective. A few more representative entries include: Excellence in education versus high-stakes testing (Hilliard, 2000); The distortion of teaching and testing: High-stakes testing and instruction (Madaus, 1998); Burnt at the high-stakes (Kohn, 2000); Judge's ruling effectively acquits high-stakes test to the disadvantage of poor and minority students in Texas (Chenoweth, 2000); and I don't give a hoot if somebody is going to pay me $3600: Reactions to Kentucky's high-stakes accountability program (Kannapel, 1996).

A short list of the main points made in the more academic critiques of high-stakes testing could begin with the work of Smith and Rottenberg (1991), published in *Educational Measurement: Issues and Practice* over a decade ago. They identified six effects—none of them positive—under the heading "Consequences of External Testing" (p. 8). The consequences included:

1. reduction of time available for ordinary instruction,
2. neglect of teaching material not covered by tests,
3. a press toward methods of instruction and assessment (frequently lower-order) in the classroom that mirror those implied by tests,
4. limits on students' instructional opportunities,
5. undesirable effects on teacher morale, and
6. imposition of "cruel and unusual punishment" on students—younger ones in particular—because of the length, difficulty, small print, time constraints, and individualistic nature of tests (p. 10).

More recent critiques have raised issues such as the potential for tests to foster negative attitudes by students toward tested content (Lattimore, 2001) or diminish students' self-esteem (Meisels, 2000).

As might be expected, the evidence put forth in various studies is of variable quality. The study design used to develop Smith and Rottenberg's (1991) list of consequences and tentative conclusions seems appropriate for initial descriptive work. From 49 classrooms in two elementary schools serving low-income students, the authors selected 19 teachers for interviews, and subsequently identified 4 teachers for more intensive observation. Typically, the conclusions suggested by such a study should be verified by more controlled, more representative, or larger scale efforts.

In the case of high-stakes testing critiques, however, the subsequent evidence appears to have become even more skimpy in support of conclusions that seem even more confident. For example, the conclusions offered in the previously cited work by Lattimore (2001) were derived from a study of three tenth graders. Meisels' (2000) suggestion that high-stakes tests do "incalculable damage to students' self-esteem" (p. 16) is not well-buttressed by any data. In Meisels' swirl of objections to multiple-choice formats, the on-demand nature of testing, and the use of a single indicator for making decisions, his conclusion that "using such tests to decide how well a child is learning is absurd" (p. 19) seems insupportable even from a rhetorical perspective.

Because the hyperbolic rhetoric of the most strident critics has failed to win much ground in the public debate, a new strategy in which testing is portrayed as a frontal assault on student learning has been introduced. Those who oppose testing claim that tests actually reduce or inhibit student achievement.

One such study that investigated the effects of testing on high school diplomas found that, although not directly affecting learning, testing might "dilute efforts to improve the education of all students" (Dorn, 2003). A second study has received much attention—both praise and approbation. This study, funded by the National Education Association, consisted of multiple analyses comparing high-stakes testing policies with achievement scores on measures such as the National Assessment of Educational Progress (NAEP) and the ACT Assessment. The study concluded "in all but one analysis, student learning is indeterminate, remains at the same level it was before the policy was implemented, or actually goes down when high-stakes testing policies are instituted" (Amrein & Berliner, 2002). The *New York Times* reported that the study had found "rigorous testing ... does little to improve achievement and may actually worsen academic performance and dropout rates" (Winter, 2002, p. A-1).

THE SKY REALLY ISN'T FALLING

In contrast to the dire pronouncements of those generally within the education profession, is the broad support for testing found just about everywhere else. A report by the Business Roundtable (2001) found that any anti-testing sentiment in the populace or "backlash" has been seriously exaggerated. In general, the American public maintains broad, consistent, and strong support for measuring all students in ways that yield accurate, comparable data on student achievement (Phelps, 1998). For example, one recent survey of 1,023 parents of school-age children found that 83% of respondents believe tests provide important information about their children's educational progress, and 9 out of 10 wanted comparative (i.e., test) data about their children and the schools they attend. Two thirds of the parents surveyed said they would like to receive standardized test results for their children in every grade; one half of those parents indicated such tests should be given twice a year and the other half said that tests should be given once a year (Driesler, 2001). There is evidence that concerns about the extent (Phelps, 1997) and cost (Phelps, 2000) of testing have been seriously overestimated.

An Achieve (2002) report, *Setting the Record Straight*, summarized popular sentiment for testing:

Despite the claims of critics, testing can and does play a vital role in improving teaching and learning. States that are serious about raising standards and achievement in schools are implementing new, more challenging tests. These tests promote better instruction and provide essential information about student performance that helps everyone in the system improve. States face significant challenges in ensuring that their standards and tests are as strong as they need to be, but the answer is to make them stronger, not get rid of them or put off using them until they are perfect. (p. 1)

Solid research evidence is also available to refute some of the most commonly encountered criticisms of high-stakes tests (see, for example, Bishop, 1998, 2000). With changes in content standards and test construction practices, few state-mandated tests can be said to be "lower order" or consist solely of recall-type questions. In fact, recent experience in states such as Washington, Arizona, and Massachusetts signals that concerns about low-level tests are being replaced by a concern that complex content is being pushed too early in students' school years, that performance expectations may be too high, and that test content is sometimes too challenging (see, e.g., Bowman, 2000; Orlich, 2000; Shaw, 1999).

The previously cited report by Amrein and Berliner (2002) has also been broadly discredited by educational researchers and the public alike with clear evidence dispelling their assertions of harm caused by testing. Some solid refutations are based on methodology (see, e.g., Braun, 2003; Carnoy & Loeb, 2002; Raymond & Hanushek, 2003; Rosenshine, 2003; Thompson, 2002).

But the public reaction has been more crisp, colorful, and to the point. For example, many newspapers across the United States quickly recognized the logical fallacies in Amrein and Berliner's arguments. In one column, a writer for the *Sacramento Bee*, illustrated the errors with an analogy involving the traffic problems endemic to California roadways:

The first and most serious [error] is its underlying assumption, that state tests aren't working if student performance isn't improving. That's a bit like saying that we ought not measure commute times because, since we started monitoring freeway traffic, commutes haven't gotten any shorter and in some cases it is actually taking people longer to get to work. If anybody suggested such a thing in transportation policy, they would be laughed out of the room. Here the study commits one of the most common errors in statistical analysis. It concludes that because one thing happened before another thing, the first probably caused the second. But that is a very dangerous conclusion. (Weintraub, 2003)

Weintraub went on to identify a second logical error—this one involving the failure to realize that a myriad of other factors besides the introduction of high-stakes testing policies have accompanied increases and decreases in test scores:

Let's return to our traffic example. Suppose the state poured a billion dollars into repairing potholes on freeways this year. The repairs are expected to make the roads smoother, causing fewer delays and shortening the commute. But next year we look at the numbers and see, unfortunately, that commutes have grown still longer. Did the repairs worsen traffic? Almost certainly not. (Weintraub, 2003)

Weintraub (2003) summarized his logical analysis of the study: "The study isn't reliable. It was conducted by avowed opponents of testing, its key assumption is suspect and its methods were flawed. Other than that, it is a fine piece of work."

Still other writers probed the immense holes in Amrein and Berliner's calculations. A writer for Denver's *Rocky Mountain News* did the math:

Amrein and Berliner themselves describe their results by saying that 67 percent of states that implemented high stakes for their tests showed a decline in fourth-grade math performance on NAEP afterward. That sounds quite alarming, but it greatly exaggerates what their data show. Their survey includes 28 states, of which 16 showed no change in NAEP scores. Of the 12 that did, eight showed declines and four showed improvement. We know they aren't big on computational skills ... but still, eight is not 67 percent of 28. On eighth-grade math the balance was almost reversed, with five states improving and three declining, while fourth-grade reading was five versus five .... How do NAEP results compare in states that don't impose high stakes? They don't say. (Seebach, 2003)

Seebach then turns to more logical errors in Amrein and Berliner's analysis:

[Amrein and Berliner] offer a hodgepodge of what they call 'unintended and negative consequences' of high-stakes testing, for instance that some teachers and school officials cheat. Well, people cheat on their income taxes too, but that is not an argument against having income taxes. If teachers cheat, they should be fired. Indeed, if people have so little faith in themselves and their students that they believe they have to cheat in order to meet expectations, they shouldn't be teaching anyway. Teachers are "teaching to the test," Amrein and Berliner complain. It may have escaped their notice that that is not an unintended consequence .... The authors also note evidence from some states that students are being kept back because they aren't ready to take high-stakes tests the following year. But what's the alternative? Surely these two can't believe that in the absence of the tests, the students would be prepared to pass them. No, they'd have been pushed forward unprepared. That's exactly what the tests are supposed to stop. (Seebach, 2003)

THE INESCAPABLE NEED TO MAKE DECISIONS

One assumption underlying high-stakes testing has received particularly scant attention: the need to make decisions. The only way to avoid many of the issues associated with high-stakes testing would be simply to avoid making any decisions at all.

By definition, decision making creates categories. If, for example, some students graduate from high school and others do not, a categorical decision has been made, even if a graduation test was not used. The decisions were, presumably, made on some basis. High school music teachers make decisions such as who should be first chair for the clarinets. College faculties make decisions to tenure (or not) their colleagues. Virtually everyone concerned embraces decision making with regard to testing in fields where public protection or personal health and safety are of concern, such as medical licensure or board examinations required for the practice of medicine.

All of these kinds of decisions are essentially unavoidable. Each should be based on sound information. And, the information should be combined with other relevant, high-quality information in some deliberate, considered, defensible manner.

In educational testing, it is currently fashionable to talk as if high-stakes tests are the single bit of information used to make categorical decisions that wreak hellacious results on both people and educational systems. But simple-minded slogans like "high stakes are for tomatoes" are, well, simple-minded.[2] And, there is a straightforward, but accurate response to the oft-repeated fiction that high-stakes tests should not be the single measure used for making important decisions such as awarding high school diplomas: Tests aren't the only piece of information and it is doubtful that they ever have been. In the diploma example, multiple sources of information are used to make decisions, and success on each of them is necessary.

Certainly, many states, over the past 25 years or so, have opted to add a test performance requirement to other requirements. But, the test is just one of several criteria that most states use. For example, for an earlier article (Cizek, 2001) I surveyed the posted graduation requirements for several states across the United States, and I looked into what the local school district in my area, Chapel Hill, North Carolina, required. It turned out that nearly every state has, first and foremost, content requirements. Wisconsin's requirements were typical:

> (a) Except as provided in par. (d), a school board may not grant a high school diploma to any pupil unless the pupil has earned: In the high school grades, at least 4 credits of English including writing composition, 3 credits of social studies including state and local government, 2 credits of mathematics, 2 credits of science and 1.5 credits of physical education; In grades 7 to 12, at least 0.5 credit of health education. (Wisconsin Statutes, Section 118.33, a, 1–2)

In addition to course requirements, Pennsylvania—like many states—included a test performance requirement, but the state also reserved authority for local boards of education to add to the requirements:

---

[2]Although it's not clear what this slogan actually means, it has become a rallying cry for many who oppose testing. The slogan was popularized in an *Atlantic Monthly* article by Schrag (2000).

> Each school district, including charter schools, shall specify requirements for graduation in the strategic plan under §4.13 … Requirements shall include course completion and grades, completion of a culminating project, and results of local assessments aligned with the academic standards. Beginning in the 2002–2003 school year, students shall demonstrate proficiency in reading, writing and mathematics on either the State assessments administered in grade 11 or 12 or local assessment aligned with academic standards and State assessments under §4.52 (relating to local assessment system) at the proficient level or better in order to graduate. (22 PA Code, §4.24, a)

Under Florida law, test performance is a requirement, and very specific requirements were spelled out for credits students must earn: For example, in addition to requiring American history, American government, and Florida government, Florida students must obtain:

> One credit in performing fine arts to be selected from music, dance, drama, painting, or sculpture. A course in any art form, in addition to painting or sculpture, that requires manual dexterity, or a course in speech and debate, may be taken to satisfy the high school graduation requirement for one credit in performing arts pursuant to this subparagraph … and one-half credit in life management skills to include consumer education, positive emotional development, marriage and relationship skill-based education, nutrition, prevention of human immunodeficiency virus infection and acquired immune deficiency syndrome and other sexually transmissible diseases, benefits of sexual abstinence and consequences of teenage pregnancy, information and instruction on breast cancer detection and breast self-examination, cardiopulmonary resuscitation, drug education, and the hazards of smoking. (Florida Statutes, Title XVI, §232.246, 2, 3, i)

Not only are highly specific course requirements and test performance mandated in order for students to obtain a high school diploma, but Florida law requires that:

> Each district school board shall establish standards for graduation from its schools, and these standards must include … achievement of a cumulative grade point average of 1.5 on a 4.0 scale, or its equivalent, for students entering 9th grade before the 1997-1998 school year; however, these students must earn a cumulative grade point average of 2.0 on a 4.0 scale, or its equivalent, in the courses required by subsection (1) that are taken after July 1, 1997, or have an overall cumulative grade point average of 2.0 or above. (Florida Statutes, Title XVI, §232.246, 5, c)

As mentioned previously, most states permit local school boards to add to the graduation requirements imposed by the state.[3] In the school district serving the area of Chapel Hill, North Carolina, those requirements include 50 hours of community service learning experience and a limit on the number of days a senior can be absent.

---

[3]An interesting exception is Idaho, which has does not have a state-issued diploma but leaves requirements and other criteria to local boards of education, each charged with issuing its own diplomas.

In conclusion, although variability surely exists across states and local districts regarding the details of graduation requirements, the picture is clear: Just one too few days attendance? No diploma. Didn't take American Government? No diploma. Not enough course credits? No diploma. Miss too many questions on a test? No diploma.

Thus, it should be obvious that to speak of a test as "single measure" is nonsensical. But the obviousness of that is not at all obvious—and too frequently critical misperceptions are held or advanced by those closest to classrooms. Profound misunderstandings, where present, have the potential to create controversy, sustain skepticism about the value of testing, and hinder educational reforms.

What is perhaps most important to understand is that tests play only one (although admittedly highly visible) part in important decisions. As has been demonstrated, across the United States similar categorical decisions are made on each of the numerous criteria enacted by legislatures and by state and local boards of education. It makes as much sense to single out a single test as a sole source of information as it does to single out civics class, attendance, or any other one of the multiple criteria as the single barrier that denies students an opportunity to graduate, or to portray testing as the lone element in any the situations typical of today's educational decision making.

Thus, given the reality that legislators have established that the awarding of a diploma should hinge on success vis-à-vis numerous criteria, policy discussions must confront the statistical truism that these conjunctive models will result in the denial of more diplomas, promotions, awards, and so on as each conjunctive element is added to the decision making model. Of course, legislatures or other regulatory bodies could decide not to require success on each of the elements. One could get a diploma by making success on, say, four out of six elements. But which four? Why not three? That decision seems somewhat arbitrary. The same three for everyone? That seems unfair, given that some people would be denied a diploma simply on the basis of the arbitrary three that were identified. And, even if all other criteria were eliminated and all that remained was a requirement that students must attend at least, say, 150 out of 180 days in their senior year to get a diploma, then what should be done in the case of an honors student who has achieved grades of A in all of her classes but has attended only 149 days?

In the end, as long as any categorical decisions must be made, and regardless of the decision making model, there is going to be subjectivity involved. And, if there is going to be subjectivity, most testing specialists— and most of the public—simply favor coming clean about the source and magnitude of the subjectivity, trying to minimize it, and engaging in open dialog about the relative costs of the false positive and false negative outcomes that result from those decisions.

TESTING AND ACCOUNTABILITY

It should be evident then, that categorical decisions such as awarding diplomas will be made with or without course requirements, with or without conjunctive models, and with or without tests. Thus, it cannot be that tests of themselves are the cause of all the consternation about high-stakes assessments. The real reasons are two-fold. One reason covers resistance to high-stakes testing within the education profession; the second explains why otherwise well-informed people would so easily succumb to simplistic rhetoric centering on testing.

On the first count, that fact that high-stakes tests are increasingly used as part of accountability systems provides a sufficient rationale for resistance. Education is one of the few professions in which advancement, status, compensation, longevity, and so on are not related to personal performance. The entire accountability movement—of which testing has been the major element—has been vigorously resisted by many in the profession. Given a choice between a new, unfamiliar system that holds one accountable for performance and a *status quo* that does not, well … what decision would most people make?

On the second count, unfortunately, with few exceptions, those who know the most about testing have been virtually absent from the public square when criticisms surface. In an attempt to provide some remedy for this and some balance to the policy debates, the following section presents 10 positive unintended[4] consequences of high-stakes testing—*good* results to be obtained from an increasing reliance on student performance data in making education administration or policy decisions.

1. Professional development. I suspect that many assessment specialists who have been involved in K-12 education painfully recall professional development in the not-too-distant past. Presentations with titles like the following aren't too far from the old reality:

- Vitamins and vocabulary: Just coincidence that they both begin with "V"?
- Cosmetology across the curriculum
- Horoscopes in the homeroom
- The geometry of hip hop: Handy hints for handling hypotenuse
- Multiple intelligences in the cafeteria

In a word, much professional development was spotty, hit-or-miss, based on questionable research, of dubious effectiveness, and thoroughly avoidable. But professional development has increasingly taken

---

[4]It is not precise to say that these positive consequences are entirely unintended. Some of the consequences listed may have been anticipated, others hoped for, still others unforeseen.

on a new face. It is more frequently focused on what works to promote student achievement. It is more curriculum-relevant and results-oriented. The press toward professional development that helps educators hone their teaching skills and content area expertise is evident. Without doubt, recent emphases on higher standards and mandated tests to measure progress toward those standards should be credited.

As clear evidence of this link, one need only consider the language and specific mandates embodied in recent federal and state department of education directives. For example, at the federal level, there is a new emphasis on focused professional development. The government publication, *Improving America's Schools: Newsletter on Issues in School Reform* reported on the need for "rethinking professional development" and stated that:

> almost every approach to school reform requires teachers to refocus their roles, responsibilities, and opportunities—and, as a result, to acquire new knowledge and skills. The success of efforts to increase and reach high standards depends largely on the success of teachers and their ability to acquire the content knowledge and instructional practices necessary to teach to high academic standards. (U.S. Department of Education, 1996)

At about the same time, the U.S. Department of Education was disseminating a list of "Principles of high-quality professional development." Among the guidelines presented for any future professional development activity in education was that it "enables teachers to develop further expertise in subject content, teaching strategies, uses of technologies, and other essential elements in teaching to high standards" (U.S. Department of Education, 1995). Rigorous, relevant professional development, designed to ensure that every pupil receives instruction from a highly qualified teacher, is also a centerpiece of the No Child Left Behind legislation. Authors such as Guskey (2000), in his book *Evaluating Professional Development,* have also begun to recognize that effects on student learning are an important component in the hierarchy of outcomes that high-quality professional development programs can foster.

A similar focus on educators' professional development has worked its way down to the state level. The following excerpt from the New Jersey Administrative Code highlights the evidence of refined focus for professional development at the state level. The Code sets "Standards for Required Professional Development for Teachers" which require that professional development activities must:

> assist educators in acquiring content knowledge within their own discipline(s) and in application(s) to other disciplines; enable classroom professionals to help students achieve the New Jersey Core Curriculum Content

Standards (CCCS); [and] routinely review the alignment of professional development content with CCCS and with the Frameworks in all disciplines. (New Jersey Administrative Code, Section 6:11–13)

2. Accommodation. Recent federal legislation enacted to guide the implementation of high-stakes testing has been a catalyst for increased attention to students with special needs. Describing the impact of legislation such as the Goals 2000: Educate America Act and the Improving America's Schools Act (IASA), Thurlow and Ysseldyke (2001) observed that, "both Goals 2000 and the more forceful IASA indicated that high standards were to apply to *all* students. In very clear language, these laws defined 'all students' as including students with disabilities and students with limited English proficiency" (p. 389). The No Child Left Behind Act reinforces the notion that the era of exceptions for exceptional students has ended. Rather, to the greatest extent possible, all pupils will be tested to obtain information about their progress relative to a state's content standards in place for all students.

In accordance with these mandates, states across the United States are scurrying to adapt those tests for all students, report disaggregated results for subgroups, and implement accommodations so that tests and accountability reporting more accurately reflect the learning of all students. The result has been a very positive diffusion of awareness. Increasingly at the classroom level, educators are becoming more sensitive to the needs and barriers special needs students face when they take tests—even ordinary classroom assessments. If not driven within the context of once-per-year, high-stakes tests, it is doubtful that such progress would have been witnessed in the daily experiences of many special needs learners.

Much research in the area of high-stakes testing and students at risk has provided evidence of this positive consequence of mandated testing. One recent example comes from the Consortium on Chicago School Research, which has monitored effects of that large, urban school district's high stakes testing and accountability program. There researchers found that students (particularly those who had some history of failure) reported that the introduction of accountability testing had induced their teachers to begin focusing more attention on them (Roderick & Engel, 2001). Failure was no longer acceptable and there was a stake in helping all students succeed. In this case, necessity was the mother of intervention.

3. Knowledge about testing. For years, testing specialists have documented a lack of knowledge about assessment on the part of many educators. The title of one such article bluntly asserted educators' "Apathy toward Testing and Grading" (Hills, 1991). Other research has chronicled the chronic lack of training in assessment for teachers and principals and has offered plans for remediation (see, e.g., Impara & Plake, 1996; Stiggins, 1999). Unfortunately, for the most part, it has been difficult to require assessment training for preservice teachers or administrators, and even more difficult to wedge such training into graduate programs in education.

Then along came high-stakes tests. What faculty committees could not enact has been accomplished circuitously. Granted, misperceptions about tests persist (e.g., in my home state of North Carolina there is a lingering myth that "the green test form is harder than the red one"), but I am discovering that, across the country, educators know more about testing than ever before. Because many tests now have stakes associated with them, it has become *de rigeur* for educators to inform themselves about their content, construction, and consequences. Increasingly, teachers can tell you the difference between a norm-referenced and a criterion-referenced test; they can recognize, use, or develop a high-quality rubric; they can tell you how their state's writing test is scored, and so on.

Along with this knowledge has come the secondary benefit that knowledge of sound testing practices has had positive consequences at the classroom level—a trickle-down effect. For example, one recent study (Goldberg & Roswell, 1999/2000) investigated the effects on teachers who had participated in training and scoring of tasks for the Maryland School Performance Assessment Program (MSPAP). Those teachers who were involved with the MSPAP overwhelmingly reported that their experience had made them more reflective, deliberate, and critical in terms of their own classroom instruction and assessment.

4 & 5. Collection and use of information. Because pupil performance on high-stakes tests has become of such prominent and public interest, an intensity of effort unparalleled in U.S. education history is now directed toward data collection and quality control. State and federal mandates for the collection and reporting of this information (and more), have also resulted in unparalleled access to the data.

Obtaining information about test performance, graduation rates, per-pupil spending, staffing, finance, and facilities is, in most states, now just a mouse-click away. How would you like your data for secondary analysis: Aggregated or disaggregated? Single year or longitudinal? PDF or Excel? Paper or plastic? Consequently, those who must respond to state mandates for data collection (i.e., school districts) have become increasingly conscientious about providing the most accurate information possible—often at risk of penalties for inaccuracy or incompleteness.

This is an unqualified boon. Not only is more information about student performance available, but it is increasingly used as part of decision making. At a recent teacher recruiting event, I heard a recruiter question a teacher about how she would be able to tell that her students were learning. "I can just see it in their eyes," was the reply. "Sorry, you are the weakest link."

Increasingly, from the classroom to the school board room, educators are making use of student performance data to help them refine programs, channel funding, and identify roots of success. If the data—in particular achievement test data—weren't so important, it is unlikely that this would be the case.

6. Educational options. Related to the increase in publicly available information about student performance and school characteristics is the spawning of greater options for parents and students. Complementing a hunger for information, the public's appetite for alternatives has been whetted. In many cases, schools have responded. Charter schools, magnet schools, home schools, and increased offerings of honors, IB and AP courses have broadened the choices available to parents. And, research is slowly accumulating which suggests that the presence of choices has not spelled doom for traditional options but has largely raised all boats (see, e.g., Finn, Manno, & Vanourek, 2000; Greene, 2001). It is almost surely the case that legislators' votes and parents' feet would not be moving in the direction of expanding alternatives if not for the information provided by high-stakes tests. And, because turnabout is fair play, the same tests are being used to gauge the success or failure of these emerging alternatives (see e.g., Miron & Nelson, 2002).

7. Accountability systems. No one would argue that current accountability systems have reached a mature state of development. On the contrary, nascent systems are for the most part crude, cumbersome, embryonic endeavors. Equally certain, though, is that even rudimentary accountability systems would not likely be around if it weren't for high-stakes tests. For better or worse, high-stakes tests are often the foundation upon which accountability systems have been built. This is not to say that this relation between high-stakes tests and accountability is right, noble, inevitable, or appropriate. It simply recognizes the reality that current accountability systems were enabled by an antecedent: mandated, high-stakes student achievement tests.

To many policy makers, professionals, and the public, however, the notion of introducing accountability—even just acknowledging that accountability is a good innovation—is an important first step. That the camel's nose took the form of high-stakes tests was (perhaps) not recognized and was (almost certainly) viewed as acceptable. Necessary and healthy debates continue about the role of tests and the form of accountability.

Although high-stakes tests have begun to help forge a path in the wilderness, the controversy clearly hinges on accountability itself. The difficult fits and starts of developing sound accountability systems should be understandable given their nascent developmental state. Understanding the importance, complexity, and difficulties as the accountability infant matures will surely be trying. How—or if—high-stakes tests will fit into more mature versions of accountability systems is hard to tell, and the devil will be in the details. But it is evident that the presence of high-stakes tests has at least served as a conversation-starter for a policy dialog that would not likely have taken place in their absence.

8. Educators' intimacy with their disciplines. Once a test has been mandated in, say, language arts, the first step in any high-stakes testing program is to circumscribe the boundaries of what will be tested. The nearly universal strategy for accomplishing this is to impanel groups of (primarily) educators who are familiar with the ages, grades, and content to be tested. These groups are usually large, selected to be representative, and expert in the subject area. The groups first study relevant documentation (e.g. the authorizing legislation, state curriculum guides, content standards). They then begin the arduous, time-consuming task of discussing among themselves the nature of the content area, the sequence and content of typical instruction, learner characteristics and developmental issues, cross-disciplinary relationships, and relevant assessment techniques.

These extended conversations help shape the resulting high-stakes tests, to be sure. However, they also affect the discussants, and those with whom they interact when they return to their districts, buildings, and classrooms. As persons with special knowledge about a particular high-stakes testing program, the participants are sometimes asked to replicate those disciplinary and logistic discussions locally. The impact of this trickling-down can be beneficial. For example, at one session of the 2000 American Educational Research Association conference, scholars reported on the positive effects of a state testing program in Maine on classroom assessment practices (Beaudry, 2000) and on how educators in Florida were assimilating their involvement in large-scale testing activities at the local level (Banerji, 2000).

These local discussions mirror the large scale counterparts in that they provide educators with an opportunity to become more intimate with the nature and structure of their own disciplines, and to contemplate interdisciplinary relationships. This is a good thing. And the impulse for this good thing is clearly the presence of a high-stakes test.

9. Quality of tests. Another beneficial consequence of high-stakes testing is the effect that the introduction of consequences has had on the tests themselves. Along with more serious consequences has come heightened scrutiny. The high-stakes tests of today are surely the most meticulously developed, carefully constructed, and rigorously reported. Many criticisms of tests are valid, but a complainant who suggests that today's high-stakes tests are "lower-order" or "biased" or "inauthentic" is almost certainly not familiar with that which they purport to critique. If only due to their long history and ever-present watchdogging, high-stakes tests have evolved to a point where they are: highly reliable; free from bias; relevant and age appropriate; higher order; tightly related to important, publicly-endorsed goals; time and cost efficient; and yielding remarkably consistent decisions.

Evidence of the impulse toward heightened scrutiny of educational tests with consequences can be traced at least to the landmark case of *Debra P. v. Turlington* (1984). Although the central aspect of that case was the legal arguments regarding substantive and procedural due process, the abundance of evidence regarding the psychometric characteristics of Florida's graduation test was essential in terms of making the case that the process and outcomes were fundamentally fair to Florida students. Although legal challenges to such high-stakes tests still occur (see the special issue of *Applied Measurement in Education* (2000) for an example involving a Texas test), they are remarkably infrequent. For the most part, those responsible for mandated testing programs responded to the *Debra P.* case with a heightened sense of the high standard that is applied to high-stakes measures. It is a fair conclusion that, in terms of legal wranglings concerning high-stakes tests, the psychometric characteristics of the test are rarely the basis of a successful challenge.

Research has demonstrated that large-scale (e.g., state-level or school system-wide) testing accounts for less than 2 days per year per student on average (Phelps, 1997). With the advent of *No Child Left Behind* regulations that every student in Grades 3 through 8 be tested annually in reading, mathematics, and science, that number of days will likely increase somewhat—particularly in states where testing in those grades and subjects had not been in place. However, it is also fair to say that one strains the gnat in objecting to the characteristics of high-stakes tests, when the characteristics of those tests are compared to what a child will likely experience in his or her classroom the other 178 days of the school year. All those genuinely committed to fair testing might appropriately refocus their attention on improving the quality of classroom assessment.

Decades of evidence have been amassed to support the contention that the quality of teacher-made tests pales compared to more rigorously developed, large-scale counterparts. Such evidence begins with the classic studies of teachers' grading practice by Starch and Elliot (1912, 1913a, 1913b) and continues with more recent studies which document that weaknesses in typical classroom assessment practices have persisted (see, e.g., Carter, 1984; Gullickson & Ellwein, 1985). It is not an overstatement to say that, at least on the grounds of technical quality, the typical high-stakes, state-mandated test that a student takes will—by far—be the best assessment that student will see all year.

A secondary benefit of high-stakes tests' quality is that, because of their perceived importance, they become mimicked at lower levels. It is appropriate to abhor teaching to the test—at least if that phrase is taken to mean teaching the exact items that will appear on a test, or limiting instruction only to those objectives that are addressed on a high-stakes test.[5] However, it is also important to recognize the beneficial effects of exposing educators to high-quality writing prompts, document-based questions, constructed-response formats, and even challenging multiple-choice items. It is not cheating, but the highest form of praise when educators then rely on these exemplars to enhance their own assessment practices.

Another version involves narrowing teaching to include only those objectives covered by the high-stakes test. Many testing professionals (and others) would also agree that exclusion of other, valuable outcomes and experiences from the curriculum is undesirable.

Finally, it is possible to align instruction with the curriculum guide, content standards, and so forth (depending on the terminology used to describe the valuable student outcomes in a particular locale). And, it is obviously desirable that any high-stakes test be closely aligned with the curriculum or content standards it purports to assess. Thus, it would neither be a coincidence—nor inappropriate—if the well-aligned instruction and testing bore a strong resemblance to each other. This is sometimes mistakenly referred to as *teaching to the test* where the more accurate (and supportable) practice should probably be distinguished by use of a different descriptor, such as *teaching to the standards* or similar.

10. Increased student learning. It is not completely appropriate to categorize increased student learning as an unintended consequence. At least in terms of the political or policy rhetoric often accompanying high-stakes tests, there are usually strong claims made regarding the effects of testing on student learning. However, not all of those concerned about educational reform would necessarily agree that increased learning should be expected. As I have argued elsewhere, a major reason that high-stakes testing was introduced in the first place may have simply been to increase the uniformity (standardize) of a state's curriculum as it is actually experienced by students (see Camilli, Cizek, & Lugg, 2001).[6]

---

[5]The phrase and practice of *teaching to the test* has come to have many different meanings. Three of these meanings are presented here. One version of the practice involves teaching students the exact (or highly similar) items that will appear on a test. Most testing professionals would agree that such behavior is both detrimental to accurate interpretation of test scores and unethical.

[6]I am sensitive to this concern as a result of an experience I had with my own children. One of our children (the youngest) has greater difficult and dislike for reading than his siblings. I attribute this, to a degree, to some of his early elementary school experiences.

One particularly vivid memory is of a parent-teacher conference we attended at the beginning of the school year. The teacher explained enthusiastically that she would be implementing a "literacy-rich curriculum" for the youngsters. Included in the children's classroom experiences would be a puppet-play (our son was in charge of making the props), a visit to a museum to learn about early paper and book making, an on-site visit from a children's book illustrator, the making of a literacy quilt, and more. The obvious—although unexpressed—question that occurred to us at the time was, "But when will our son actually learn how to *read*?"

This experience was instructive because, in other classrooms (even in the same school district) other students at the same grade level experienced a much different curriculum—a curriculum decidedly leaning toward instruction in letters, sounds, comprehension, oral and silent fluency, and so forth. The kind of early reading program experienced by any given student depended in large measure on the teacher to whom the student happened to be assigned.

Some critics of high-stakes testing have suggested that these assessments may increase students' *test scores*, but not students' *learning*. However, that argument has not been made clearly. More importantly, a clear method for or logic regarding how to measure increases in learning in ways that would *not* show up in test score gains has not been put forward.

The most cynical observers have suggested either that *no effects* of testing are likely (as in the commonly heard metaphor that frequent temperature taking has no effect on reducing a fever) or that testing has adverse effects on learning (as in the previously cited publication of Amrein and Berliner, 2002). Thus, at least in some quarters, increased student achievement attributable to the presence of high-stakes tests would qualify as an unexpected consequence.

Through the fog of negative assertions from education insiders, though, some astute observers have been able to see the effects of testing clearly. A recent article in the *Virginian-Pilot* reported on an evaluation of Virginia's rigorous accountability testing system [called the "Standards of Learning" (SOL)] over the period since the SOL program was instituted in 1998. The evaluation revealed that:

- 4th- and 6th-grade Virginia students' scores on the norm-referenced *Stanford Achievement Tests* in reading, language, and mathematics had increased over the time frame studied (scores for ninth grade students remained stable);
- statewide average SAT-Verbal and SAT-Mathematics scores rose; and
- "more students have taken Advanced Placement tests and enrolled in rigorous International Baccalaureate programs since the SOL program began" (Study Shows, 2003, p. 1).

Another recent example reports on increasing student achievement in Massachusetts. *USA Today* cites a review of that state's standards-based reforms by Achieve, "the state using the nation's highest regarded test is reaping some of the most impressive gains." The article concluded that "testing can improve student performance, especially when states serve up high-quality education standards backed by relevant, high-quality tests" (Schools sharpen testing, 2001, p. A–14).

The news from Massachusetts is particularly enlightening, as that state has a relatively long track record with high-stakes testing. The Massachusetts Comprehensive Assessment System (MCAS) is also one of the most transparent and scrutinized programs of its kind. Recent news reports indicate that students are learning more of what that state hopes for students to achieve as measured by its high school examinations. In 2002, 1 year after pass rates on the MCAS exam rose significantly—a gain that was viewed skeptically by opponents of that high-stakes testing program—

- overall achievement increased again. In spring 2002, 86 percent of sophomores passed the MCAS English exam (up from 82% in 2001), whereas 75% passed the math exam (the same as in spring 2001) and 69% of sophomores passed both sections (Hayward, 2002a);
- achievement gaps narrowed. On the 2002 tests, the percentage of African-American students passing the English section increased by 7% (although the pass rate for that group on the math exam slipped by 3 points). "The pass rate for Hispanics high-schoolers on the English exam jumped from 52 percent to 61 percent" (Hayward, 2002a); and
- dropout rates remained stable. According to the Boston *Herald* newspaper, "The state's high school dropout rate remained stable at 3.5% during the 2000–2001 school year, countering theories that the MCAS tests would lead to an exodus" (Hayward, 2002b). The 3.5% rate was the same as for the 1999–2000 school year, and 1% less than for the 1998–1999 school year.

These rosy outcomes related to student learning and related concerns are corroborated by testimony from students themselves. For example, in a recent study (Mass Insight Education, 2002) interviews were conducted with 140 randomly selected urban high school students regarding their perceptions about the MCAS. The results revealed that:

- 67% of students who failed the MCAS the first time they took it said that, as a result, they are working harder in school; 65% said that they pay more attention in class since failing the MCAS;
- 74% of students interviewed said that missing too much school is a "big reason" why students don't pass MCAS; 64% said that not working hard enough in school and on homework is a big reason;

- 74% reported that they consider themselves to be more able in math, reading or writing because they have to pass the MCAS in order to graduate; and
- 53% said that they get more help and attention from teachers since getting their MCAS results.

Taken together, these results are not dispositive, of course, with respect to questions about the consequences of high-stakes testing in general, or with respect to effects on student learning in particular. However, the results are reasonably positive—and markedly more positive than most opponents of high-stakes testing seem willing to admit.

ACCOUNTABILITY REDUX

Why the apparent reluctance of some educators to embrace high-stakes testing? As an insightful colleague of mine has observed, "the crux of the matter is not the broad issue of testing, but *high stakes* testing (Camilli, 2003, p. 36).

In my own experience teaching university courses on testing to in-service teachers, many of them have articulated to me precisely the same conclusion as Camilli has offered, though in somewhat different terms. It's not the tests exactly that they sometimes dislike so much, but the fact that the tests have consequences. Some kids fail. Others don't get a diploma. Some suffer negative self-perceptions.

There's a catch-22 here, however. On the one hand, there is a distinctive moniker that we apply to instructors who hold the unflagging belief that all students can succeed, who have the unfailing penchant for anticipating positive outcomes for their students, and who display antipathy toward any roadblock that might thwart a child's pursuit of personal aspirations and goals. Among other characteristics, these are a few of the qualities possessed by what we call *a good teacher*. On the other hand, it is perhaps precisely these predilections and the possibility of realizing an outlet for these noble notions that attracts people into the teaching profession in the first place. It is surely unrealistic to expect them to abandon those values during the second week in October of every year. Although this is merely speculation on my part, there may also be essential differences in world views or in philosophies regarding human nature that account for what makes some people comfortable with consequences and others not. There may also be other reasons why persons might oppose standards with consequences as we currently see that impulse playing out in the education policy arena (see Mehrens & Cizek, 2001).

Regardless, it is indeed the stakes that are the heart of the matter. It can be hoped that the presence, severity, and diffusion of consequences can be tenuously negotiated in whatever the future of accountability systems holds.

No current system is without blemish. But it would be unwise to sacrifice the good on the altar of the perfect.

An analogy comes to mind. I recall that, when I was in high school, the marquee outside the gymnasium would annually announce, "Boys Fall Sports Physicals, Tuesday, 7:00pm." Basically this meant the following: If you wanted to participate in a fall sport, you would have to show up on Tuesday night, strip down with dozens of other guys, and permit a local volunteer physician to poke, prod, and prompt you to "turn your head and cough" when directed to do so. If the doctor didn't discover anything dangerous, you'd be permitted to compete with one of the fall sports teams. If the doctor found a heart murmur, you'd be out.

Accountability systems seem to me to be just like those high school sports physicals: potentially embarrassing; done by an external entity; somewhat invasive; carrying the potential to deny some individuals access to an opportunity; but, in the main, necessary and beneficial for the people involved.

Of course, in the field of education, as in the field of medicine, it's what we do with test results within the accountability system that makes all the difference. If a kid is thought to have a heart murmur, we generally acknowledge that he or she has a problem and we do something about it. In education, if a student fails a proficiency test, there is a tendency to invoke concerns about bias or possible random fluctuations in test results. Now, we all know that achievement tests are not perfect. But neither are medical tests. Pregnancy tests are sometimes wrong. Blood pressure readings are subjective and variable within an individual. Even with the miraculous DNA tests, experts can only make statements like "there is 99.93% chance that the DNA is a match." Yet, blood pressure is not reported as 120/80 with an associated standard error. Maybe I don't really have high blood pressure. Maybe my pressure is 120/80 plus or minus 17. Maybe I just don't have good blood pressure taking skills.

As Camilli (2003) observed, the underlying issue really is accountability itself. I think that we are inclined to accept medical measurements as highly accurate and error-free because there's no finger pointing, only therapy. Maybe my blood pressure is high because I failed to heed the physician's orders to lay off the blueberry pancakes and lose some weight. Maybe the pregnancy test was positive because I was sexually active. It may not matter. The physician's response is simply to prescribe the healthiest next step.

In education, if a student doesn't perform well on a test, there are a lot of possible (and confounded) explanations. Bad teaching, lack of persistence, distracting learning environment, dysfunctional home environment, and so forth. We know that all of these (and more) exist to a greater or lesser extent in the mix. Who should be accountable? The teacher for the quality of instruction? Sure. The student for effort and persistence? Yes. The administration for providing safe learning environment? Yep. The parents for establishing a supportive home environment? Yessiree. The only limitation is that, in education, we can only make policies to address any of those (or other) factors that are legitimately under governmental control.

Now let's compare medical tests and educational achievement tests. Today's medical tests are pretty good. When a defective medical measuring device is identified, it gets pulled by the FDA. If there were intolerable error rates in home pregnancy test kits, it would create a stir, and the product would be improved, or fall out of use. The quality of today's educational measurements is also quite high. By accepted professional standards, we have better assessments than ever. I can't think of a large-scale, high-stakes test that doesn't have a reliability estimate near .90 or above, a bushel of content validity evidence, outstanding decision consistency indices, cutscores that minimize false negative decisions, and multiple opportunities for students to take them. It's no exaggeration to say—especially compared to the tests a student will be exposed to all year in his or her classroom—that a state-mandated student proficiency test is probably the highest quality test that the kid will see all year ... maybe over his or her entire school career.

Again, can those tests be any better? Of course. But the bottom line is that, if we were to compare all of the measures used to gauge student performance—e.g., attendance, course credits, high-stakes test score, grades, etc., the murmur is most reliably identified by the high-stakes test. I think it's about time people stopped wringing their hands over the exceptions, started providing the interventions necessary, and quit shying away from identifying and addressing the sources of the problems *wherever* they lie.

KEEPIN' IT REAL

Just as all achievement tests—high-stakes or otherwise—can be improved, we must also recognize the limitations of such tests, particularly those of the state-mandated, large-scale variety that are currently the focus of research and the center of vigorous political debates. Contrary to what many policy makers and advocates of testing would state or imply, *the current generation of high-stakes tests is incapable of delivering on the promise of providing high-quality information that teachers can use for individualizing instruction for any particular student.*

I realize that the preceding disclosure might brand me as a whistleblower among assessment advocates. But it's true. Policy makers and others have touted large-scale achievement tests as having great instructional relevance. However, the utility of the product has been vastly overstated. Hopes have been unrealistically inflated. Expectations have been fostered that (very shortly) following the administration of the state-wide test, Ms.

Jones will have delivered to her detailed diagnostic information for each student in her class.

Unfortunately, the reality is that (a) current tests are not designed to be individually diagnostic, (b) the amounts of time generally allocated to testing preclude gaining fine-grained information about any individual student, and (c) even results based on comparative clustering of course content are of doubtful assistance to teachers. (For example, suppose a test reveals that a student was *Below Basic* on the subtest, *Mathematics Applications*; how could a teacher possibly incorporate that information into tomorrow's lesson?). We must all get past the fiction that current large-scale achievement tests of the state-mandated variety are, in the near term, going to provide much at all in the way of instructional relevance for individual students or specific guidance for teachers.

The reality of the matter is that current large-scale high-stakes tests function best as fairly good indicators of an individual student's overall status and as broad indices of systemic educational health. This does not lessen their value, however. For example, no serious investor would make a decision about what to do regarding a specific stock (the individual case) based solely on where the Dow Jones Industrial Average (the broad index) happens to be on a given day. Does this mean that the coarse indicator is useless? Of course not. No serious investor would suggest doing away with the Dow Jones average, either. It performs the task it was designed to do remarkably well.[7]

And so it is with current high-stakes, state-mandated assessments. The results give policy makers, educators, and parents some very useful—although limited—information. As macrolevel gauges, aggregated results

---

[7]I invoked the Dow Jones average example because, although I have little to no knowledge about the stock markets, I thought that the context would be familiar to many readers. Perhaps a better analogy—and one more familiar to me as a father of three children—is the Apgar scoring for newborns system for providing an overall indicator of the health of newborn children.

Named after Dr. Virginia Apgar, the scale is used to express an infant's physical condition minutes after birth. The APGAR acronym represents five characteristics of newborns that are each scored on a 0–2 point continuum: *A*ppearance (skin color); *P*ulse; *G*rimace (reflex irritability); *A*ctivity (muscle activity); and *R*espiration. A score on each of the characteristics is assigned to a newborn at one minute and five minutes after birth, with a total possible score ranging from 0 of 10. A total score of 7 to 10 is considered normal; a score of 4 to 7 indicates that the infant may be in need of some resuscitative measures; a score of 3 or below indicates immediate resuscitation needs. Dr. Apgar reportedly developed the scale in 1952 to prompt medical personnel to pay more attention to newborns in the first critical minutes of life, and her work is considered to have been a major impulse in the formation of the perinatology specialty (Apgar Scoring for Newborns, 2002).

Like a student's score or classification on a high-stakes achievement test, the Apgar score does not directly reveal any specific diagnosis or prescribe definitive individual treatments. Nonetheless, the Apgar score is now widely recognized as an indispensable indicator of an individual health.

provide essential data for monitoring general educational progress or re-gress across often large and complex systems in a given state. Perhaps the greatest instructional utility can be realized if the units of analysis are groups of students. For example, current tests yield reasonably confident conclusions about broad areas of strength and weakness for school build-ings and districts. To the extent that test results are reviewed, analyzed, and result in curricular and instructional changes, they are certainly useful.

Finally, for individual students, the state of the art in large-scale testing permits fairly confident conclusions about a student's proficiency, though at a level that most educators would not find readily amenable to classroom use. For example, most state achievement testing programs yield highly ac-curate conclusions about a student's overall competence in reading com-prehension; none is capable of supporting a confident conclusion that Tabitha knows a simile from a metaphor.

Just as accountability systems have not reached developmental matu-rity, neither have testing programs. A complete assessment system would have numerous desirable components: it would provide general monitor-ing functions; it would give teachers diagnostic information for individual students; it would supply administrators with data for refining curriculum and instruction; it would yield evidence for evaluations of teacher and school effectiveness, and others. Is such a system going to be cheap? Perfect out of the blocks? Right around the corner? No. No. No.

However, embryonic manifestations of an integrated system that serves both macrolevel and microlevel concerns are beginning to emerge in various locales. One such example is the well-articulated and coordinated system of local benchmarks, curriculum, teacher supports, assessments, remediation avenues, and local accountability mechanisms found in the Gwinnett County (GA) Public Schools (see www.gwinnett.k12.ga.us/). At the state level, Ohio is currently developing a system of pupil assessments, linked to system-wide content standards, that serves state-level accountability and monitoring concerns. Concurrently, developmental work is proceeding to design and promote complementary assessment strategies that teachers can use to obtain diagnostic information for individual students, along with the recognition that extensive professional development will be necessary to en-hance educator facility with diagnostic assessment to inform instruction in the classroom. These examples (and others) portend more useful assessment and accountability systems down the road.

CONCLUSION

It would be foolish to ignore the shortcomings and undesirable conse-quences of high-stakes tests. Current inquiry along these lines is essential, productive, and encouraging. However, in the context of some consternation about high-stakes tests, particularly within the education profession, it is equally essential to consider the unanticipated positive consequences, and to incorporate these into any cost-benefit calculus that should characterize sound policy decisions.

Passionate debates about the nature and role of high-stakes tests and accountability systems are healthy and necessary. To these frays, the stakeholders may bring differing starting points and differing conceptualizations of the meaning and status that should be afforded to issues ranging from technical adequacy, to educational goals, to social justice. It is an exhilarating time of profound questioning about context, content, and consequences of testing. High-stakes tests: we don't know how to live with them; we can't seem to live without them. The oft-quoted first sentence of Charles Dickens' *A Tale of Two Cities* ("It was the best of times, it was the worst of times") seems especially relevant to the juncture at which we find ourselves. The remainder of Dickens' (1859) opening paragraph merely extends the piquant metaphor: "It was the age of wisdom, it was the age of foolishness, it was the epoch of belief, it was the epoch of incredulity, it was the season of Light, it was the season of Darkness, it was the spring of hope, it was the winter of despair, we had everything before us, we had nothing before us, we were all going direct to Heaven, we were all going direct the other way" (p. 3).

ACKNOWLEDGMENT

This chapter is based in large part on the author's previously published writings, including "More Unintended Consequences of High-Stakes Testing" (2001), "E" (2003), and "Standard Setting and the Public Good: Benefits Accrued and Anticipated" (with W. A. Mehrens, 2001).

REFERENCES

Achieve. (2000, Summer). *Achieve policy brief. Testing: Setting the record straight.* Cambridge, MA: Author.

Amrein, A. L., & Berliner, D. C. (2002, March 28). High-stakes testing, uncertainty, and student learning. *Education Policy Analysis Archives [on-line], 10*(18). Available: http://epaa.asu.edu/epaa/v10n18/

Applied Measurement in Education. (2000). *Special issue on Texas high-school graduation test. 13*(4).

Apgar scoring for newborns. (2002). Retrieved December 27, 2002 from http://apgar.net/virginia/

Banerji, M. (2000, April). *Designing district-level classroom assessment systems.* Paper presented at the annual meeting of the American Educational Research Association, New Orleans, LA.

Beaudry, J. (2000, April). *The positive effects of administrators and teachers on classroom assessment practices and student achievement*. Paper presented at the annual meeting of the American Educational Research Association, New Orleans, LA.

Bishop, J. H. (1998). The effect of curriculum-based external exit exam systems on student achievement. *Journal of Economic Education, 29*(2), 171–182.

Bishop, J. H. (2000). Curriculum-based external exit exam systems: Do students learn more? How? *Psychology, Public Policy, and Law, 6*(1), 199–215.

Bowman, D. H. (2000, November 29). Arizona poised to revisit graduation exam. *Education Week [on-line]*. Available: http://www.edweek.org/ew/ewstory.cfm?slug=13ariz.h20

Bracey, G. (1989, April 5). Advocates of basic skills 'know what ain't so'. *Education Week, 8*(28), 24, 32.

Bracey, G. (2002, January 23). International comparisons: An excuse to avoid meaningful educational reform. *Education Week, 21*(19), 30, 32.

Braun, H. (2003). Reconsidering the impact of high-stakes testing. *Education Policy Analysis Archives [on-line], 12*(1). Available: http://epaa.asu.edu/epaa/v12n1

Brooks, S. S. (1922). *Improving schools by standardized tests*. Boston: Houghton-Mifflin.

Business Roundtable. (2001). *Assessing and addressing the 'testing backlash.'* Washington, DC: Author.

Camilli, G. (2003). Comment on Cizek's 'More Unintended Consequences of High-Stakes Testing'. *Educational Measurement: Issues and Practice, 22*(1), 36–39.

Camilli, G. A., Cizek, G. J., & Lugg, C. A. (2001). Psychometric theory and the validation of performance standards: History and future perspectives. In G. J. Cizek (Ed.), *Setting performance standards: Concepts, methods, and perspectives* (pp. 445–475). Mahwah, NJ: Lawrence Erlbaum Associates.

Carnoy, M., & Loeb, S. (2002). Does external accountability affect student outcomes? A cross-state analysis. *Educational Evaluation and Policy Analysis, 24*, 305–331.

Carter, K. (1984). Do teachers understand principles for writing tests? *Journal of Teacher Education, 35*(6), 57–60.

Chenoweth, K. (2000). Judge's ruling effectively acquits high-stakes test: To the disadvantage of poor and minority students. *Black Issues in Higher Education, 51*, 12.

Cizek, G. J. (2001). More unintended consequences of high-stakes testing. *Educational Measurement: Issues and Practice, 20*(4), 19–27.

Cizek, G. J. (2003). E. *Educational Measurement: Issues and Practice, 22*(1), 40–44.

Debra P. v. Turlington. (1984). 730 F. 2d 1405.

Dickens, C. (1859). *A tale of two cities*. London: Chapman and Hall.

Dorn, S. (2003). High-stakes testing and the history of graduation. *Education Policy Analysis Archives [on-line], 11*(1). Available: http://epaa.asu.edu/epaa/v11n1/

Driesler, S. D. (2001). Whiplash about backlash: The truth about public support for testing. *NCME Newsletter, 9*(3), 2–5.

Finn, C. E., Jr., Manno, B. V., & Vanourek, G. (2000). *Charter schools in action: Renewing public education*. Princeton, NJ: Princeton University Press.

Florida Statutes, Title XVI, 232.246, 2, 3, I.

Goldberg, G. L., & Roswell, B. S. (1999/2000). From perception to practice: the impact of teachers' scoring experience on performance-based instruction and classroom assessment. *Educational Assessment, 6*(4), 257–290.

Greene, J. P. (2001). *An evaluation of the Florida A-plus accountability and school choice program*. Tallahassee, FL: Florida State University.

Gullickson, A. R., & Ellwein, M. C. (1985). Post-hoc analysis of teacher-made tests: The goodness of fit between prescription and practice. *Educational Measurement: Issues and Practice, 4*(1), 15–18.

Guskey, T. R. (2000). *Evaluating professional development*. Thousand Oaks, CA: Corwin.

Hayward, E. (2002a, August 30). MCAS scores improve as minorities narrow gap. *Boston Herald [on-line]*. Available: www2.bonstonherald.com/news/local_regional/mcas08302002.htm

Hayward, E. (2002b, August 27). Dropout rates remain stable despite MCAS. *Boston Herald [on-line]*. Available: www2.bonstonherald.com/news/local_regional/mcas08262002.htm

Hilliard, A. (2000). Excellence in education versus high-stakes testing. *Journal of Teacher Education, 51*, 293–304.

Hills, J. (1991). Apathy toward testing and grading. *Phi Delta Kappan, 72*, 540–545.

Impara, J., & Plake, B. (1996). Professional development in student assessment for educational administrators. *Educational Measurement: Issues and Practice, 15*(2), 14–20.

Kannapel, P. (1996, April). *I don't give a hoot if somebody is going to pay me $3600: Local school district reaction to Kentucky's high-stakes accountability system*. Paper presented at the Annual Meeting of the American Educational Research Association, New York. (ERIC Document No. 397 135).

Kohn, A. (2000). Burnt at the high stakes. *Journal of Teacher Education, 51*, 315–327.

Kohn, A. (2001). Fighting the tests: A practical guide to rescuing our schools. *Phi Delta Kappan, 82*(5), 349–357.

Lattimore, R. (2001). The wrath of high-stakes tests. *Urban Review, 33*(1), 57–67.

Madaus, G. (1998). The distortion of teaching and testing: High-stakes testing and instruction. *Peabody Journal of Education, 65*, 29–46.

Mass Insight Education. (2002, March). *Taking charge: Urban high school students speak out about MCAS, academics and extra-help programs*. Boston: Author.

Mehrens, W. A., & Cizek, G. J. (2001). Standard setting and the public good: Benefits accrued and anticipated. In G. J. Cizek (Ed.), *Setting performance standards: Concepts, methods, and perspectives* (pp. 477–486). Mahwah, NJ: Lawrence Erlbaum Associates.

Meisels, S. J. (2000). On the side of the child. *Young Children, 55*(6), 16–19.

Miron, G., & Nelson, C. (2002). *What's public about charter schools? Lessons learned about choice and accountability*. Thousand Oaks, CA: Corwin.

New Jersey Administrative Code, 6, 11–13.

Ohanian, S. (2001). News from the test resistance trail. *Phi Delta Kappan, 82*(5), 363–366.

Orlich, D. C. (2000). Education reform and limits to student achievement. *Phi Delta Kappan, 81*, 468–472.

Phelps, R. P. (1997). The extent and character of system-wide student testing in the United States. *Educational Assessment, 4*(2), 89–122.

Phelps, R. P. (1998). The demand for standardized student testing. *Educational Measurement: Issues and Practice, 17*(3), 5–23.

Phelps, R. P. (2000). Estimating the cost of standardized student testing in the United States. *Journal of Education Finance, 25,* 343–380.

Raymond, M. E., & Hanushek, E. A. (2003). High-stakes research. *Education Next,* 3(3), 48–55.

Roderick, M., & Engel, M. (2001). The grasshopper and the ant: Motivational responses of low achieving students to high-stakes testing. *Educational Evaluation and Policy Analysis, 23,* 197–227.

Rosenshine, B. (2003, August 4). High-stakes testing: Another analysis. *Education Policy Analysis Archives [On-line], 11*(24). Available: http://epaa.asu.edu/epaa/v11n24/

Schools sharpen testing. (2001, October 17). *USA Today,* A–14.

Schrag, P. (2000, August). High stakes are for tomatoes. *Atlantic Monthly, 286*(2), 19–21.

Seebach, L. (2003, January 11). All the marbles. *Rocky Mountain News [on-line].* Available: http://www.rockymountainnews.com/drmn/news_columnists/article/0,1299,DRMN_86_1666617,00.html

Shaw, L. (1999, October 10). State's 4th-grade math test too difficult for students' development level, critics say. *Seattle Times [on-line].* Available: http://seattletimes.nwsource.com/news/local/html98/test_19991010.html

Smith, M. L., & Rottenberg, C. (1991). Unintended consequences of external testing in elementary schools. *Educational Measurement: Issues and Practice, 10*(4), 7–11.

Starch, D., & Elliot, E. C. (1912). Reliability of the grading of high school work in English. *School Review, 21,* 442–457.

Starch, D., & Elliot, E. C. (1913a). Reliability of the grading of high school work in history. *School Review, 21,* 676–681.

Starch, D., & Elliot, E. C. (1913b). Reliability of grading work in mathematics. *School Review, 22,* 254–259.

Stiggins, R. (1999). Evaluating classroom assessment training in teacher education programs. *Educational Measurement: Issues and Practice, 18*(1), 23–27.

Study shows SOLs improving students' performance. (2003, February 27). *Virginian-Pilot [on-line].* Available: www.pilotonline.com/breaking/br0227sol.htm

Thompson, B. (2002, November). A Response to Amrein and Berliner. *In Defense of Testing Series [on-line].* Available: www.EducationNews.org

Thompson, S. (2001). The authentic testing movement and its evil twin. *Phi Delta Kappan, 82*(5), 358–362.

Thurlow, M. L, & Ysseldyke, J. E. (2001). Standard setting challenges for special populations. In G. J. Cizek (Ed.), *Setting performance standards: Concepts, methods, and perspectives* (pp. 387–410). Mahwah, NJ: Lawrence Erlbaum Associates.

United States Department of Education. (1995). *Principles of high-quality professional development [on-line].* Available: http://www.ed.gov/G2K/bridge.html

United States Department of Education. (1996). *Improving America's Schools: Newsletter on Issues in School Reform [on-line].* Available: http://www.ed.gov/pubs/IASA/newsletters/profdev/pt1.html

Weintraub, D. (2003, January 23). Research damning tests draws a flawed conclusion. *Sacramento Bee [on-line].* Available: http://www.sacbee.com/content/politics/columns/weintraub/v-print/ story/5964487p-6923701c.html

Winter, G. (2002, December 28). Make-or-break exams grow, but big study doubts
    value. *New York Times*, A–1.
Wisconsin Statutes, 118.33, a, 1–2.

3

The Rich, Robust Research Literature on Testing's Achievement Benefits

Richard P. Phelps
Third Education Group

As Assistant District Attorney, Jack McCoy said to his boss, "It isn't easy to prove a negative." Real-life prosecutors, on whom the U.S. Constitution places the burden of proof in criminal court cases, would concur with their television counterpart. Generally, it is far easier to prove that something exists than that it does not. Proving the former requires looking only until a thing is found; proving the latter requires looking everywhere a thing could possibly be found.

Nonetheless, one finds research reporting replete with statements like "there is no research on ..." or "little research evidence exists that would support ..." "my study is the first to ...." Statements of this sort beg the question: Have they really looked everywhere they could? Or, as would often be appropriate: Have they done anything more than a perfunctory key-word search?

Such is the case with research on the achievement effects of standardized testing. Peruse the press coverage and the more prominent education journals over the past decade and one can find numerous statements like "despite the long history of assessment-based accountability, hard evidence about its effects is surprisingly sparse, and the little evidence that is available is not encouraging."[1]

Unfortunately, many folk who know no better may believe such proclamations. So, I have decided to compile a list of studies that have uncovered empirical evidence of achievement benefits from testing with stakes.

TYPES OF TESTING BENEFITS

For the sake of both brevity and clarity, I divide the benefits of testing into three groups. First, there is the benefit of information used for *diagnosis* (e.g., of a student's or teacher's problems or progress). Standardized tests may reveal weaknesses or strengths that corroborate or supplement a teacher's or principal's analysis. Information for diagnosis, however, may be obtained from no-stakes standardized tests. For that, and other reasons, virtually no one disputes this benefit, and so it is not a part of the literature review here.

Second, some standardized tests are designed to provide information used in personnel *selection* (e.g., of job applicants by employers, in admissions by universities). This information is typically measured in predictive validity coefficients—usually simple Pearson correlation coefficients of test performance against some future performance measure (e.g., first-year college grades, supervisor job ratings)—or allocative efficiency coefficients (which would be more difficult to illustrate).

Although these selection benefits are disputed by some of those who oppose university admissions and employment testing, there exists a mass of empirical evidence supporting the existence and significance of these benefits. Indeed, there are so many empirical studies verifying the benefits of employment testing that meta analyses have been conducted of the many meta analyses. These studies, conducted mostly by personnel (i.e., industrial/organizational) psychologists, number in the thousands (see, e.g., Hunter & Hunter, 1984; Hunter & Schmidt, 1982; Hunter and Schmidt, 1983; Hunter, Schmitt, Gooding, Noe, & Kirsch, 1984; Schmidt & Hunter, 1998; Schmidt, Hunter, McKenzie, & Muldrow, 1979). The number of studies supporting the existence and significance of benefits to university admissions testing may not be as numerous but these studies are, nonetheless, quite common (see, e.g., Willingham, Lewis, Morgan, & Ramist, 1990; College Entrance Examination Board, 1988; and Cole & Willingham, 1997), and have quite a long history. According to Manuel (1952):

---

[1]This particular quote comes from a long-time opponent of high-stakes standardized tests, and many other, similar statements have been uttered by him and other testing opponents. The past several years, however, have witnessed a small group of alleged testing supporters, affiliated with the Republican Party-aligned think tanks, also asserting a paucity or absence of such research, then declaring themselves to be pioneers when they conduct such research.

In 1930 … George Stoddard in the 1930 *Yearbook of the National Society of College Teachers of Education*, referring to the use of tests of scholastic aptitude for predicting first-semester and first-year scholarship of freshmen, that "the writing thereon has assumed huge proportions." In 1949 Robert Travers in a paper published in *School and Society* stated that "during the past 15 years over 1,000 studies have appeared which have attempted to evaluate one or more tests for the purpose of predicting some aspect of scholastic achievement." It is still a favorite topic. The current (November 1952) number of *Psychological Abstracts* lists three articles dealing with prediction at the college level. (p. 75)

Third, there remain those benefits that accrue from the changes in behavior induced by the presence of a test, usually a standardized test with stakes. Those behavior changes typically include increases in motivation (on the part of students, teachers, administrators, or others), the incorporation of feedback information from tests, an associated narrowing of focus on the task at hand, and increases in organizational efficiency, clarity, or the alignment of standards, curriculum, and instruction.[2] Most any parent or taxpayer likely would consider increases in any of these behaviors to be positive, to clearly be benefits. Many education researchers, however, consider them to be negative, and sometimes count them as costs.

This review, then, focuses on this third group of testing benefit studies—those finding evidence of improved achievement, motivation (which would induce improved achievement), or organizational clarity and alignment (which, presumably, would also induce improved achievement). It is this third group—studies showing evidence of achievement gains from testing—that does not exist, the censorious naysayers assert.

HOW A LARGE NUMBER OF STUDIES BECAME "SPARSE" AND WIDE-RANGING RESEARCH BECAME "THIN"

Let's get this out of the way—I believe that many testing critics who declare there to be a paucity of studies in the third group do so because they are biased against high-stakes standardized testing. Their declarations represent wishful thinking. Moreover, as one does not normally look for that which one does not wish to find, mainstream education research lacks anything other than fairly superficial literature reviews of the topic. Ergo, this effort here.

There are, however, other, more respectable reasons for not knowing the research literature on standardized testing's achievement benefits. First

---

[2]Many studies verify that tests with stakes for student, teacher, or school change the behavior of teachers. Many other studies verify that tests without stakes for student, teacher, or school do not.

among them, of course, is the simple fact that so many researchers have declared that the literature does not exist. Why would one spend time looking for something that does not exist?

The Lost Art of the Literature Review

Second, I would argue that the skill of literature searching, in general, may be approaching extinction. One would think that the wonderful improvements in data bases and computer search engines over the past quarter century would have dramatically improved literature searching. Instead, they may have made it worse. My conclusion derives from reading several too many research articles on standardized testing with a wholly erroneous assessment of the research base on the topic.

Too often nowadays, researchers content themselves with a superficial computer search on the most obvious keywords, typically relegating even that mundane task to research assistants or librarians who may have little understanding of the topic. Even worse, other researchers may do nothing more than cite the conclusions of one of these casual, superficial reviews, making no effort whatsoever to familiarize themselves with the research base directly.

A complete reliance on keyword searches is inadequate to the task for several reasons. First is the matter of which keywords to choose. Different folk can attribute different keywords to identify the same concept. Sometimes, the differences in wording are subtle; sometimes they are dramatic. Moreover, different research disciplines can employ entirely different vocabularies to the same topic. A *net benefit* to an economist, for example, may be called *consequential validity* by psychometricians, *positive effects* by program evaluators, or *positive washback* by education planners.

It is telling, moreover, that research articles based on extraordinarily superficial literature searches seem to have no trouble getting published in the same scholarly journals that minutely scrutinize analytic methodologies. Methodology seems to matter quite a lot; an even minimal effort to understand the literature almost not at all. Some quantitative methodologists believe that they are immune from the research disease common in the softer social sciences and humanities of respecting complexity for complexity's sake. The reader may have heard the story of the scientist who sent a research article to several humanities journals that was entirely made up and full to bursting with mostly unexplained technical terms, that was accepted at most of those journals, ... or, of the quasiexperimental study that compared the journal acceptance rate of articles that were exactly the same in content but different in terms of the technical difficulty and denseness of the prose (the more difficult to read and understand, the better chance an article had of being accepted for publication, the content held equal).

But, some quantitative researchers seem to have their own blind spots, revering complex analytic methodology, and almost completely disregarding the value of quality work in any or all of the many other essential aspects of a research project, such as the literature search. It almost seems that, although good literature searches require organization, persistence, and a wide familiarity with terms, concepts, and classifications because they are unchallenging in terms of analytic methodology, it is simply not considered important to do them well.

Second, a large proportion of the studies uncovering testing benefits were focused primarily on other results, and it is those foci and those results that determined which keywords were supplied to the research data base. When testing benefit findings are coincidental to a study, a simple computer search probably will not find them.

Third, many, if not most, studies finding testing benefits are simply not to be found stored in the more common research literature data bases. Research data bases tend to be biased toward the work of academic researchers, and academic researchers may be biased against testing. Researchers with a predisposition against testing are more likely to work in academe, where they are not required to perpetuate a practice of which they disapprove. Researchers with more favorable dispositions toward testing are more likely to work in the field, for testing companies or state education agencies, for example.

Getting one's work published in an academic journal and listed in a widely available research literature data base is far less important for the latter folk than for the former. Academics' perceived worth, promotion, and tenure are largely determined by the quantity and status of their publications. Practitioners, by contrast, respond to a quite different set of incentives. They must contribute to the mission of their organization, where spending the time to run the gauntlet of academic journal review could be considered nothing more than a diversion.

Many research studies conducted by private firms are considered proprietary and never released. Testing program evaluations conducted by or for state governments are typically addressed to state legislatures or state boards and are not written in the standard academic journal style. They end up on a shelf in the state library, perhaps, and included in a state government database, perhaps, but no where else. Many busy psychometricians write up their findings briefly, enough to get them on the program of professional meetings where they can update their skills and keep in touch with their friends and colleagues. But, as practitioners, they no more need to polish up those papers for academic journal publication than would your neighborhood doctor or dentist, who likely treats research in a similar way.

Fourth, some studies documenting positive effects to high-stakes testing report some negative effects at the same time. For example, in the golden age of minimum-competency testing (MCT)—the 1970s and 1980s—many researchers expressed a concern that MCTs might raise achievement for the weakest students only at the expense of more advanced students, as system resources would be diverted to bringing the slowest students up to the minimum threshold. Studies conducted then and since have shown that MCTs do accelerate the weakest students' achievement and, not always, but sometimes at the expense of more advanced students. Several of these studies are included in the following list of studies.

A researcher looking only at the average gains, however, would see little to no positive effect from an MCT. A researcher looking at all levels of student achievement, by contrast, could see the positive effect when a high-stakes test is set at a reachable threshold higher than a student's current achievement level, and might recommend a multiple-target high-stakes testing system—which is what most other countries in the world employ.

Finding Positive Effects From Testing. Oh, the Shame!

Some research studies finding positive achievement effects from high-stakes testing have been altered or covered up by their own progenitors. I include in the following list several studies that produced clear, statistically significant evidence of positive achievement effects from high-stakes testing, which can only be found by reading the data tables or the technical appendix of the report, as the author's text suggests just the opposite result.

One study, for example, which found generally positive results, was reported in an article whose text was critical of testing entitled *Statewide testing and local improvement: An oxymoron?* Another study that used a multistate teacher survey as its primary source of evidence, reported strongly positive results in a book chapter but, tagged on at the end of the narrative, one of the authors added a section entitled "Reconsideration," which included sentiment such as:

> We are not satisfied with the data presented here. We do not believe these data tell us what is happening to schooling in America. Regardless of the role of standardized testing, we believe that this teachers' portrayal is crude and misleading. ... The sample was contrived, insufficiently urban, and perhaps resulted in an unduly optimistic picture, but we think a random sample of teachers from these states would have said pretty much the same things. The instrument ... has a certain charm, but is crude and failed to develop real insights into how curricular priorities are changing. ... It is important to study carefully the views of teachers, but important also to examine what teachers may not yet be able to tell us. (Stake and Theobald, 1991, pp. 200–201)

The survey instrument that this fellow, a highly respected evaluator, and a co-author had developed was fine; it simply did not produce the results he desired. Other results from the study, more negative toward testing, were featured most prominently in the study's summary and abstract.

So Students Learn More; So What?

Fifth, a surprising number of studies—indeed, some of the most celebrated —whose summaries and conclusions report negative results, reveal mostly positive results to the more intrepid reader willing to sift through the details. To find the positive results, one must ignore the researchers' interpretations, read the fine print, and peruse the data tables on one's own. For example, at least several studies exist that claim mostly negative results from the introduction of a high-stakes test, essentially because the test induced a change in curriculum and instruction, a change some teachers, administrators, or the researchers themselves did not like. A closer look at the study results, however, reveal that all concerned—teachers, administrators, students, and parents—observed students working harder and learning more as a result of the test.

In other words, study conclusions often depict as negative results that only some education insiders would find objectionable. Most parents and taxpayers would focus on the increased student motivation and learning as the only relevant outcomes ... and applaud.

Indeed, many testing program evaluations do not even broach the topic of student achievement gains, instead focusing solely on teacher and administrator reactions to the test. A consumer advocate, however, might conclude that teachers who do not like a testing program that is successful in raising student achievement may be ill-suited to the job and, perhaps, should pursue another profession. Mainstream education research usually recommends dropping a testing program if teachers and administrators do not like it.

I have read several dozen testing program studies that employed surveys in their research design. I have encountered only two in which some respondent group claimed that students did not learn more as a result of a testing program.

Moreover, most of these testing program evaluations are conducted just after a new testing program has been implemented, when teachers are most likely to resent the change and disruption. Talk to a teacher in a system that has had a test for 20 years and adapted to it, and the opinion might be even more positive.

Finally, I argue, based on personal experience and that of several colleagues, that studies revealing testing benefits are not as likely to be published in many mainstream education journals simply because the editors and their boards prefer not to publish such studies. Corroborating this suspicion is my experience in finding few testing benefit studies in the more mainstream, policy-oriented education journals, and many in the more technical, pure research journals.

LITERATURE REVIEW OF RESEARCH ON THE ACHIEVEMENT BENEFITS OF TESTING

Despite some educators' lack of interest in, or outright censorship of, the evidence demonstrating high-stakes testing's beneficial achievement effects, some studies have managed to find their way into print, and I have started to build a record of them. Thus far, I have looked in fairly accessible locations that can be found through computer searching and, even then, only in education research sources. I have not searched the scholarly Psychology or Sociology literature, or (mostly proprietary) business reports, where the largest body of relevant information is likely to be found. And, would anyone like to wager against finding an abundance of reports demonstrating high-stakes testing's beneficial achievement effects in the military's research files?

I have not looked for sources from any of the more than 100 countries outside North America, where education researchers are, for the most part, more accepting of and less hostile to high-stakes testing. I include here mention only of those evaluations I found coincidentally through my search of U.S. sources. One might well surmise, of course, that other countries' testing program evaluations have tended to find positive results, as the number of high-stakes testing programs across countries remains large and is increasing (Phelps, 1996, 2000).

Moreover, I have not yet made the effort to uncover any U.S. state or district testing program evaluations not listed in the standard data bases. Such an effort would require a separate search in each state's archives. In cases in which I have found a citation to a state report more than several years old, I have been unsuccessful in obtaining the report just by contacting current state education department employees.

Those critics who proclaim a dearth of studies revealing net benefits to testing programs, by implication, must believe that governments do not evaluate their testing programs. Among the hundreds of jurisdictions worldwide where high-stakes testing has been implemented, few to none have bothered to evaluate the programs (or, at least, to evaluate their effect on achievement)? This, despite the fact that many, if not most, of these jurisdictions are required by law to evaluate new programs? That is pretty difficult to believe.

Even with the superficial (although, granted, rather tedious and time consuming) effort I have made thus far, I seem to have had far more success than have some who claim to speak for all the literature on the subject. I believe that I have done only a little more than scratch the surface of the research base. As one psychologist, writing in the 1980s wrote: "Research studies about the influences of tests began to appear in the literature in the early 1930s" (Milton, 1981, p. 11).

I've found a few older than that, but I was unable to secure most of those he cited from the 1930s, which included such works as *An examination of examinations, Assessing students: How shall we know them?*, *The effect on recall and recognition of the examination set in classroom situations, How students study for three types of objective tests*, and *An experimental study of the old and new types of examination: The effect of the examination set on memory.*

Indeed, there are more studies, whose titles suggest they might show evidence of testing's achievement effects, that I was *not* able to obtain than studies I was able to obtain. Moreover, I have about a dozen long, detailed bibliographies of testing studies, going back decades, that I have not yet begun to process. Peruse the education research literature back in time and one can find hundreds of articles with titles including phrases such as "the effects of testing on ...," "the impact of testing on ...," "the consequences of testing for ...."

Look a little deeper and one finds bibliographies such as:

- a review of research entitled *The effects of tests on students and schools* with 240 citations (Kirkland, 1971);
- a *Compendium of educational research, planning, evaluation and assessment activities* with 60 citations that describes then-current research being conducted in state education departments (New Jersey Department of Education, 1977);
- *Minimal competency testing: Issues and procedures, an annotated bibliography*; with 28 entries (Wildemuth, 1977);
- *Annotated bibliography on minimum competency testing*, with 52 citations, that seems to have been compiled by ERIC staffers (1978);
- *Competency testing: An annotated bibliography* with hundreds of citations to research just from the mid-1970s (Jackson & Battiste, 1978); and
- *Competency testing: Bibliography*, with 240 citations (Hawisher & Harper, 1979).

And, that's just the 1970s. To be sure, there is some duplication across these bibliographies, but not that much. Moreover, not all the citations refer to work that investigated the achievement benefits of minimum competency testing, but some of them did, and many of them might have. I have been able to obtain only a small proportion of the studies listed.

Also written in the 1970s is an edited volume containing descriptions of seven state evaluations of their minimum competency testing programs

(Gorth & Perkins, 1979). And, those were conducted prior to the wave of adoptions of both "sunshine" and "sunset" laws across the states in the 1980s, when many states for the first time began to require that all state programs be formally evaluated periodically. The number of state-government sponsored testing program evaluations has surely increased since the 1970s, but one will find few of them in standard education research data bases.

Those who have claimed a paucity of evidence for testing's achievement effects either have not looked very hard, or did not wish to find it.

SEARCH METHODS

For this literature review, I conducted keyword computer searches of academic journals. But, I went back further in time than most have, used more keywords than most would, and consulted more data bases than most do (e.g., Dissertation Abstracts, several independently constructed bibliographies).

I found many studies of testing benefits, however, by more conventional means, including word-of-mouth suggestions, library catalog searches, browsing library bookshelves, and, most important, following citation chains. Studies on a topic often cite other studies on the same topic (as they should) that, in turn, cite still more studies on the topic.

TYPES OF ACHIEVEMENT BENEFIT STUDIES

Some of the studies found in this literature review observed improvements in motivation or organizational alignment directly, typically through case-study interviews, observations, or survey questionnaires. Most of the other studies attempted to measure an improvement in student achievement without necessarily knowing the mechanism inducing the improvement (which could be increased motivation, organizational alignment, both, or something else), typically through multivariate analysis, prepost studies, or interrupted time series analysis against a shadow measure. These methods are described in the following.

Evidence of positive achievement effects from a high-stakes testing program could take the form of improved student scores, for part or all of the student population, on a separate test by comparison with a control group of students not in a high-stakes testing program, or on the same test administered before the implementation of the high-stakes testing programs, with as many other influential factors as possible held constant. Or, evidence of positive achievement effects from a high-stakes testing program might take the form of higher wages or improved job performance or stability later for graduates of school systems with high-stakes testing programs, by comparison with other students.

Indirect evidence of achievement effects would take the form of improvements in factors that we know lead to improved student achievement, such as a greater motivation to achieve or more time or effort devoted to studying, and improved organizational alignment for academic achievement. That alignment can be vertical—increased correlation of efforts among state, district, school, and teacher efforts—or horizontal—increased correlation of efforts across districts, schools, and classrooms.

Appendix B lists all the studies showing achievement effects from testing that I have organized thus far, arranged by type of methodology used.

Controlled Experiments

The goal of an experiment is to create two or more groups of people as similar as possible and treated the same except for the variation in a single treatment factor. Ideally, persons are assigned to their groups randomly. There exist an abundance of studies testing the effects of a wide variety of "extrinsic motivators," usually revealing that extrinsic motivators tend to increase motivation. Some of these studies involved tests (Cameron & Pierce, 1994, 1996; Tuckman, 1994).

For example, one group, or "classroom," might be given graded tests throughout the period of a course while the other group is not. Then, the two groups' achievement gains at the end of the course would be compared.

For another example, one group might be told that the final exam counts and the other group that it does not. Or, one group might be told that the final exam counts for much or all of the course grade, the other that it counts for little of the course grade.

In all but one of the controlled experiments that I have read (and listed in Appendix B) the introduction or suggestion of stakes seemed to induce greater academic achievement.

Quasiexperimental Designs

This type of study models an experiment as closely as is practical. Large-scale studies, such as those involving entire states or nations, cannot be conducted under strictly controlled conditions, so some liberties must be taken with the requirements of a pure experiment. Often, the *control* and *treatment* groups already exist, thus random assignment is not possible. At best, the researcher can try to summarize the background characteristics of each group or try to statistically control them in the analysis of the data.

In the studies listed in Appendix B, then, typically two or more groups are compared on some outcome measure, one of the groups having been exposed to high-stakes testing conditions and one of them not.

Multivariate Analysis

Typically using data sets created by national or international test administrations (e.g., National Assessment of Educational Progress [NAEP], Third International Mathematics and Science Study [TIMSS]) or by federally funded longitudinal studies (e.g., National Education Longitudinal Study [NELS], High School and Beyond [HSB]), researchers attempt to isolate the effect of a high-stakes testing program (thus mimicking an experimental design) on some outcome (e.g., academic achievement, wages or job security later in life), by statistically "controlling" many other factors, some of which may also influence the outcome factor.

These analyses tend to employ cross-sectional (e.g., students from states or countries with high-stakes tests compared to their counterparts in the other states and countries) and, sometimes, also longitudinal (e.g., change over time in achievement of each student or each student cohort) aspects. The statistical algorithms typically used for such studies are some forms of multiple analysis of variance or multiple regression.

Some researchers hold that multivariate statistical studies represent the only legitimate research model short of large-scale randomized field trials. Economists, in particular, are fond of criticizing case studies and, especially, surveys as too subjective to be meaningful. Then, apparently without noticing, they typically work their statistical magic on data sets provided by federal government statistical agencies that obtained their data largely or entirely ... you guessed it ... from surveys. They tend to be well-done surveys, mind you, but they are still surveys.

Moreover, multivariate analysis suffers from another profound shortcoming, that one might call the "black box effect." Often, and perhaps usually, the researchers analyzing the data sets do not really know the data sets very well. The organization of research most common in the United States these days seems to have adopted an unfortunate labor specialization that completely separates data collection from data analysis. This labor organization is mirrored by an equivalent social organization, in which analysts are usually considered more authoritative than collectors. Sadly, though, the analysts too often analyze data sets they do not understand very well—misinterpreting the meaning and character of variables, and ascribing levels of validity and reliability to variables that any collector would know are unrealistic. As the saying goes "garbage in, garbage out," and many analysts simply do not have sufficient familiarity in the data they analyze or the environment in which the data are generated to discern which are garbage and which are not.

If there is a kernel of truth to the claims that little to no research has been done on the achievement benefits of standardized tests in general, or high-stakes standardized tests in particular, it would relate to the structure of the federal government's education data bases. Until the advent of the "State NAEP" in the 1990s, it was not possible for an outsider to definitively determine the state of a respondent in the data base. The state of residence, or of origin, of each respondent was suppressed, due to concerns about inadequate numbers of respondents for most states in a sample that was nationally, but not regionally, representative. Some of these data sets include respondents' claims about the existence or nonexistence of mandated state tests, or high-stakes tests. But, those responses are not all that reliable; some respondents—even when they are teachers or administrators—get that question wrong, thinking a test they use is state-mandated when it is not, or not state-mandated when it is. That is why some of the only large-scale multivariate studies on the effects of state mandated testing, prior to the mid-1990s, were conducted by researchers with inside access to the confidential records of these data sets (e.g., Linda Winfield or Norman Fredericksen, when each worked at the Educational Testing Service).

Just because national data sets with reliable information on the presence of, or an easily determined, value for state mandated testing did not exist prior to 1990 does not mean that studies of the effects of state mandated testing were not conducted. Indeed, many were. They were of a different type—done within the confines of one or a small group of states or districts. Moreover, for those snobby academics who dismiss surveys, cases studies, and program evaluations as inadmissible in the court of research, many were multivariate studies, with prepost or interrupted time series designs which, in this chapter, are grouped into their own, separate categories.

Interrupted Time Series With Shadow Measure

This research design is possible when a jurisdiction has maintained, and continues to maintain, some measure of achievement different than a newly introduced high-stakes measure. In the most typical case, a state or district will continue the annual administration of a no-stakes, national norm-referenced test even after the introduction of a separate high-stakes test. They then might observe an abrupt and sustained improvement in scores on the no-stakes test. The "interruption" in the time series is the moment when the high-stakes requirement was introduced.

If the researchers can detect a significant jump in the performance on the no-stakes test at or around the time of the start of the high-stakes regime, the evidence suggests that achievement is improving because of the newly introduced stakes (due to increased motivation or organizational alignment). The more similar the two tests are in content and structure, the larger the jump is likely to be.

The method is quite similar to one popular among financial economists for gauging the impact on stock prices of singular events. A temporal window of plus or minus a day or two frames the day of a key event concerning a firm, and changes in the firm's stock price within that window is observed. The price change for the one stock will be compared to coincident movements in the overall market and industry to remove the effect of larger trends and, what is left is the change in a single firm's price, presumably due to the singular event in question.

Although the typical study employing this method uses test scores as measures, other measures of achievement can be used as well. One study listed in Appendix B (Fontana, 2000), for example, examined the change in the number of New York schools reaching a minimum state student performance standard once the threat of a restructuring was added to the status of a school as "under review" by the state. Another (Task Force on Educational Assessment Programs, 1979), observed the abrupt change in student course selections (and student course offerings) toward core subjects and higher levels, after a state test was instituted as a graduation requirement.

Prepost Studies

Unlike the previous method, which looks for a change over time in a measure other than the one with high stakes attached to it, simple prepost studies look at the change in a single measure after stakes are attached to it. For this method to be feasible, a jurisdiction must have employed a measure without stakes and then, at some point, attached stakes to it. Say a school district administers a standardized test annually for years with no stakes (e.g., test performance is simply used for student or instructional diagnosis), and then 1 year makes performance on the test above a certain threshold a graduation requirement. An average of student scores taken before the requirement was set can be compared to the equivalent afterwards, to see if the requirement itself made a difference in test performance.

One must be careful in simple pre-post studies to control for background trends that may also influence the measure, however. Standardized test scores, for example, do not usually stay flat over time even without changes in stakes. The factors that determine that background trend—in the previously mentioned example, the trend one would have expected in the test scores if it had remained a no-stakes test—must be accounted for so that the effect of the high-stakes requirement is isolated.

Case Studies

Case studies typically involve an intense examination of a single to several jurisdictions. Also typically, case studies of high-stakes testing programs are conducted a short time after the program's introduction. A laudable, if unusually thorough, case study would also collect information before the introduction of a program (so as not to depend exclusively on subjects' memories of the state of things before the event) and then again only after the program had become well established (so as not to confound subjects' opinion of the new program with their attitude toward change itself).

Several types of research methods may be embedded in a case study, although interviews, surveys, and reviews of administrative records are probably the most common.

True, case study designs are so flexible, and so much of their essential information is created and controlled by the researcher, that they can be easily manipulated to achieve predetermined results in the hands of the unscrupulous.

Case studies conducted by honest, skilled, and inquisitive researchers, however, may offer more explanatory power than any other research method. Although experiments may provide the most trustworthy evidence, that evidence often emanates from highly artificial situations in very small scale. While multivariate analyses can approach the experimental design (by including many explanatory variables) and cover a large scale (i.e., national or international data sets), they can never include all the explanatory factors, and it takes a true data expert to intimately understand the details and intricacies of large-scale data sets.

Given all the imperfections of multivariate analysis, to which too few multivariate analysts will admit, it can be highly refreshing and enlightening to read well-done case studies. I recommend, for example, those conducted of high school academic programs by the Southern Regional Education Board in the mid-1990s or those of secondary school examination systems in eight countries by Eckstein and Noah. Reading them is an education in itself.

Program Evaluations

The most common type of study designs found in this search are program evaluations. Really, *program evaluation* is a catch-all term used to describe a study that incorporates a variety of methods. By implication, evaluations are holistic; many or all aspects of a program are studied, which is why and how a variety of methods comes into play. Probably most commonly included in program evaluations are surveys (written and oral), interviews, reviews of administrative records, and site visits. Indeed, program evaluation's inclination to use any and all methods appropriate to the task at hand is probably its greatest strength.

The ideal program evaluation, however, is a randomized experiment conducted on a large-scale under conditions as natural as is practical. That the ideal type makes up only a tiny portion of all program evaluations is testament to the difficulty and high cost of implementing the ideal.

Polls and Surveys

Studies solely incorporating surveys are included in this compilation (Appendix B) only if they inquired about increases in student achievement, or in student, teacher, or administrator motivation. There are other surveys that focused on other effects of a standardized testing program, but did not pose any question on these essential topics.

Opinion polls, too, are included in the list, but only if they included items on the relation between testing and increases in student achievement, or in student, teacher, or administrator motivation.

Benefit-Cost Studies

Benefit-cost studies attempt to estimate the real world (e.g., dollar) value of identified and measurable benefits and costs. The total amount of benefit minus the total amount of cost equals the net benefit.

It is, perhaps, true that most any project or program can be successful at some price. Spend enough money and one can make even poorly designed programs work. But, of what use is that? Public spending oblivious of the cost-effectiveness of projects and programs would soon deplete the public purse.

It is not enough, then, to simply demonstrate the statistical likelihood of achievement benefits to a testing program, as have most of the studies included here. One must also demonstrate that these benefits can be achieved in a cost effective manner.

Honest benefit-cost studies tend to find huge net benefits to testing programs. That is, the benefits greatly outweigh the costs. The huge difference between benefits and costs is as much a function of very low costs as of apparently large benefits.

Theoretical Models and Literature Reviews

Often used as an antecedent to an empirical study, indeed often as an aide to help design the empirical study, theoretical models describe in a rigorous, holistic manner how a system should work, under a set of reasonable assumptions. These models can be think piece narratives, or conceptual models, usually constructed by experts with considerable experience in the field who know how school systems work in practical terms. Or, they can be logical, abstract mathematical exercises, as is popular with economists. The latter, for example, might draw a linear programming graphic on a Cartesian plane, represent benefits with integral calculus, and locate the most beneficial feasible outcome as a Calculus maxima.

Studies Left Out

In order to be concise, I eliminated from inclusion the largest swaths of ground in the field of testing benefit research. Among the other categories of research with a substantial quantity of empirical research on the benefits of testing, and particularly high-stakes testing, are:

1. *Studies conducted in other countries that would require translation* and studies conducted by or for other countries' governments that found achievement benefits to high-stakes standardized testing.
2. *Studies of the predictive validity and/or allocative efficiency of U.S. university admissions tests,* such as the SAT and ACT. (See, for example, Willingham, Lewis, Morgan, & Ramist; Cole; College Entrance Examination Board.)
3. With only some of the more easily obtained studies excepted, *program evaluations of testing programs* conducted by or for state or local education agencies.
4. Industrial/Organizational (a.k.a., Personnel) psychologists' *studies of the relative advantages of the use of various types of tests compared to other measures commonly available to employees or employers in job selection.* These studies number in the thousands.[3]
5. Most studies measuring the benefits or demonstrating the efficacy of "opting out" tests—tests that allow a student to avoid or skip past coursework, costly in money and time, by demonstrating, on a test, mastery of the required material, skill, or aptitude (see, e.g., Aber, 1996; Jones, 1993; Morgan & Ramist, 1998; Olmsted, 1957; Pressy, 1954; Stanley, 1976; Terman, 1954; Wedman, 1994).
6. Most of what John Bishop called "the vast literature" on effective schools, from the 1970s to the present, for which testing is an essential component.
7. Most of the equally vast literature on mastery learning, mostly from the 1960s through the 1980s, for which testing is an essential component.

LITERATURE REVIEWS, META ANALYSES, AND RESEARCH SYNTHESES

Meta analysis is a calculation method popular among researchers for summarizing the impact of a group of studies on the same topic. Generally, it is used with experimental or quasiexperimental studies. The size of the effect

---

[3]See for example: Bishop (1988a), Boudreau (1988), Hunter and Hunter (1984), Hunter and Schmidt (1982), Gooding, Noe, and Kirsch (1984) and Schmidt and Hunter (1998).

in each experiment is added to those of the other studies in the group to accumulate an overall "effect size." Effect size calculations take into account not only the strength of the effect, but the size of the sample in each study. A very strong effect from an experiment involving two classrooms of fourth graders should not be considered equally against a weaker effect found in an experiment involving all the fourth graders in two states.

Naturally, effect size calculations make more sense in quantitative research. With qualitative studies, however, nominal or ordinal measures can sometimes be used to approximate. For example, all the case studies in a group arriving at a positive assessment of a certain type of program can be given a plus, and all those arriving at a negative assessment can be given a minus, and the overall balance can represent something of a vote, at least as to the direction of sentiment, if not its magnitude.

Fortunately for this author, meta analyses or research syntheses on some of the topics highlighted in this chapter have already been conducted by other researchers. Among *experimental studies*, they include:

- Locke and Latham's (2002) meta-analysis of three decades' experiments on *motivation and productivity* (conclusion: Clear performance targets and goal-setting to reach them substantially increase productivity);
- Bangert-Drowns, Kulik, and Kulik's (1991) meta-analysis of 35 studies on the achievement effects of varying *frequency of testing* (conclusion: Achievement gains are almost always higher with testing than without; the optimal amount is more than weekly);
- Kulik and Kulik's (1989) meta-analysis of 53 studies of the achievement effects of varying types and frequencies of *feedback* to students on their performance, tests being the most common form of feedback information (conclusion: The feedback from tests improves achievement substantially, not only by identifying and clarifying weaknesses but also in disabusing those students complacent due to overconfidence);
- Kulik and Kulik's (1987) meta-analysis of 49 studies of the achievement effects of *mastery testing* (i.e., testing as a part of mastery learning programs, conclusion: Mastery learning, and the testing that is an essential part of it, produces substantial achievement gains);
- Guskey and Gates' (1986) research synthesis of 25 studies on *mastery learning* (conclusion: Mastery learning produces substantial achievement gains);
- Natriello and Dornbusch's (1984) review of studies on the achievement effect of *standards* (conclusion: In general, higher standards lead to greater effort, in part because students tend to not take seriously work that adults do not seem to take seriously, but there are limits; set the standards too high and some students may not try);

- Staats's (1973) review of experiments on classroom reinforcement programs, some of which involved testing; and
- Carroll's (1955) review of experiments on language learning in the military, in government, and at universities (conclusion: The more intense the experience, the more rapid the learning, and testing helps to intensify the experience).

Two wonderful literature reviews—one by Crooks (1988) and another by Kirkland (1971)—survey some of the above terrain.

The large body of research literature most pertinent to *program evaluation* studies of testing is that for effective schools. The phrase *effective schools* pertains to a combination of traits, typically isolated in mixed-mode program evaluations. As such, effective schools studies do not lend themselves well to the experimental design. Nonetheless, a "vast literature" has, indeed, developed on the topic, continues to grow, and has reached a remarkable degree of consensus—effective schools focus strongly on academics, have strong principals who see themselves as academic leaders, maintain high academic standards, monitor academic progress closely and continuously, hold themselves accountable for academic achievement, and test frequently.

Many fairly thorough reviews of the literature date to around the early 1980s, and include those by Purkey and Smith (1983), Murnane (1981), Averch, Carroll, Donaldson, Kiesling, and Pincus (1971), Edmonds (1979), MacKenzie (1983), Clark, Lotto, and Astuto (1984), Rosenshine (1983), Northwest Regional Laboratory (1990), and Cotton (1995). Much of the more recent study has fractured among various different subtopics and often is labeled differently and more difficult to find. Indeed, one frequently encounters education program evaluations that reproduce the results of the effective schools studies of two decades ago without their authors realizing it. The number of studies finding, essentially, the same several traits that make "effective schools" producers of high achievement gains must now number in the several hundreds, at least.

Because he is personally responsible for so many of them, John Bishop's curriculum vita serves as a solid base for building the research literature on *quantitative large-scale multivariate* studies on testing. He has translated the results from his studies into grade-level equivalent gains for students from jurisdictions with high-stakes testing programs. Translate in a similar fashion for the other multivariate studies, and one has a quantitative summary of the literature.

This author's unique contribution to the meta-analytic literature is to quantitatively summarize the direction and magnitude of public opinion on the question of whether testing promotes achievement. The question has been asked more than a few times in *polls and surveys,* and asked of several respondent groups—students, teachers, administrators, parents, and the general public.

The Achievement Effect of Testing, as Measured in Reviews of the Experimental Literature

As I don't believe that I can improve on the informative research reviews of Crooks and Kirkland, I will not try.

Following is Crooks' (1988) summary of the Bangert-Drowns, Kulik, and Kulik (1991) meta-analysis of the research literature on testing frequency (which incorporates the test/no test choice).

> The review by Bangert-Drowns et al. (1988) used data from 31 studies which: (a) were conducted in real classrooms, (b) had all groups receiving the same instruction except for varying frequencies of testing, (c) used conventional classroom tests, (d) did not have serious methodological flaws, and (e) used a summative end-of-course examination taken by all groups as a dependent variable. The course length ranged from 4 weeks to 18 weeks, but only 9 studies were of courses shorter than 10 weeks. Bangert-Drowns et al. reported their results in terms of effect size (difference in mean scores divided by standard deviation of the less frequently tested group).

> Overall, they found an effect size of 0.25 favoring the frequently tested group, representing a modest gain in examination performance associated with frequent testing. However, the actual frequencies of testing varied dramatically, so the collection of studies was very heterogeneous. In 12 studies where the low frequency group received no testing prior to the summative examination, the effect size increased to 0.43. It seems reasonable to hypothesize that, in part, this large increase may have come about because students who had at least one experience of a test from the teacher before the summative examination were able to better judge what preparation would be most valuable for the summative examination. On average, effect sizes were smaller for longer treatments, probably because most longer treatments had included at least one intermediate test for the less frequently tested group.

> Bangert-Drowns et al. were surprised to find that the number of tests per week given to the high frequency group was not significantly correlated with the effect size. Rather, the effect size was best predicted from the frequency of testing for the control group. This suggests that the prime benefit from testing during a course comes from having at least one or two such tests, but that greater frequencies do not convey much benefit. One further analysis they conducted, however, raises some doubts about this conclusion. They identified eight studies which had groups with high, intermediate, and low frequencies of testing. Compared to the low frequency groups, the high frequency groups had a mean effect size of 0.48, whereas the intermediate frequency groups had a mean effect size of 0.22. The difference between 0.48 and 022 was statistically significant. This finding must be treated with caution, however, because of the small proportion of the total sample included in this analysis.

Overall, the evidence suggests that a moderate frequency of testing is desirable, and more frequent testing may produce further modest benefits. Groups that received no testing during the course were clearly disadvantaged, on average. Only four studies reported student attitudes towards instruction, but all favored more frequent testing, with a mean effect size of 0.59, a large effect. (Crooks, 1988, pp. 448–449)

Following is Crooks' (1988) summary of the Kulik and Kulik meta-analysis of the research literature on mastery testing.

Kulik and Kulik (1987) conducted a meta-analysis of studies of testing in mastery learning programs, analyzing data from 49 studies. Each study took place in real classrooms, provided results for both a class taught with a mastery testing requirement and a class taught without such a requirement, and was judged free of serious experimental bias. The studies varied in length from 1 to 32 weeks, with about half shorter than 10 weeks ....

The mean effect size on summative, end-of-course examination performance was 0.54, a strong effect. Kulik and Kulik note that this mean effect size is substantially lower than the figure of 0.82 reported recently by Guskey and Gates (1986) in another review of studies on mastery learning. They rightly point out, however, that 9 of the 25 studies used by Guskey and Gates calculated effect sizes using combined scores from the instructional quizzes (which the mastery groups had multiple opportunities to pass) and the final examination, thus biasing the results in favor of the mastery group. The mean effect size for the 16 studies which avoided this bias was 0.47, a figure much more consistent with the Kuliks' findings.

Effect sizes varied markedly in relation to three features of the studies. Studies that had the same frequency of testing in both groups had a mean effect size of 0.48, whereas studies in which the test frequency was not controlled (usually higher in the mastery testing group) had a mean effect size of 0.65. This difference was not statistically significant, but it is worthy of note that the extra benefit for more frequent testing is similar to the 0.25 reported in the earlier section on frequency of testing.

A statistically significant difference was found between effect sizes from studies in which similar levels and types of feedback were given to students in both groups, and those from studies in which this was not the case (in these cases, the mastery testing groups could be expected to have received more feedback). The two mean effect sizes were 0.36 and 0.67, suggesting that a major component of the effectiveness of mastery testing arises from the additional feedback that it usually provides.

Thus the results of research on mastery testing suggest that the sizable benefits observed largely represent the combined effects of the benefits described in earlier sections from more frequent testing, from giving detailed feedback on their progress on a regular basis, and from setting high but attainable standards. One further effect that is probably important is the benefit of allowing repeated opportunities to attain the standard set. This feature might have considerable benefits in increasing motivation and a sense of self-efficacy, while reducing the anxiety often associated with one-shot testing (Friedman, 1987). Kulik and Kulik (1987) reach a similar conclusion to Abbott and

Falstrom (1977): the other features often included in courses based on mastery learning models do not appear to add significantly to the effects described here. (Crooks,1988, pp. 457–458)

Following is Crooks' (1988) summary of the Natriello and Dornbusch (1984) review of the research literature on the achievement effects of varying classroom evaluation techniques.

> ... higher standards generally led to greater student effort and to students being more likely to attend class. Students who perceived standards as unattainable, however, were more likely to become disengaged from school. Natriello has suggested there may well be a curvilinear relationship between the level of standards and student effort and performance, with some optimal level for each situation. This optimal level would probably depend on other aspects of the evaluation arrangements, such as whether or not students are given opportunities to get credit for correcting the deficiencies of evaluated work, or the nature of the feedback on their efforts. The weaker students, who are most at risk in high demand classrooms, may need considerable practical support and encouragement if they are to avoid disillusionment.
>
> Not surprisingly, ... if students thought the evaluations of their work were not important or did not accurately reflect the level of their performance and effort, they were less likely to consider them worthy of effort.
>
> When student performance on achievement tests is the criterion, research has generally shown that higher standards lead to higher performance (e.g., Rosswork, 1977), although again a curvilinear relationship may be predicted. Most of the relevant classroom-based research derives from studies of mastery learning, ... (Crooks, 1988, pp. 449–450)

Now, I pull excerpts from the marvelously thorough research review, *The effects of tests on students and schools*, compiled by Marjorie C. Kirkland (1971). Her review is not segmented in the same manner as Crooks', since the literature was somewhat less developed (although, surprisingly vigorous, contrary to some current claims) in 1971. I present her review in snippets, parcels relevant to the discussion of standardized testing's achievement benefits, that were scattered around her article.

> Studies showed that systematic reporting of test results assisted students (ninth grade) in developing greater understanding of their interests, aptitudes, and achievements. This improvement in self-estimates of ability was greater for students who were characterized as having high self-regard than for those having low self-regard. An improvement in self-estimates of ability was observed 14 days after the test report (Barrett, 1968) and one month later (Westbrook, 1967). (Kirkland, 1971, pp. 309–310)
>
> In line with the above studies and others which he reviewed, Bloom (1968) concluded that learning must include both the student's subjective recognition of his competence and public recognition by the school or society. (Kirkland, 1971, p. 312)

Three studies (Keys, 1934; Kirkpatrick, 1934; Ross & Henry, 1939) indicated that the less able student profited more from frequent testing than the more able student. The less able student seemed to profit mainly from direction of his learning to specifics and from practice in selecting correct responses .... One finding would seem to encourage the continuance of periodic testing: at least 70% of the students in the Turney (1931), Keys (1934), and Ross and Henry (1939) studies favored frequent tests and felt the test helped them to learn more. (Kirkland, 1971, p. 312)

... where standardized testing was suddenly introduced, as in the Navy (Cronbach, 1960; Stuit, 1947), an impact could be seen. The Navy program clearly demonstrated that tests are a powerful instrument for administrative control of a classroom. The tests showed which teachers were bringing their groups "up to the standard" so that administrators could take prompt remedial action. Such tests present a threat to the teacher. Even without the threat of discharge or reprimand, the desire to make a good impression would cause the teacher to make a greater effort to teach effectively and, in turn, result in the teacher putting pressure on students to work harder. (Kirkland, 1971, p. 332)

The Achievement Effect of Testing, as Measured in Large-Scale Quantitative Multivariate Studies

As the labor economist John Bishop has done the most in this group of methodologies, and knows the data sets the best, it is convenient to start with his work. Most of his studies used large multistate or multicountry data sets with which he would compare long-term outcomes (e.g., adults wages, job security), or students' performance on a common test, between two sets of students—one from jurisdictions with curriculum-based external exit examination requirements, and one from jurisdictions without. He summarizes the results of his studies that used performance on a common test as the outcome variable in Table 3.1.

In Table 3.2 the effect sizes from some other studies. For brevity's sake, I include only some of the recent national or international studies; many state and local studies are, of course, listed in Appendix B.

The Achievement Effect of Testing, as Measured in Polls and Surveys

Many researchers argue that polls and surveys, at best, measure only "perceptions." Strictly speaking, that is true, but some information is very difficult to obtain any other way. Take, for example, the factor of motivation. We would like to know if standardized testing motivates students to work harder, pay better attention in class, take their school work more seriously, and so on. Some surveys have asked them, their parents, and their teachers for their observations. But, technically, those observations are just perceptions. They could be misperceptions, or they could be reported falsely.

TABLE 3.1
Studies Show That Students in Countries and States That Require Students to Pass Curriculum-Based External Exit Exams in Order to Graduate Learn More Than Their Peers Who do not Take Such Exams

Studies Show That Students in Countries and States That Require Students to Pass Curriculum-Based External Exit Exams in Order to Graduate Learn More Than Their Peers Who do not Take Such Exams	Grade-Level Equivalent Gains for Students Who Took Exit Exams
National Assessment of Educational Progress, Math (New York and North Carolina as compared with other states, 1998)	0.4
National Assessment of Educational Progress, Science (New York and North Carolina as compared with other states, 1998)	0.5
National Assessment of Educational Progress, Reading (New York and North Carolina as compared with other states, 1998)	0.7
Third International Math and Science Study, Math (40 nations, 1995)	1.0
Third International Math and Science Study, Science (40 nations, 1995)	1.3
International Assessment of Educational Progress, Math (15 nations, 1991)	2.0
International Assessment of Educational Progress, Science (15 nations, 1991)	0.7
International Assessment of Educational Progress, Math & Science (Canadian Provinces, 1991)	0.5
International Assessment for the Evaluation of Educational Achievement, Reading (24 nations, 1990)	1.0

Note. All results were significant at the $p < 0.05$ level, with the exception of the International Assessment of Educational Progress, Science. Numbers are rounded to the nearest 0.1

Yet, try to imagine what might be better. Can motivation be defined physiologically, perhaps? Could we, for example, attach electrodes to students in a randomized experiment to see if the electrical impulses of the tested students were different from those of the non-tested students? And, if they were, would that mean they were more motivated, more stressed, or what?

Most of the data used in social science research is derived from surveys, accepting the observations of respondents as valid and accurate, as they perceive it. Some of the more sophisticated survey research organizations double check samples of responses against some independent measure, when

TABLE 3.2
Some Recent National or International Mutlivariate Studies

Winfield, 1990 (U.S. NAEP Reading)

"No advantages of MCT programs were seen in grade 4, but they were in grades 8 and 11" Presence of minimum-competency effect in grade 8 represented about an 8 (.29 s.d. effect size) point advantage for white students and a 10 (.38 s.d. effect size) point advantage for blacks in mean reading proficiency as compared to their respective counterparts in schools without MCTs. At grade 11, the effect represented a 2 (.06 s.d. effect size) point advantage for white students, a 7 (.26 s.d. effect size) advantage for blacks, and a 6 (.19 s.d. effect size) advantage for Hispanics. (p. 1)

Jacobson, 1992 (minimum competency tests, U.S. states, using NLS data set)

rise of 12.6% in math scores of students in the lowest ability quintile; - decline of 12.7% in math scores of students in the middle three quintiles (p. 1)

Bishop, 1992 (U.S. NELS:88 and HS&B data sets)

the presence of minimum competency tests had a 5.1% per year positive effect on the future earnings of women, no effect on males' future earnings

Mullis, Jenkins, Johnson, 1994 (U.S. NAEP Mathematics)

[among] the three strongest variables related to gains in mathematics achievement were: "a moderate amount of testing (i.e., weekly or monthly)" (p. 70)

Frederickson, 1994 (U.S. NAEP)

1978 to 1986 gains in NAEP scores were 7.9 percentage points higher for 9-year olds, 3.1 points higher for 13-year olds, and 0.6 points higher for 17-year olds in high-stakes states than in low-stakes states; the respective higher point gains unique to "higher-order" NAEP items were 4.5, 4.6, and 1.9. All the gain differences were statistically significant, except for the 0.6 points for 17-year olds.

Woessman, 2000 (TIMSS classroom-level data)

The presence of "centralized exams" equals a .16 standard deviation increase in performance on the 8th-grade mathematics test of the Third International Mathematics and Science Study, and a .11 standard deviation increase in science.

Grissmer, Flanagan, Kawata, Williamson, 2000 (State NAEP)

[did not come to conclusion by means of direct test, but by process of elimination (i.e., did not explain NAEP gain scores by means of background or resource variables; attributes them to high accountability reform governance structures)]

Phelps, 2001

(TIMSS, plus many other data sources) The average number of [high-stakes] decision points of the bottom-performing group [of countries] is statistically significantly different from that of the top-performing group, as determined by a t test ($t = 7.69$; $p < 0.0001$) between the two means (p. 414)

(continued)

TABLE 3.2   (continued)

Wenglinsky, 2001

(1996 NAEP Mathematics) Standardized coefficients in structural equation model were .37, .57, and .65, respectively for "take tests," "assess through multiple-choice tests," and "assess through extended response tests." "… input factors with statistically significant effects in increasing achievement include "take tests," "assess through multiple-choice tests," and "assess through extended response tests. … avoiding reliance on authentic assessments [is] positively related to student achievement." (pp. 23–30)

Thompson, 2002 (State NAEP)

Regression p-values for 4th grade Reading, Math and 8th grade Math are +0.16, +0.04, and +0.14. Respective Analysis of Variance p-values are 0.11, 0.015, and 0.13. "… there is a positive relationship between high stakes and changes in scores on the NAEP. There is a negative relationship between high stakes and changes in ACT scores. There is no evidence of relationships between high stakes and changes in scores on either the SAT or Advanced Placement tests." (p. 1)

Carnoy, Loeb, Smith, 2002 (State NAEP)

a "two step move" (along the state accountability index scaled 1 to 5, from low to high accountability) for White 8th graders means 2.8 percentage points more gain in the proportion scoring at the basic skill level or above; "Gains for other racial/ethnic groups are even greater … For African-Americans, the potential gains on the 8th grade test from increased accountability are approximately five percentage points for every two step increase in accountability, … the gain for Hispanic 8th graders is almost nine percentage points. The mean of the gains is 6.1 percentage points. … so a two-step increase makes a large difference." (p. 1)

Rosenshine, 2003 (State NAEP)

"states that attached consequences outperformed the comparison group of state on each of the three NAEP tests for the last four-year period" Average four-year increase in clear (i.e., not Texas or North Carolina) high-stakes states: 4th grade mathematics (1996–2000) 3.45 (n = 11 states); 8th grade mathematics (1996–2000) 3.42 (n = 7 states); 4th grade reading (1994–1998) 3.44 (n = 9 states). Average four-year increase in control states: 4th grade mathematics (1996–2000) 2.40 (n = 15 states); 8th grade mathematics (1996–2000) 1.63 (n = 13 states); 4th grade reading (1994–1998) 1.21 (n = 14 states). (p. 1)

Braun, 2003 (State NAEP)

"For each grade, when we examine the relative gains of states over the period, we find that the comparisons strongly favor the high-stakes testing states. … At grade 4, the difference in means between the high-stakes and low-stakes states is 4.3 score points and at grade 8 it is 3.99 score points. Note that in computing the difference in means, the gain of the nation over the period 1992 to 2000 is eliminated. … On the other hand, when we follow a particular cohort … , we find the comparisons slightly favor the low-stakes testing states." (p. 1) that is possible, as quality control. But, most pollsters trust respondents to tell the truth, and in cases in which there is no conflict of interest and the respondents' identities are kept anonymous, usually there is little reason to doubt.

Among the hundreds of polls and surveys on education over the past several decades, some have included items that focused specifically on testing programs' benefits or, rather, the observation or perception of benefits. I classify those items into two groups—questions about improving teaching or instruction, and questions about improving learning, education, or the motivation of students. I further divide the items between those posed to "education provider" group respondents (i.e., teachers, administrators, board members) and "education consumer" group respondents (i.e., the public, students, parents, employers).

Two measures are used to represent the direction and magnitude of responses:

- *the percentage point differential*, which is calculated by subtracting the unfavorable response percentage from the favorable response percentage for any poll or survey item, and discarding the neutral responses and nonresponses (e.g., no opinion, don't know, refusal to respond); and
- *the 95% confidence interval*, around a survey proportion, is computed by dividing 0.5 by the square root of the number of survey respondents, then multiplying by 2 (i.e., the pollster's standard).

Questions of this type never received a negative response. Even in studies with decidedly negative perspectives toward standardized testing, most respondents thought instruction had improved, which has to be considered a benefit. The negative studies tend to argue that the instruction, improved or not, is accompanied by a "narrowed curriculum," "teaching to the test," or similar alleged demons.

One can see from Table 3.3 that the tilt toward positive responses is rather strong. The +50 point differential one finds in polls of both producer and consumer respondent groups suggests that favorable responses must be at least triple the number of unfavorable responses. A +50 differential, for example, could result from a sample response of 75% yes, 25% no, ... from a sample response of 70% yes, 20% no, and 10% no opinion, ... or from a sample response of 60% yes, 10% no, and 30% no opinion.

The typical national public opinion poll will capture a sample of about 1,100 respondents, and produce results with a margin of error of plus or minus 3.5 or 4 percentage points. The positive difference for the polls summarized above of around +15, measured in 95% confidence interval units, represent positive responses fifteen times a typical ninety-five percent confidence interval, leaving little doubt as to the majority's opinion.

TABLE 3.3
Has *Teaching or Instruction* Improved Because of the Standardized Testing
Program?: U.S. and Canada Survey and Poll Items, 1960 to 2003

	Provider Respondent Groups (e.g., teachers, administrators)			Consumer Respondent Groups (e.g., students, parents, the public)		
	Number of Items	Mean Percentage Point Differential	Confidence Intervals	Number of Items	Mean Percentage Point Differential	Confidence Intervals
Surveys	11	+36.2	+6.9	–	–	–
Polls	3	+52.0	+14.3	12	+50.8	+15.8
TOTAL	14	+39.6	+10.6	12	+50.8	+15.8

Table 3.4 presents poll and survey observations regarding standardized testing's benefits on the other side of the classroom—in student learning, effort, or motivation. Pollsters and researchers posed questions about learning improvement more than twice as often as questions about instructional improvement.

The responses summarized in Table 3.4 are similarly positive and robust as those in Table 3.3. One may notice from both tables, however, that consumer groups tend to respond more positively than provider groups to either set of questions. One may also notice, moreover, that responses in public opinion polls tend to be more positive toward testing than those in research study surveys, which are typically conducted by education professors.

There can be little doubt, however, that respondents—be they education provider or education consumer—strongly believe that standardized tests induce improvements in teaching and learning.

BUT, WHAT ABOUT SPECIFIC STUDIES OF A SPECIFIC PROGRAM BEING PROPOSED NOW?

Studies of programs being proposed do not exist; one can only study programs that have already existed. Some researchers are fond of arguing that one should read (or fund) their work because they "are the first" to study some aspect of a program or the program in a certain situation. Often, the claims are simply not true. Often, the unique aspect or situation is picayune or ephemeral and provides little new information of any general interest.

Just as often, this tactic is used as blanket condemnation of an entire research literature. Indeed, it is, essentially, the tactic that has virtually banned

TABLE 3.4
Has *Learning, Education, Student Effort or Student Motivation* Improved
Because of the Standardized Testing Program?: U.S. and Canada Survey
and Poll Items, 1960 to 2003

	Provider Respondent Groups (e.g., teachers, administrators)			Consumer Respondent Groups (e.g., students, parents, the public)		
	Number of Items	Mean Percentage Point Differential	Confidence Intervals	Number of Items	Mean Percentage Point Differential	Confidence Intervals
Surveys	31	+34.3	+5.9	12	+34.8	+12.3
Polls	4	+50.3	+12.6	21	+48.5	+14.2
TOTAL	35	+36.2	+6.6	33	+43.5	+13.5

the use of general ability tests in employment decisions despite the evidence from, literally, thousands of experimental studies demonstrating that such tests are one of the best predictors of work performance. Testing opponents have used the argument, successfully, that general tests cannot be valid for specific jobs; employment tests must be developed and validated for each unique job. Naturally, this requirement is not imposed on any of the other pieces of evidence that employers use in hiring decisions, most of which are less reliable than general mental ability tests. It is just another way that the use of standardized tests are specially restricted in our society.

Taken to its extreme, the tactic would ban the use of all standardized testing. If tests could only be used after they were developed and validated for each situation and each person, they would no longer be standardized.

Yet, even if one cannot find a specific research study of a specific program at a specific place at a specific time under specific conditions, the vast research literature on standardized testing covers in each and every one of the essential characteristics of high-stakes standardized testing's relationship to achievement, for example:

- the effect of setting high standards on achievement;
- the effect of testing on achievement, rather than not testing;
- the relationship between the frequency of testing and achievement;
- the effect of detailed feedback on achievement;
- the effect of high-stakes testing on student, teacher, and administrator motivation;
- the effect of high-stakes on student, teacher, and administrator behavior, by contrast to low-stakes' effect;

- the effect of high-stakes testing on the alignment of curriculum and instruction;
- the effect of setting clear targets for performance on achievement;
- the learning effect of test-taking itself; and
- the firm conviction of all concerned—students, parents, the public, teachers, administrators, employers—that high-stakes testing induces students to study and learn more.

All the aforementioned are generally and strongly positive, based on an abundance of research studies from the 1920s to the present.

BUT, WHAT ABOUT THE "OTHER SIDE" OF THE ISSUE?

Testing critics who bother to read this are likely to assert that I only looked for studies that show positive effects of testing and that, for all anyone knows, the number of studies showing negative effects greatly outnumber those I have found.

They would be wrong on all counts. I looked for any studies that examined effects of testing, and I did find some that found little or no effect and a tiny number that found negative effects ... on achievement.

That is not to say that some students who genuinely suffer from test anxiety are not adversely affected by school programs that rely on testing. That is not to say that some students who perform poorly on tests will not feel bad. That is not to say that some students denied admission to programs or institutions due to a poor test performance are not denied opportunities they seek.

On average, however, the use of testing tends to improve academic achievement. The evidence for this proposition is overwhelming and voluminous. Many articles written acclaiming the contrary begin with statements like "Much research has shown that standardized testing, particularly when it is high-stakes, produces mostly negative consequences." Follow the references and look at the details, however, and one is likely to find, as I have, that the articles cited may consist of little more than unsupported declarations, and most of the rest found positive effects on student achievement, but education administrators, and maybe teachers, disliked the test for other reasons, such as the limits that standards and tests impose on their freedom.

Granted, then, I am ignoring the most popular complaints of testing critics. If a testing program clearly improves student achievement, but teachers or administrators do not like it simply because they are made to change the manner and content of their work from that which they personally prefer, I admit that I really don't much care, and neither should any taxpayer or parent.

The public schools do not exist so that education professionals can spend their workdays in a manner that optimizes their personal pleasure and preferences. They exist to educate students.

DENIAL OF THE OBVIOUS?

If one were to relate the claims of some testing critics, that research has found no achievement benefits to testing, to the average Joe on the street one would likely elicit bewilderment. How could research show that incentives don't matter? How could research show that students do not study any more or any harder when a test that counts looms before them?

The general public favors high-stakes standardized testing, in overwhelming numbers, and has for at least four decades. Public-school parents are even stronger advocates than nonparents, even when reminded that their own children might risk being held back a grade or from graduation if they do not pass. Low-income parents are even stronger advocates than high income parents, even when reminded that their own children might risk being held back a grade or from graduation if they do not pass.

Every poll of adult public opinion is a survey of experienced, former students. Why would adults be so emphatically in favor of high-stakes testing if they knew, based on their own student experience, that there were no positive achievement effects? They want to make their children suffer just as they suffered? Not likely. They support high-stakes tests because they believe, based on their own abundant experience, that students study harder in the face of tests with consequences.

Observe, for example, the results of this September 2000 question posed to parents of K–12 public-school parents by interviewers from Public Agenda:

> **Q.** Students pay more attention and study harder if they know they must pass a test to get promoted or to graduate. Do you agree or disagree?
> **A.** Strongly or somewhat agree   75%
>   Strongly or somewhat disagree   23%
>   Don't know/No opinion   3%

A majority—54%—*strongly* agreed with the statement.

The common assumption that people respond to incentives—sometimes called *extrinsic motivators* in the education literature—indeed forms the foundation of classical liberal economics. If not true, one might as well erase most economics professors' classroom diagrams from the blackboard. An abundance of experimental evidence, however, supports the classical economic assumptions.

Much of the experimental evidence in education was accumulated in the hundreds of studies of mastery learning and effective schools from the 1970s into the 1990s. Mastery learning incorporates testing in a big way. Students are given structured assignments with a schedule and a clear goal to accomplish, and tests may be used to monitor progress toward, or mastery of, that goal which is, most often, measured by a standardized test with stakes. (see, e.g., Bangert-Drowns, Kulik, & Kulik, 1988; Guskey & Gates, 1986; Kulik & Kulik, 1987). Moreover, some experts have argued that, of all the characteristics typical of mastery learning programs, the substantial positive effects in the experimental evidence are consistently found only from the testing and the feedback provided by the testing (Abbott & Falstrom, 1977; Friedman, 1987; Kulik & Kulik, 1987).

Likewise, much of the program evaluation evidence has been accumulated in the effective schools research literature, which advocates frequent monitoring of student progress through testing. (see, e.g., Clark, Lotto, & Astuto, 1984; Cotton, 1995; Northwest Regional Educational Laboratory, 1990; Purkey & Smith, 1983; Taylor, Valentine, & Jones, 1985).

The testing used in the mastery learning and effective schools studies was not always large-scale or high-stakes, but usually it was. Moreover, large-scale and high-stakes tests possess all the characteristics found in those studies to make the difference in improving achievement.

The currently common strident refusal of some testing critics to cut high-stakes testing any slack started in the 1980s, I believe, shortly after the publicity surrounding the *A Nation at Risk* report. Denials of testing benefits have since become increasingly frequent, increasingly insistent, and increasingly wrong.

In earlier decades, criticisms of standardized tests were more muted (and less far-fetched). External standardized tests may have been disliked by some education researchers, but they were not hated and loathed by so many, as is true now. Indeed, most references to high-stakes standardized testing three or more decades ago just assumed that it had positive motivational, alignment, and achievement effects. Their existence was widely accepted as fact, as being simply obvious.

CONCLUSION

A large number of testing researchers have insisted that there exists no, or hardly any, evidence that the use of standardized testing produces any benefits. Indeed, one group of (mostly education professors) hired by the National Research Council over a decade ago declared there was no evidence there were any benefits to the use of employment testing, despite the fact that over a thousand controlled experiments had been conducted finding that the benefits were pronounced and persistent.

Some of these nay-sayers probably don't want you to know the truth; some just do not bother to read the research literature. Both traits could be attributed to some others.

The research literature on testing's achievement effects—the subject of this chapter—is likely not as vast as that for testing's predictive (or, selection) effects (the kind produced by employment or college admission tests). But, the latter literature exceeds a thousand studies. The former certainly exceeds a few hundred studies, and that seems like a lot to me.

How some researchers can get away with telling the world that the work of hundreds or thousands of other scholars simply does not exist or, even if it did, it couldn't be any good (because it wasn't done by them), is itself a worthy topic for study on the ethics of research conducted in universities, think tanks, and government funded research centers.

ACKNOWLEDGMENTS

The author thanks the Educational Testing Service, whose research fellowship freed up the time necessary to conduct this study, and acknowledges the able assistance of the librarians at ETS's Brigham Library and the support of Richard Coley, Linda DeLauro, Carla Cooper, and Drew Gitomer.

REFERENCES

Abbott, R. D., & Falstrom P. (1977). Frequent testing and personalized systems of instruction. *Contemporary Educational Psychology, 2*, 251–257.

Aber, J. (1996). *Getting a college degree fast: Testing out & other accredited short cuts.* New York: Prometheus Books.

Annotated bibliography on minimum competency testing. (1978). ERIC ED156186.

Averch, H. A., Carroll, S. J., Donaldson, T. S., Kiesling, H. J., & Pincus, J. (1971). *How effective is schooling? A critical review and synthesis of research findings.* Santa Monica, CA: Rand.

Bangert-Drowns, R. L., Kulik, J. A., & Kulik, C. C. (1991). Effects of frequent classroom testing. *Journal of Educational Research, 85*(2), 89–99.

Bishop, J. H. (1988). *The economics of employment testing.* Working Paper #88-14, Cornell University, School of Industrial and Labor Relations, Center for Advanced Human Resource Studies.

Boudreau, J. W. (1988, December). *Utility analysis for decisions in human resource management.* Working Paper 88-21, New York State School of Industrial and Labor Relations, Cornell University.

Braun, H. (2003). *Reconsidering the impact of high-stakes testing.* Research Implications Bulletin. Educational Testing Service.

Cameron, J., & Pierce, W. D. (1994). Reinforcement, reward, and intrinsic and extrinsic motivation: A meta-analysis. *Review of Educational Research, 64*(3), 363–423.

Cameron, J., & Pierce, W. D. (1996). The debate about rewards and intrinsic motivation: Protests and accusations do not alter the results. *Review of Educational Research, 66*(1), 39–51.

Carroll, J. B. (1955). The Harvard Foreign Language Aptitude Tests. In the *12th Yearbook of the National Council on Measurement Used in Education, Part 2.* Cleveland.

Clark, D. L., Lotto, L. S., & Astuto, T. A. (1984). Effective schools and school improvement: A comparative analysis of two lines of inquiry. *Educational Administration Quarterly, 20*(3), 41–68.

Cole, N., & Willingham, W. (1997). *Gender and Fair Assessment*. Princeton, NJ: ETS.

College Entrance Examination Board. (1988). *Guide to the College Board Validity Study Service*. New York: Author.

Cotton, K. (1995). *Effective schooling practices: A research synthesis 1995 update*. Northwest Regional Education Laboratory.

Crooks, T. J. (1988). The impact of classroom evaluation practices on students. *Review of Educational Research, 58*(4), 438–481.

Edmonds, R. R., & Frederiksen, J. R. (1979). *Search for effective schools: The identification and analysis of city schools that are instructionally effective for poor children*. Washington, DC: Educational Resources Information Center.

Fontana, J. (2000, June). New York's test-driven standards. In A. A. Glatthorn & J. Fontana (Eds.), *Coping with standards, tests, and accountability: Voices from the classroom*. Washington, DC: NEA Teaching and Learning Division.

Frederiksen, N. (1994). *The influence of minimum competency tests on teaching and learning*. Princeton, NJ: Educational Testing Service.

Friedman, H. (1987). Repeat examinations in introductory statistics. *Teaching of Psychology, 14*, 20–23.

Gorth, W. P., & Perkins, M. R. (Eds.). (1979). *A study of minimum competency programs: Final comprehensive report (Vols. 1–2)*. Amherst, MA: National Evaluation Systems.

Grissmer, D. W., Flanagan, A., Kawata, J., & Williamson, S. (2000, July). *Improving student achievement: What NAEP state test scores tell us*. Los Angeles: RAND.

Guskey, T. R., & Gates, S. L. (1986). Synthesis of research on the effects of mastery learning in elementary and secondary classrooms. *Educational Leadership, 43*(8), 73–80.

Hawisher, M. F., & Harper, M. J. (1979). *Competency testing: Bibliography*. Winthrop College, Rock Hill, SC: Competency Testing Project.

Hunter, J. E., & Schmidt, F. L. (1982). Fitting People to Jobs: The Impact of Personnel Selection on National Productivity. In M. D. Dunnette & E. A. Fleishman (Eds.), *Human Performance and Productivity: Human Capability Assessment* (Vol. 1, pp. 233–284). Hillsdale, NJ, Lawrence Erlbaum Associates.

Hunter, J. E., & Schmidt, F. L. (1983, April). Quantifying the effects of psychological interventions on employee job performance and work-force productivity. *American Psychologist, 473–478*.

Hunter, J. E., & Hunter, R. F. (1984). Validity and utility of alternative predictors of job performance. *Psychological Bulletin, 96*(1), 72–98.

Jackson, M., & Battiste, B. (1978). *Competency testing: An annotated bibliography*. Unpublished manuscript, ERIC: ED167503.

Jacobson, J. E. (1992, October 29). Mandatory testing requirements and pupil achievement. PhD dissertation, Massachusetts Institute of Technology.

Jones, J. B. (1993). Effects of the use of an altered testing/grading method on the retention and success of students enrolled in college mathematics. EdD dissertation, East Texas State University.

Kirkland, M. C. (1971). The effects of tests on students and schools. *Review of Educational Research, 41*, 303–350.

Kulik, C.-L., & Kulik, J. A. (1987). Mastery testing and student learning: A meta-analysis. *Journal of Educational Technology Systems, 15*, 325–345.

Kulik, J. A., & Kulik, C.-L. (1989). The concept of meta-analysis. *International Journal of Education Research, 227–340*.

Locke, E. A., & Latham, G. P. (2002, September). Building a practically useful theory of goal setting and task motivation: A 35-year odyssey. *American Psychologist.*

Mackenzie, D. E. (1983). Research for school improvement: An appraisal of some recent trends. *Educational Researcher, 12*(4), 5–17.

Manuel, H. T. (1952). Results of a half-century experiment in teaching a second language. *Modern Language Journal, 36,* 74–76.

Milton, O. (1981). *Will that be on the final?* Springfield, IL: Thomas.

Morgan, R., & Ramist, L. (1988, February). *Advanced placement students in college: An investigation of course grades at 21 colleges.* Educational Testing Service, Report No. SR-98-13. Princeton: ETS.

Mullis, I. V. S., Jenkins, F., & Johnson, E. G. (1994, October). *Effective schools in mathematics: Perspectives from the NAEP 1992 assessment.* U.S. Education Department, National Center for Education Statistics.

Murnane, R. J. (1981). Interpreting the evidence on school effectiveness. *Teachers College Record, 83*(1), 19–35.

Natriello, G., & Dornbusch, S. M. (1984). *Teacher evaluative standards and student effort.* New York: Longman.

New Jersey Department of Education. (1977, November). *Compendium of educational research, planning, evaluation, and assessment activities: USA & Canada.* Division of Research, Planning & Evaluation, Bureau of Research & Assessment. Trenton, NJ.

Northwest Regional Educational Laboratory. (1990, April). *Effective schooling practices: A research synthesis, 1990 update.* Portland, ME: Author.

Olmsted, J. W. (1957). Tests, examinations, and the superior college student. In *The effective use of measurement in guidance: The Sixth Annual Western Regional Conference on Testing Problems.* Educational Testing Service, Los Angeles, CA, pp. 17–20.

Phelps, R. P. (1996). Are U.S. students the most heavily tested on earth? *Educational Measurement: Issues and Practice, 15*(3), 19–27.

Phelps, R. P. (2000). Trends in large-scale, external testing outside the United States. *Educational Measurement: Issues and Practice, 19*(1), 11–21.

Phelps, R. P. (2001). Benchmarking to the world's best in mathematics: Quality control in curriculum and instruction among the top performers in the TIMSS. *Evaluation Review, 25*(4), 391–439.

Pressey, S. L. (1954). Acceleration: Basic principles and recent research. In A. Anastasi (Ed.), *Testing problems in perspective: Twenty-fifth anniversary volume of topical readings from the invitational conference on testing problems* (pp. 96–101). Washington, DC: American Council on Education.

Public Agenda Online. (2000, September). *Survey finds little sign of backlash against academic standards or standardized tests.* New York: Author.

Purkey, S. C., & Smith, M. S. (1983). Effective schools: A review. *The Elementary School Journal, 84*(4), 427–452.

Rosenshine, B. (1983). Teaching functions in instructional programs. *The Elementary School Journal, 83*(4), 335–351.

Rosenshine, B. (2003). High-stakes testing: Another analysis. *Educational Policy Analysis Archives, 11*(24). Retrieved August 7, 2003, from http://epaa.asu.edu/epaa/v.11n24

Schmidt, F. L., & Hunter, J. E. (1998). The validity and utility of selection methods in personnel psychology: Practical and theoretical implication of 85 years of research findings. *Psychological Bulletin 124,* 262–274

Schmidt, F. L., Hunter, J. E., McKenzie, R. C., & Muldrow, T. W. (1979). Impact of valid selection procedures on work-force productivity. *Journal of Applied Psychology, 64*(6), 609–626.

Schmitt, N., Gooding, R. Z., Noe, R. D., & Kirsch, M. (1984). Meta-analysis of validity studies published between 1964 and 1982 and the investigation of study characteristics. *Personnel Psychology, 37*(3), 407–422.

Staats, A. (1973). Behavior analysis and token reinforcement in educational behavior modification and curriculum research. In C. E. Thoreson (Ed.), *72nd Yearbook of the NSSE: Behavior modification in education.* Chicago: University of Chicago Press.

Stanley, J. C. (1976). Identifying and nurturing the intellectually gifted. *Phi Delta Kappan, 58*(3), 234–237.

Task Force on Educational Assessment Programs. (1979). *Competency testing in Florida: Report to the Florida cabinet, Part 1.* Tallahassee.

Taylor, A., Valentine, B., & Jones, M. (1985, December). *What research says about effective schools.* National Education Association.

Terman, L. M. (1954). The discovery and encouragement of exceptional talent. *American Psychologist, 9,* 221–230.

Thompson, B. (2002, November). High stakes testing and student learning: A response to Amrein and Berliner. *Educational News Org., Commentaries and Reports.*

Tuckman, B. W. (1994, April 4–8). *Comparing incentive motivation to metacognitive strategy in its effect on achievement.* Paper presented at the Annual Meeting of the American Educational Research Association, New Orleans, LA. ERIC ED368790.

Wedman, I. (1994). The Swedish Scholastic Aptitude Test: Development, use, and research. *Educational Measurement: Issues and Practice, 13*(2), 5–11.

Wildemuth, B. M. (1977). *Minimal competency testing: Issues and procedures, an annotated bibliography.* ERIC ED150188.

Wenglinsky, H. (2001, September). *Teacher classroom practices and student performance: How schools can make a difference.* Princeton, NJ: Educational Testing Service.

Willingham, W. W., Lewis, C., Morgan, R., & Ramist, L. (1990). Implications of using freshman GPA as the criterion for the predictive validity of the SAT. *Predicting College Grades: An Analysis of Institutional Trends over Two Decades.*

Winfield, L. F. (1990, March). School competency testing reforms and student achievement: Exploring a national perspective. Research report. Princeton, NJ: Educational Testing Service.

Woessman, L. (2000, December). *Schooling resources, educational institutions, and student performance: The international evidence.* Kiel Institute of World Economics. Kiel Working Paper No. 983.

4

Some Misconceptions About Large-Scale Educational Assessments

Dean Goodman
Ronald K. Hambleton
University of Massachusetts at Amherst

Today, educational reform is affecting just about every school administrator, teacher, and public school child in this country. With the No Child Left Behind (NCLB) federal legislation in the United States, states have little choice but to embark upon major educational reforms, especially in the areas of reading and mathematics. But many of the educational reform initiatives extend well beyond those required by the NCLB legislation with many states conducting curriculum and educational assessment reform at all grade levels and subjects. The reforms extend to higher expectations for teacher proficiencies, curricula with more emphasis on higher level thinking skills, more commitment and increased resources to after-school programs and summer school programs, careful attention to the instructional needs of children with learning disabilities, and much more. No two states appear to be proceeding in exactly the same way to design and implement their educational reform initiatives but in most states the initiatives are substantial and comprehensive.

Despite the many dissimilarities, however, many of the criticisms heard about the assessment components of these state educational reform initiatives are very much the same: For example, high-stakes state assessments set students up for failure, too much time and money is being taken up with the assessments, many of the test items in these state assessments are biased against minority students and students from lower socioeconomic backgrounds, and the performance standards set on these educational assessments are too high, dooming many children to failure. We have worked with many departments of education in both the United States and Canada, and all of the criticisms (and more) have been heard at one time or another, wherever we might be. At the same time, our experiences suggest that these criticisms are often based on misconceptions about these large-scale high-stakes assessment programs and how they are conceptualized, designed, implemented, and evaluated.

The purpose of this chapter is to address what we believe are five widely held misconceptions about large-scale high-stakes assessment programs. These include (a) that high-stakes assessments set up students, teachers, and schools for failure; (b) that large-scale assessments are too costly; (c) that state assessments are filled with biased test items; (d) that the performance standards are often set too high; and (e) that policymakers, educators, and members of the general public actually understand the test results they are presented with. What follows is a consideration of each of the misconceptions.

HIGH-STAKES ASSESSMENTS SET UP STUDENTS, TEACHERS, AND SCHOOLS FOR FAILURE

An unfortunate assumption that seems to fuel opposition to state assessments in America's Kindergarten to Grade 12 (K to 12) education systems is that the use of statewide tests, and the high stakes that are typically attached to them, are setting up students for failure. Several criticisms and perceptions that fuel this assumption warrant discussion. These include the criticism that state tests do not measure what is important in K to 12 education, the belief that a single test score is used to determine grade promotion and high school graduation, and the perception that educational accountability systems only involve assessment.

State Assessments Do Not Measure What is Important in K to 12 Education

A common criticism of state assessment programs is that they do not measure what is most important in K to 12 education. Critics argue that these assessments focus on a limited part of the curriculum and assess only lower order skills and knowledge such as factual recall. Clearly, it is not possible for one assessment to measure all important skills and concepts that are taught over one or more years of instruction, and some processes may be better assessed in the context of the classroom. As with all forms of assessment, decisions must be made regarding the skills and knowledge that will be assessed by a state's educational assessments. Fortunately, those responsible for developing statewide assessment programs often engage in a number of important activities that inform these decisions, some of which will be outlined next.

In the past decade, one of the most fundamental shifts in statewide assessments has been the concerted effort to develop assessments that are based on state content standards. Content standards outline what students should know and be able to do in a given subject area. These standards provide a common focus for both instruction and assessment (National Research Council, 1999), offering direction to teachers about what to teach students in the classroom, and to state testing programs about what to assess in statewide assessments.

The most recent survey of state assessment programs by *Education Week* (2003a) reveals an increasing commitment by states to administer criterion-referenced assessments that are designed to measure student mastery of state content standards. Expanded uses of constructed response questions and writing tasks are two ways that states are taking to address their content standards. This is an important trend. In 2002, 42 states administered these types of assessments at the elementary, middle, and high school levels, up from 37 states in 2001 (Education Week, 2003a). In stark contrast, in 1995 only 19 states administered criterion-referenced assessments that were aligned with state standards (Education Week, 1997).

With the enactment of the *No Child Left Behind Act of 2001 (NCLB)*, there is an even greater commitment to ensure that large-scale tests or assessments reflect the knowledge and skills expected to be learned by all students in a state. To comply with this federal law, states must adopt "challenging academic content standards and challenging student achievement standards" (NCLB, 2002, Sec. 1111[b][1][A]) and administer state or local assessments that are aligned with these standards (Sec. 1111[b][3][C]). States that cannot demonstrate they have satisfied these requirements will not be eligible for substantial federal funding.

As outlined in technical reports and related documents produced by state testing programs (e.g., Massachusetts Department of Education, 2003; New York State Department of Education, 2003; North Carolina Department of Public Instruction, 2003), states engage in a rigorous set of activities to align their educational assessments to the state content standards. Using the state standards as their framework, test developers work with subject-matter experts to develop test blueprints that specify the types of skills, concepts, and cognitive processes that will be assessed by the state tests. Item-writers create pools of test items that align with these blueprints, typically using multiple item formats (e.g., multiple choice, constructed-response items, and writing tasks) to tap into the wide range of knowledge and skills to be assessed. These pools of test items are reviewed by committees of subject-matter experts, assessment experts, and members of key stakeholder groups to ensure that the items assess the constructs of interest in a fair and developmentally appropriate manner. At this stage, potentially problematic items are revised or removed from the item pools. Items are then field tested under test-like conditions, and student responses to the items are evaluated by review committees to ensure that any remaining problematic items are removed or revised. Following this evaluation process, the test developers then compile the items into test forms, which are subjected to further reviews (and, often, additional field tests) to ensure that the final tests are effective measures of the skills and knowledge students are expected to possess at a given grade.

Now, it must surely be true that not all states are completely successful in aligning their assessments with their content standards, but the methodology is certainly in place for aligning curriculum and assessment, and evaluating that the alignment is present (see, e.g., work by Bhola, Impara, & Buckendahl, 2003; O'Neil, Sireci, & Huff, in press; and Webb, 1999, in investigating the alignment of test content and state content standards). It behooves each state to make available information regarding curriculum-assessment alignment in their technical reports, and where there are gaps, to do something to fix them. But to malign states for not being sensitive to curriculum-assessment alignment is not consistent with the facts.

To address concerns about "teaching to the test," state assessment programs typically administer different forms of a test within and across each testing cycle. These forms often share a sufficient number of items to ensure that the forms can be placed on a common scoring metric through a statistical equating process (see Cook & Eignor, 1991; Kolen, 1988; and Kolen & Brennan, 1995; for discussions of ways different test forms can be equated). The test forms also contain unique sets of items that enable reliable information to be collected on a wide range of skills and concepts taught throughout the course of study. Ironically, when curriculum and assessment are in alignment, "teaching to the test" is exactly what teachers should be doing because the test or assessment will contain a sampling of questions from the curriculum, and so the only way to effectively prepare students to perform well on the tests is to teach the curriculum to which the tests are matched.

Problems can still arise in "teaching to the test" if teachers are conscious of the sometimes arbitrary ways in which a state assesses particular skills (e.g., with a particular item format, and/or a particular scoring rubric) and begin to teach students to simply try to score better on the assessments (e.g., encouraging students to "beat" the tests by capitalizing on flaws in the test items or the scoring rubrics) without necessarily mastering the content standards. Gains in assessment results can be expected, especially early in the history of a testing program. But after that time, the best way to show achievement gain is for teachers to help students master the content standards because there are only so many points achievable (and hopefully few) from capitalizing on those test-taking skills that inflate scores due to shortcomings in the test construction process. The likely long-term payoff in achievement gain is much greater from teaching the content standards than making all students "test-wise."

Too Much Emphasis is Placed on a Single Test Score

Another misconception of state assessments is that states are placing too much emphasis on a single test score. In their condemnation of state assessments, critics are eager to detail the plight of students who cannot graduate or move on to the next grade based on the results of a single test. Critics rarely point out, however, when it comes to graduation tests, that scores on statewide tests are only one piece of information that must be considered when making graduation or promotion decisions: school grades (measures of ability that are by no means infallible), credits in core subject areas, and attendance records also play an important role in the decision making process.

Moreover, critics often fail to acknowledge that students are given multiple opportunities to pass these tests. In Massachusetts, for example, students have five opportunities to pass the state graduation test, and students who do not obtain passing scores by the end of their senior year may demonstrate the requisite skills and knowledge in other ways (e.g., in 2002, 7 of the 19 states with graduation contingent on performance on statewide exams also provided alternative routes for students who failed the exams; Education Week, 2003b). In Massachusetts, too, there is an appeals process for students who are close to the passing score on the mathematics and English language arts tests, have high attendance at school, and have taken the state graduation test at least twice. The appeals are accepted if the students' school grades in core subjects are comparable or better than the grades of students who were just above the passing score on the state test. This system appears to be working well. Surprisingly, the public does not seem to be aware of the appeals process because rarely is this feature mentioned in public discourse about the state graduation requirement.

Educational Accountability Systems Only Involve Testing

The myth that high-stakes testing is setting students up for failure is also fed by the belief that educational accountability systems only involve testing. Although tests play an important part in state accountability systems, they do not represent the only part. A key goal of any accountability program is to improve student learning, not to only measure it. Test results provide a standardized way to identify students who may need additional support to gain the skills and knowledge that all students in the state should possess, according to the Board of Education in each state. Remediation programs are typically in place to offer extra support to those students who are not able to pass the tests or assessments. For example, in 2002, of the 20 states where student promotion or graduation were contingent on statewide examinations, 16 states required remediation for students that failed these exams (Education Week, 2003b). In most of these states (14 out of 16), this remediation was financed at the state-level (Education Week, 2003b).

A study by Mass Insight Education and Research Institute (Mass Insight, 2003) indicates that students who do not pass the state tenth-grade assessments take advantage of available remediation programs, and have reacted positively to them. Four out of five high school students from the three largest urban school districts in Massachusetts who did not pass the Massachusetts Comprehensive Assessment System (MCAS) tests reported having participated in remediation programs for extra help (Mass Insight, 2003). Students reported high levels of satisfaction with these extra-help programs. More than three quarters of participating students would recommend them to other students needing help (Mass Insight, 2003) and 65% of students who participated in remediation programs credited the programs for their success on a subsequent retest.

TESTS ARE TOO COSTLY

Another common criticism of large-scale state assessments is that they are too costly. Critics of state assessment programs argue that students and teachers are spending too much time on these assessments, and that too much money is being spent as well. In the past decade, however, a body of evidence has been compiled that shows the costs associated with large-scale assessment are really not as high as some critics have charged.

Costs Associated With Standardized Testing: Evidence From the Early-1990s

Studies conducted by the National Commission on Testing and Public Policy (NCTPP, 1990) and the U.S. General Accounting Office (GAO, 1993) offer early insight into the costs of standardized testing in the United States, and illustrate the importance of placing these costs in a meaningful context.

After 3 years of investigating trends, practices, and impacts of the use of standardized tests, the NCTPP (1990) offered the blunt appraisal that U.S.

students "are subjected to too much standardized testing" (p. 14). This judgment was informed by the NCTPP's conservative estimate that U.S. elementary and secondary students spent the equivalent of more than 20 million school days per year simply taking standardized tests. Without doubt, this estimate is large, but only if considered out of context. As noted by Phelps (1997), when the 40 million U.S. students who take the tests are considered, this imposing figure reduces to only "one-half day of testing per student per year" (p. 96), a figure that does not seem to support the assertion that students are overtested.

A markedly different appraisal of the extent and cost of standardized testing in U.S. schools was offered by the GAO (1993). After conducting a comprehensive investigation into the costs of standardized testing, the GAO concluded that U.S. students do not seem to be overtested. The GAO reported that, on average, students spent 3.4 hours in 1990 and 1991 taking systemwide tests (tests that were administered to all students, or a representative sample of students, at any one grade level in a district or state), or "less than one-half of 1 percent of a student's school year" (p. 18). After other types of standardized tests (e.g., Chapter 1 tests, state advanced-subject-area tests, and college entrance exams) were considered, the per-student average was still just 4 hours per year (pp. 74–76). (As noted by the GAO, this value seemed consistent with estimates provided in earlier studies [e.g., Anderson, 1982; U.S. Congress Office of Technology Assessment, 1992], and the approximately one-half day of testing figure that was derived from the NCTPP, 1990, data.) Even after activities such as test preparation were considered, the total amount of time students spent on test-related activities on standardized tests averaged less than 7 hours for the year (p. 18). These findings appear to suggest that American students have not been subjected to an onerous amount of testing in the past, although it obviously seems that way to the critics.

Also, important to consider beyond the time students spend taking tests or assessments, are the uses to which that information collected during testing is put. In Massachusetts, for example, assessment results are considered by each school in assisting students and used to modify school instructional practices, and where necessary, they influence the design of after-school programs, and impact on in-service training programs for teachers. The additional time required of students to take tests or assessments needs to be weighed against these additional uses of the test information and its value in the instructional process.

It is common for critics when confronted with the reality that test time on a per-student basis is not unreasonable to remind the public that students spend an inordinate amount of time preparing for tests. Although extra time is definitely spent by students in preparing for tests, according to the GAO study, this amount of time appears less than the critics would suggest, and it must be noted that these additional uses of the test results need to be factored into the discussions as well. A teacher learning from the test results that students in her class were especially weak in fractions might use the information to improve instruction on that topic in the future and improve student learning for a whole classroom of children. Clearly, this area of trade-offs between the amount of student preparation and testing time versus the instructional value to teachers of results from tests needs to be further studied.

The GAO (1993) also collected data on how much time school and school district staff spent on test-related activities. Unfortunately, the data reported by the GAO (i.e., that, on average, each district spent 1,500 personnel hours on system-wide testing) were aggregated to a level that was not very meaningful for our purposes here. Subsequent analyses of GAO data by Phelps (1997) showed that the average amount of time school and school district personnel directed to test-related activities was quite low: less than 6 hours per year. The largest proportion of this time was devoted to administering the test (40%). Less than 30% of this time was spent preparing students for the test. Twelve percent of this time was devoted to analyzing or reporting the results of the tests, and the remaining time was directed toward "test development, training (either getting trained or training others), scoring, collecting, sorting, mailing or other activities" (p. 101). Phelps (1997) also reported that teachers, on average, spent no more than 7 hours per year on system-wide test-related activities, offering compelling evidence that large-scale assessments historically have not been very costly in terms of teachers' time.

The GAO study (1993) also showed that the monetary costs of large-scale testing are not excessive. The estimated cost for all test-related activities in 1990–1991 was approximately $15 per student, which included $4 in direct costs and more than $10 in state and local staff time. The least expensive types of tests were multiple choice, which averaged approximately $14 per student. Tests with at least some performance component averaged approximately $20, and tests consisting of 20% to 100% performance-based questions averaged $33 per student. On average, the overall costs associated with testing represented about one half of 1% of school district budgets, and less than 2% of state education agency budgets, figures that seem far from excessive. The Massachusetts Department of Education reported in 1999 that state assessments were costing $15 per student per assessment and approximately 50% of the assessments required constructed responses by the students and need to be scored by graders. Cheaper off the shelf tests were available to the state but they noted that (1) the off-the-shelf tests could not be released (Massachusetts releases the state assessments within 3 months of administration on their Web site), (2) they would not meet the content standards nearly as well, (3) they would be less useful diagnostically, and (4) test security is a much greater problem with off-the-shelf tests because only two or three forms exist (whereas with the state's assessments, a new assessment is constructed every year). In this instance, the reduced cost of off-the-shelf tests was definitely not judged as a saving that was worth the loss of valuable information to students and their teachers.

Current and Future Costs of Educational Assessment

Although past criticisms regarding the amount of time and money spent on large-scale state assessments seem largely unwarranted, how valid are current criticisms? Recent research shows that the amount of assessment in U.S. schools has increased noticeably since the early-1990s. For example, Education Week (2001) reported that, on average, students spent approximately 5.3 hours taking state tests in 2001–2002. This represented a 1.9 hour increase from the 3.4 hours of systemwide testing reported by the GAO (1993) in 1990–1991.

With the enactment of NCLB, the amount of assessment that will occur in the United States seems destined to increase over the next several years. Under this federal law, states are required to test all of their students annually in Grades 3 through 8 in mathematics and reading or language arts, and at least once in Grades 10 through 12 by the 2005–2006 school year (NCLB, 2001, § 1111[b][3][C][v][I]). To comply with the law, states must also test students in science at least once in Grades 3 through 5, Grades 6 through 9, and Grades 10 through 12 by 2007–2008 (NCLB, 2001, § 1111[b][3][C][v][II]). In total, each state will be required to administer 17 large-scale assessments under NCLB, almost triple the number previously required under federal law.

Clearly, NCLB will increase the number of legislated large-scale assessments administered in the United States. However, because most existing assessments will be adapted to satisfy NCLB requirements, the resulting amount of time that each student will spend on assessments in many states as a result of this legislation may not be much different from what has been reported in the past. For example, if one assumes that each NCLB test will take 2.5 hours to administer, students in the relevant grades will only spend between 5.0 hours and 7.5 hours annually on NCLB tests (values that are not much different from the 5.3 hours of annual testing reported by Education Week [2001] in 2001–2002). This amount of testing is approximately equivalent to only 1 school day per year (less than 1% of an average school year of 180 days).

Recent estimates of the costs of testing also indicate that the amount of money spent on tests is not excessive. Expanding on the GAO (1993) study, Phelps (2000) reported that the all-inclusive cost associated with systemwide testing in the United States (including up-front development costs and opportunity costs that consider time taken away from instruction) was about $16 per year per student in 1998 dollars (a figure that seems far from excessive given that the average per-student expenditure in the United States at that time was about $6,739 per year!).

While not as comprehensive as the all-inclusive costs reported by Phelps (2000), it is worthwhile to consider more recent estimates of state expenditures for accountability-related activities. In her analysis of costs associated with 25 state accountability systems, Hoxby (2002) reported that states spent between $1.79 to $34.02 per pupil on accountability-related activities in 2001–2002, and that no state spent *even 1 percent* of its elementary and secondary school budget on accountability" (p. 69). In Massachusetts, we have estimated that the state currently spends approximately one-third of 1% (or about $1 of every $300) of the educational budget on testing. This does not seem like unreasonable expenditure of educational dollars to inform the public, policymakers, teachers, and students about the progress students are making in relation to the state curricula.

In a recent report to Congress, the GAO (2003) estimated the cost of testing under NCLB will be between $1.9 billion to $5.3 billion for 2002 through 2008 (these differences are largely explained by the method by which assessments will be scored, with the lower estimate reflecting multiple-choice assessments that can be machine scored and the higher estimate reflecting the use of a combination of multiple-choice questions and open-ended questions that are hand scored). Although admittedly large, these estimates become far less daunting when averaged across the seven-year time frame reported by GAO: the average estimated costs of all state testing (including new and existing assessments) will be between $271 million and $757 million annually from 2002 to 2008. When the number of students that will be tested are considered (approximately 21.6 million, using enrollment figures provided by Rebarber & McFarland, 2002), these costs reduce to only about $13 to $35 per student, figures that align with other recent per-pupil cost estimates.

LARGE-SCALE EDUCATIONAL ASSESSMENTS ARE FULL OF BIASED TEST ITEMS

The charge that educational assessments contain test items that are unfair or biased against groups of students such as Blacks and Hispanics is regularly heard from test critics. That minority groups often perform less well on educational assessments in many states has been widely reported and is correct. Whether looking at ACT and SAT scores, nationally standardized achievement test results, NAEP results, or state indicators of educational achievement, Blacks and Hispanics often perform at least one standard deviation below the majority group of students. But are these results because of shortcomings in the educational assessments due to stereotyping of minority groups and/or the uses of inappropriate concepts, vocabulary, situations, terminology, test speededness, and so forth? Or, are the achievement gaps due to the existence of real differences in educational accomplishments? We strongly suspect that the achievement gap has little to do with any bias in the educational assessments themselves and has a lot to do with many other educational and social factors.

What is the psychometric definition of *item bias*? Item bias is the presence of some characteristic (e.g., unusually difficult language), which results in differential performance for two individuals with the same level of proficiency but who are from different designated groups of interest (e.g., males or females; African Americans or Caucasians). For example, a situation such as motor car racing may be introduced in a mathematics test item that is intended to address the concepts of speed, distance, and time. Motor car racing may even be introduced to make the test item itself more interesting and relevant to students. Unfortunately, motor car racing may be substantially less familiar to females than males. This lack of familiarity with motor car racing could result in lower item scores for females than males, on the average, due to a feature of the test item (i.e. placing the math item in the context of a motor car racing scenario) that is not actually central to the skill being assessed. The fix is easy in this example—rework the mathematics problem to focus on, say, a person going for a walk, or a ride in a car. These activities would be common to all students.

Test publishers and state departments of education are relentless in their search for potentially biased test items by reviewing items for potential gender, racial/ethnic, cultural, religious, regional, or socioeconomic disparities in understanding or performance. Consider the steps taken routinely by many testing agencies and state departments of education to remove bias from educational assessments:

1. Item writers who are members of multicultural and multiracial groups are among those who are used to write the assessment material—directions, questions, scoring rubrics, etcetera.
2. Item sensitivity committees representing diverse minority groups are established to focus on aspects of educational assessment material that might be unfair to minority students, or may represent stereotyping of minority groups.
3. Item reviewers, prior to any field testing of assessment material, are instructed to identify aspects of test items that might be unfair to minority groups or represent stereotyping.
4. Statistical analyses are carried out on field-test data searching for assessment material that is potentially problematic for minority groups.
5. All test publishers and most state departments of education have a document that is used by item sensitivity committees and other reviewers to spot potentially problematic or biased assessment material.

6. At the final stages of test and assessment development, content committees are sensitive to the inclusion of material that is not assessing the content standards or may be biased against minority groups.

Normally item writers and reviewers would be asked to avoid or identify a variety of potential sources of item bias that might distinguish majority and minority groups of students: content that may not have the same meaning across groups, test items that contain vocabulary that may not have the same meaning in all groups, clues in items that might give an unfair advantage to students in one group over another, items that because of student prior knowledge may advantage one group over another, and so on. Often, item writers are asked to avoid 25 to 30 potential sources of item bias in their work, and just in case they slip up, item *reviewers* are given the same list of potential sources of item bias to see if they can spot these problems or any others in items that have been written.

In addition to judgmental reviews, it is common to compile statistical data (e.g., using logistic regression or the Mantel-Haenszel procedure) to compare students in majority and minority groups (at least for males and females, and Blacks, Hispanics, and Whites). For several years, the Center for Educational Assessment at the University of Massachusetts has been conducting studies to identify potentially biased test items on seven of the state's educational assessments. Black–White, Hispanic–White, and Male–Female analyses are routinely carried out. In the year 2000, for example, potential item bias was studied in 696 items and only 24 items were identified for additional investigation. This is a rate of 3.5% of the test items with a combined potential bias of a small fraction of a point (on a 40 point test) if all of the potentially biased test items were actually biased against a single minority group. Items are flagged for further investigation if majority and minority groups matched on overall ability show a .10 or greater difference on a per point basis. (This means that there would need to be 10 of these potentially biased items in a test to result in an actual one point difference between the majority and minority group due to potentially biased test items.) Clearly the amount of bias that is appearing on educational assessments is likely to be small because of the efforts that are being made to spot and eliminate problems early. There is simply little or no evidence to claim that item bias is a serious problem today on state assessments.

PERFORMANCE STANDARDS ARE SET TOO HIGH

In Massachusetts, one of the popular explanations for the high failure rate among tenth grade students has been that the passing scores were set too high. In fact, the same criticism is heard in many states. It might be expected that critics could point to specific flaws in the procedure that was used to set

4. LARGE-SCALE EDUCATIONAL ASSESSMENTS

the performance standards. Perhaps uninformed panelists were involved in the process of setting the performance standards, panelists did not understand the process they used to set performance standards, or the performance standards were simply pulled "from the air." The reality, however, is that critics rarely know how performance standards were set despite the fact that details are usually provided in technical manuals, and instead they base their opinions on the numbers themselves—that too many students are failing, or not enough students are in the top performing category, for example. Reasonableness of the results is certainly one criterion that can be applied in practice and is a basis for rejecting some results, such as when *everyone* fails an assessment. But there are many other criteria to use, too.

The fact is that there are well-developed methods for setting performance standards, and most states try hard to apply those methods well (see, e.g., Cizek, 2001). It is not uncommon to involve 15 to 25 educators (called *panelists* in standard-setting studies) in the process. These panelists include teachers, curriculum specialists, administrators, and sometimes even the public. The typical standard-setting study might take 2 to 3 days of deliberation and includes sufficient training to enable panelists to carry out the standard-setting process with confidence.

Panelists, for example, might be asked to sort through student work and classify as *Failing, Basic, Proficient*, or *Advanced*. From their classifications of student work, performance standards or cut-off scores to classify students into four categories of performance can be identified (see, e.g., Cizek, 2001). Via discussion, student performance data on the assessment itself, and consequential data (e.g., information about the percent of students passing with particular performance standards), panelists in a standard-setting study are given the opportunity to revise their classifications of student work. Eventually, based on panelists' final classifications of student work, performance standards are determined based on the averages of the performance standards set by individual panelists in the standard-setting process.

Today, three related methods for setting performance standards are in place: Bookmark, Body of Work, and either the Angoff or extended Angoff (Cizek, 2001). All are popular with states, and research evidence is available to justify the use of the methods in practice. But the methods should not be judged solely by whether the results (e.g., percent of passing students) are consistent with expectations. In the main, the validity of performance standards should be judged by:

1. the qualifications and demographics of the panelists who were given the task of setting the performance standards,
2. the clarity and suitability of the performance descriptors that were used,

3. the reasonableness of the process the panelists used to arrive at the performance standards,
4. the confidence the panel members had in the process itself and the final performance standards, and
5. the compilation of validity evidence available to support the performance standards.

Very often, the setting of performance standards on state assessments is one of the most challenging steps in the assessment process, and considerable resources are used in making sure that the process is done well. On those occasions when it is not done well, the process can be repeated as it was recently in New York State. All in all, although clearly judgment is involved in setting performance standards, the process itself has substantial merit. Let those critics who think performance standards were set too high in a state find the flaw in the process itself.

POLICY-MAKERS, EDUCATORS, AND MEMBERS OF THE GENERAL PUBLIC UNDERSTAND TEST RESULTS

A goal of every K–12 assessment program is to provide information that can be used to improve student learning. To achieve this goal, assessment data must be accurately interpreted by the intended users of the data. It is commonly assumed that typical users of assessment results, such as policy-makers, educators, and members of the general pubic, understand the information that is typically included in test results reports. However, a body of research has been compiled in the past decade that indicates this assumption is, unfortunately, untrue. The problem falls squarely in the laps of test publishers and state departments of education and must be addressed before test scores can be used appropriately.

The Importance of Score Reporting

Score reporting is one of the most important features of all large-scale assessments. Score reports act as the primary vehicles for disseminating results on these assessments. They serve as key reference documents in discussions about how students performed on a given assessment, and how student performance can be improved. They are undoubtedly one of the highest profile components of the assessment process, publicly available in a variety of forms and reviewed in detail by many individuals who may never see a copy of the actual assessment from which the reports are based (e.g., newspaper reporters, policymakers, and parents).

Despite the obvious importance of score reports, they are afforded relatively little attention in relation to other aspects of the large-scale testing process. Issues regarding test design, data collection, scoring, and data analysis are subjected to intense scrutiny and debate by all sorts of experts, including those who are or are not part of the testing program. To dissuade criticisms about a test or the data derived from it, the various steps that were taken to resolve complex technical issues are routinely outlined in technical manuals that accompany each assessment. Regrettably, steps to ensure the validity of the interpretations made by the intended users of test results are typically not carried out or documented. Reviews of proposed score reports are often limited to members of technical advisory committees. Although these reviews can be very helpful, they do not provide insight into the problems that users with little experience in interpreting test score reports (e.g., policymakers, parents, and a large number of teachers) may encounter when reading these reports. Recent research on this topic shows that these problems can be great. A national study of adults showed that quantitative literacy was shockingly low in this country with other half the sample, for example, not able to even read a bus schedule (see, Kirsch, Jungeblut, Jenkins, & Kolstad, 1993).

Misunderstandings Users May Have About Test Score Reports

Research by Hambleton and Slater (1997), Impara, Divine, Bruce, Liverman, and Gay (1991), and Wainer, Hambleton, and Meara (1999) provide valuable insight into some of the common misunderstandings users of test results may have when interpreting test score reports.

Hambleton and Slater (1997) found that many policymakers and educators made fundamental mistakes when interpreting results contained within the executive report for the 1992 National Assessment of Educational Progress. Statistical jargon in the report (e.g., statistical significance, variance, standard error) confused and even intimidated some of the adult interviewees (all of whom were educational policymakers). One common mistake was to assume "statistically significant differences" were "big and important differences" (p. 10).

Tables and graphs were more problematic than the text for participants in the Hambleton and Slater (1997) study. Symbols (e.g., < and > to denote statistically significant differences) and technical footnotes were misunderstood or ignored by many users of the reports. Unfamiliar chart formats were very difficult and intimidating for many of the participants, and required too much time to interpret. Footnotes offered little help in explaining the tables and charts; they were often lengthy and contained statistical details that the policy makers and educators did not understand or ignored. Reporting results in terms of cumulative percents (i.e., the percentage of students *at or above* each proficiency category) was also a major source of confusion, a finding that was also reported by Wainer et al. (1999).

Impara et al. (1991) investigated the extent to which teachers were able to interpret results provided on a student-level report from one state, and to what extent interpretive information that accompanied the report helped improve teacher understanding. Although many teachers provided reasonable interpretations of test score data, Impara et al. found that some types of information were frequently misinterpreted (e.g., scale scales, normal curve equivalent scores, and grade-equivalent scores). Impara et al. noted that interpretive information helped facilitate understanding of test scores, but even with this information some problems remained (e.g., even with interpretive material, three-fourths of the teachers did not understand the meaning of overlapping bands in a percentile band performance profile).

Wainer et al. (1999) showed that problems associated with data displays in score reports can be addressed with the application of some simple reporting principles (e.g., reducing the amount of information conveyed in a single display, eliminating judgments about statistical significance, and grouping the data into meaningful rank-ordered clusters). They also showed the value of field testing the reports with intended users to identify potential strengths and weaknesses, as well as the benefits of using empirical methods to evaluate alternate displays. Based on their discovery that the preferences of users did not always lead to the most accurate interpretations, Wainer et al. also made the important recommendation that user preference should not be the sole basis for determining how to report assessment results. This recommendation is not well-known and therefore does not impact significantly on today's test score reporting practices, unfortunately.

Resources for Improving Score Reports

Although score reporting has not been afforded the same level of attention as other aspects of the test development and data analysis process, there is growing recognition of its importance. A body of work is now available that can help inform and enhance current test reporting practices. Test developers are encouraged to become familiar with this literature and the guidelines and principles contained within. Literature on the visual display of quantitative information offers some excellent design principles that can improve the quality of test score reports (the work of Tufte, 1983, and Wainer, 1997, are particularly enlightening). Hambleton (2002) outlined some key research-based guidelines for making test score reporting scales and reports more understandable (e.g., making charts and figures understandable without reference to the text, creating specially designed reports for each intended audience), and discusses several important advances in the area of score reporting (e.g., Mislevy's concept of market basket reporting and the use of item response theory and item mapping procedures to add meaning to reporting scales). A publication by Forte Fast and the Accountability Systems and Reporting State Collaborative on Assessment and Student Standards (2002) will be especially helpful to states and local agencies that are striving to meet the reporting requirements of NCLB. It provides some excellent guidelines and illustrations that will help state and local agencies improve their reporting practices, and communicate accountability, assessment, and other educational indicators in an easily understood manner.

Finally, Goodman and Hambleton (2004) discussed the different ways student-level results are currently being reported, and offer some recommendations for reporting this information in a more effective manner (e.g., providing an easy-to-read narrative summary of the student's results at the beginning of the student score report; including essential information about the assessment in the score report and complementing this information with a more detailed, but easy-to-understand interpretive guide; and personalizing the score reports and interpretive guides to make them less intimidating to parents and students).

CONCLUSION

In this chapter we have carefully considered what we believe to be five common misconceptions of large-scale educational assessments. These misconceptions result from a general lack of understanding about large scale assessments and assessment in general. Criticisms about setting students up for failure with state assessment programs, and about the high costs for assessments and student time, seem to be grossly inflated based upon our review of the available literature. The evidence we could find does not support the criticisms. Criticisms about the preponderance of biased test items, and performance standards that are too high, appear to be overstated as well. In most states, these technical aspects of state assessment programs are being carefully addressed, although admittedly they are technically challenging problems. Finally, we do agree that there is much work to be done concerning the way test results are reported to the public, policymakers, and educators. At least some of the criticisms we hear are due to persons simply misunderstanding the meaning of the test scores and their implications for instructional improvement and school accountability. More research about score reporting, and more field-testing of possible reports, should reduce the problems that have plagued this aspect of large scale assessments.

Many of the criticisms we hear about educational assessments appear to be based on misconceptions. Critics sometimes misrepresent the available information, if they have any at all, and the public hears it and often believes the criticisms to be true. After all, educational assessments are easy to dislike.

Recently, for example, it was reported by a researcher and picked up by the newspapers that the high school drop-out rate had increased by 25% due to the Massachusetts high school graduation requirement. First, the 25% increase was misleading because the researcher's statistics indicated that the actual increase was from 4% to 5%, which would represent an increase of only one more drop out per 100 students in the educational system. The 25% increase was the most sensational way to highlight the 1% change (from 4% to 5%), and is quite misleading. Second, the validity of the increase of even 1% could not be confirmed. Finally, and most importantly, the assumption made by the researcher was that there was a causal link between the increase in the drop-out rate and the presence of the high school graduation test. The link may be there but it remains to be shown. Other factors could explain the increase in the drop-out rate too. More research would be needed to pin-down the explanation. It may even be due to several factors.

Compounding the problem of negative press for testing is just a dislike for taking tests on the part of many persons. Probably most of us don't like taking tests, and so criticisms are easy to accept. Newspapers are not always the most accurate conveyer of test results either, and so they too can confuse and mislead. Then there are just some problems that are hard to understand like the detection of item bias and the setting of performance standards. We are certainly not suggesting here that all criticisms are invalid, and that all educational assessments have merit. What we are suggesting is that many state educational assessments have worthy goals, and that the information from state assessments provides a framework for improving classroom instruction, and for providing some educational accountability. What's really needed now are more serious validity studies of the assessment programs and their consequences. In states such as Maryland, Virginia, Massachusetts and others, educational reform has been underway for many years. It seems time now to put aside the rhetoric, and really find out what is going on with students and our schools, and what the assessments measure and don't measure, and what are their consequences—both positive and negative. The many misconceptions that persist about large scale educational assessments serve only to confuse. Valid information obtained from large scale assessment programs should be the goal now because it can inform the public, policymakers, and educators, and lead to improvements in American education.

REFERENCES

Anderson, B. (1982). *Test use today in elementary schools and secondary schools*. In A. K. Wigdor & W. R. Garner (Eds.), *Ability testing: Uses, consequences, and controversies* (pp. 232–285). Washington, DC: National Academy Press.

Bhola, D. S., Impara, J. C., & Buckendahl, C. W. (2003). Aligning tests with states' content standards: Methods and issues. *Educational Measurement: Issues and Practice, 22*, 21–29.

Cizek, G. (Ed.). (2001). *Setting performance standards: Concepts, methods, and perspectives.* Mahwah, NJ: Lawrence Erlbaum Associates.

Cook, L. L., & Eignor, D. R. (1991). IRT equating methods. *Educational Measurement: Issues and Practice, 10*(3), 37–45.

Education Week. (1997). *Quality counts: A report card on the condition of public education.* Retrieved September, 17, 2003, from http://www.edweek.org/sreports/qc97/indicators/tables/sta-t1.htm

Education Week. (2001). *Quality counts 2001: Testing time.* Retrieved October 19, 2003, from http://www.edweek.org/sreports/qc01/articles/qc01chart.cfm?slug=17test-c2.h20

Education Week. (2003a). *Quality counts: If I can't learn from you.* Retrieved September, 17, 2003, from http://www.edweek.org/sreports/qc03/templates/article.cfm?slug=17sos.h22

Education Week. (2003b). *Quality counts: If I can't learn from you.* Retrieved October, 10, 2003, from http://www.edweek.org/sreports/qc03/reports/ standacct-t1.cfm

Forte Fast, E., & the Accountability Systems and Reporting State Collaborative on Assessment and Student Standards. (2002). *A guide to effective accountability reporting.* Washington, DC: Council of Chief State School Officers.

Goodman, D. P., & Hambleton, R. K. (2004). Student test score reports and interpretive guides: Review of current practices and suggestions for future research. *Applied Measurement in Education, 17*(2), 145–220.

Hambleton, R. K. (2002). How can we make NAEP and state test score reporting scales and reports more understandable? In R. W. Lissitz & W. D. Schafer (Eds.), *Assessment in educational reform* (pp. 192–205). Boston: Allyn & Bacon.

Hambleton, R. K., & Slater, S. (1997). *Are NAEP executive summary reports understandable to policy makers and educators?* (CSE Technical Report 430). Los Angeles, CA: National Center for Research on Evaluation, Standards, and Student Teaching.

Hoxby, C. M. (2002). The cost of accountability. In W. M. Evers & H. J. Walberg (Eds.), *School accountability* (pp. 47–73). Stanford, CA: Hoover Institution Press.

Impara, J. C., Divine, K. P., Bruce, F. A., Liverman, M. R., & Gay, A. (1991). Does interpretive test score information help teachers? *Educational Measurement: Issues and Practice, 10*(4), 16–18.

Kirsch, I., Jungeblut, A., Jenkins, L., & Kolstad, A. (1993). *Adult literacy in America.* Washington, DC: National Center for Education Statistics.

Kolen, M. J. (1988). Traditional equating methodology. *Educational Measurement: Issues and Practice, 7*(4), 29–36.

Kolen, M. J., & Brennan, R. L. (1995). *Test equating: Methods and practices.* New York: Springer-Verlag.

Massachusetts Department of Education. (2003). *Massachusetts Comprehensive Assessment System: 2002 MCAS Technical Report.* Malden, MA: Massachusetts Department of Education.

Massachusetts Insight Education and Research Institute. (2003). *Seizing the day: Massachusetts' at-risk high school students speak out on their experiences at the front lines of education reform.* Boston: Author.

National Commission on Testing and Public Policy. (1990). *From gatekeeper to gateway: Transforming testing in America.* Chestnut Hill, MA: Author.

National Research Council. (1999). *Testing, teaching, and learning: A guide for states and school districts.* Washington, DC: National Academy Press.

New York State Department of Education. (2003). *New York State Testing Program English Language Arts Grade 8 Technical Report 2002.* New York: New York State Department of Education.

No Child Left Behind Act of 2001, Pub. L. No. 107-110, § 1111, 115 Stat. 1449-1452 (2002).

North Carolina Department of Public Instruction. (2003). *North Carolina testing program: The multiple-choice test development process.* Retrieved October, 20, 2003, from http://www.ncpublicschools.org/accountability/testing/policies/mcTestDevelopment/

O'Neil, T., Sireci, S. G., & Huff, K. (in press). Evaluating the consistency of test content across two successive administrations of a state-mandated science assessment. *Educational Assessment.*

Phelps, R. P. (1997). The extent and character of system-wide student testing in the United States. *Educational Assessment, 4*(2), 89–121.

Phelps, R. P. (2000, Winter). Estimating the cost of standardized student testing in the United States. *Journal of Education Finance, 24,* 343–380.

Rebarber, T., & McFarland, T. W. (2002, February). *Estimated cost of the testing requirements in the No Child Left Behind Act.* Paper presented at the Education Leaders Council Test Summit.

Tufte, E. R. (1983). *The visual display of quantitative information.* Cheshire, CT: Graphics Press.

U.S. Congress Office of Technology Assessment. (1992). *Testing in American schools: Asking the right questions* (OTA-SET-519). Washington DC: U.S. Government Printing Office.

U.S. General Accounting Office. (1993). *Student testing: Current extent and expenditures, with cost estimates for a national examination* (GAO/PEMD-93-8). Washington, DC: Author.

U.S. General Accounting Office. (2003). *Characteristics of tests will influence expenses; Information sharing may help states realize efficiencies* (GAO-03-389). Washington, DC. Author.

Wainer, H. (1997). *Visual revelations: Graphical tales of fate and deception from Napoleon Bonaparte to Ross Perot.* New York: Copernicus Books.

Wainer, H., Hambleton, R. K., & Meara, K. (1999). Alternative displays for communicating NAEP results: A redesign and validity study. *Journal of Educational Measurement, 36*(4), 301–335.

Webb, N. L. (1999). *Alignment of science and mathematics standards and assessments in four states* (Research Monograph No. 18). Madison, WI: National Institute for Science Education.

5

The Most Frequently *Unasked* Questions About Testing

Stephen G. Sireci
University of Massachusetts Amherst

Many people ask questions about tests, but they frequently ask the wrong ones. Many people criticize tests, but their criticisms often display their lack of knowledge about the strengths and limitations of tests. Currently, tests are a critical part of educational reform movements throughout the world. However, the testing enterprise is complex and involves scientific and psychological concepts that are not readily accessible to lay audiences. This complexity, in part, may foster a mistrust of educational testing. Most people do not like to take tests, and for many people, test results consistently provide bad news. For these reasons, educational tests are popular targets of criticism.

I am a psychometrician, which means I help build and evaluate tests. My specialty area is educational testing, which includes tests that children take in school, college admissions tests, and tests adults take to get licensed to work in a profession. Many people may find it hard to believe that I justify my work by saying it contributes to the educational process. I believe tests, if properly developed, scored, and interpreted, can improve instruction and help people to achieve their goals. However, I realize that many people do not see things as I do.

One day, as I was driving home from work feeling good about my psychometric self, I saw a bumper sticker with the acronym MCAS stricken out and the caption "These tests hurt kids!" To give you some background,

111

MCAS stands for the Massachusetts Comprehensive Assessment System, which is a set of tests administered to public school students in Massachusetts. I teach at the University of Massachusetts and assist the state in MCAS research from time to time. As I stared at the bumper sticker I had the terrible thought that these people were out to get me. Why do they think these tests hurt kids, and why would they go to the trouble of printing bumper stickers to voice their outrage? Soon after, *I* became outraged when I learned that the union to which I belong, and to which I pay $600 annual dues, spent $600,000 on anti-MCAS commercials.

From these experiences, I decided to try and find out what the criticisms were all about. I began to ask people with these bumper stickers (and t-shirts!) why they thought these tests hurt kids. Some reasons seemed well founded (e.g., administering these tests takes up valuable instructional time) and some did not (e.g., these tests are just used to make minority students look bad). I also followed debates in the popular press and the news. Soon, one thing became very clear. There were fundamental problems with many of the criticisms because the general public has very little knowledge about the qualities of a good test. It appears that many of the criticisms of tests are based on half-truths, at best. I admit there are good tests and there are bad tests. I also know that sometimes, good tests are put to bad uses. However, distinguishing between appropriate and inappropriate test uses is not easy. To do it properly, one must ask the right questions. Unfortunately, the right questions are frequently unasked.

In this chapter, I focus on questions about tests that are rarely asked, but if answered, provide a strong foundation for understanding test quality. By answering these unasked questions, we empower the general public to properly scrutinize the tests that end up on their children's desks. The purpose of this chapter is to discuss important questions that should be raised when critiquing any test that has important consequences for the individuals who take it or for those who use test scores to make "high-stakes" decisions. It is only after consideration of these issues that we can form intelligent opinions about the quality and appropriateness of tests.

THE SIX MOST FREQUENTLY UNASKED QUESTIONS

There are at least six questions that are critically important for understanding test quality that are rarely asked. These questions are:

1. What is a *standardized* test?
2. What is the difference between a norm-referenced test and a criterion-referenced test?
3. What is *reliability*?
4. What is *validity*?

5. How are passing scores set on a test?
6. How can I get more information about a test?

These questions may seem basic to some and technical to others. In either case, answers to these questions must be well understood to properly critique a particular test for a particular purpose. Therefore, let us ask and answer these questions in turn.

What is a Standardized Test?

The term *standardized test* has quite possibly made more eyes glaze over than any other. Standardized tests have a bad reputation, but it is an undeserved one. People accuse standardized tests of being unfair, biased, and discriminatory. Believe it or not, standardized tests are actually designed to promote test fairness. *Standardized* simply means that the test content is equivalent across administrations and that the conditions under which the test is administered are the same for all test takers. Thus, standardized tests are designed to provide a level playing field. That is, all test takers are given the same test under the same conditions. I am not going to defend all standardized tests, for surely there are problems with some of them. The point here is that just because a test is standardized does not mean that it is "bad," or "biased," or that it measures only "unimportant things." It merely means it is designed and administered using uniform procedures. Standardized tests are used to provide objective information. For example, employment tests are used to avoid unethical hiring practices (e.g., nepotism, ethnic discrimination, etc.).

If an assessment system uses tests that are not standardized, the system is likely to be unfair to many candidates. Those of you who had the pleasure of viewing the old film *Monty Python and the Holy Grail* saw an excellent example of a nonstandardized assessment. In this film, a guardian protected a bridge by requiring that three questions be answered before a traveler was permitted to cross. Answering any question incorrectly resulted in being catapulted into the abyss. Thus, this was a high-stakes test. The three questions asked of the first traveler were: What is your quest?, What do you seek?, and What is your favorite color? The second traveler was asked the same first two questions, but was then asked for the air speed velocity of a swallow. Clearly, the two assessments were not of equal content or difficulty. The second traveler who plummeted into the abyss had a legitimate claim of test bias.

On the other hand standardized tests are designed to be as similar as possible for all test takers. The logic behind standardization stems from the scientific method. Standardize all conditions and any variation across measurements is due to differences in the characteristic being measured, which in educational testing is some type of knowledge, skill, or other proficiency. To claim that a test is standardized means that it is developed according to carefully designed test specifications, it is administered under uniform conditions for everyone, the scoring of the test is the same for everyone, and different forms of the test are statistically and qualitatively equivalent. Thus, in testing, standardization is tantamount with fairness.

Before leaving our discussion of standardized tests, there are two common misconceptions about standardized tests that need to be dismissed. The first misconception is that standardized tests contain only multiple-choice items. Obviously, uniform content, test administration, and scoring conditions pertain to all item types, not just multiple-choice items. The second misconception is that standardized tests measure only lower level thinking skills. That is simply not true, and if you do not agree, sign up to take the Graduate Records Exam or the Law School Admissions Test.

At this juncture, it should be clear to what the term *standardized test* refers and to what it does not refer. Thus, we will now ask and answer the second most frequently unasked question.

What is the Difference Between Norm-Referenced and Criterion-Referenced Tests?

The terms *norm-referenced* and *criterion-referenced* are technical and represent one reason why people accuse psychometricians of speaking in an incomprehensible language. These terms refer to very different ways in which meaning is attached to test scores. That is, they refer to different ways in which the tests are *referenced* to something.

In norm-referenced testing, a person's test score is compared to (referenced to) the performance of other people who took the same test. These other people are the "norm group," which typically refers to a carefully selected sample of students who previously took the test.

There are several types of norm groups, the most common being national, local, and state. *National norms* refer to a nationally representative sample of test takers. This sample of students is carefully selected to represent key demographic characteristics of our nation. Local norms usually refer to the entire population of students within a school district. For example, local norms on an eighth-grade test would be used to compare one eighth-grade student's score with all other eighth-grade students in the district who took the same test. State norms are used in the same manner, with students' scores being referenced to all other students across the state who took the same test.

Many scores reported on norm-referenced tests focus on percentiles, which reflect the percentage of students who scored at or below a specific score. For example, if Fiona achieved a national percentile rank of 94, she performed as good as or better than 94% of the national norm group to whom the test was initially administered. Another way of describing her test performance is that she scored in the top 6% of the national norm group. If her local percentile rank were 87, then she scored as good as or better than 87% of the students in her district who took the same test (in the same grade level, of course). Other scores associated with norm-referenced tests include grade equivalent scores, which represent the average score of students in a particular grade at a particular point in time. For example a grade equivalent score of 3.0 represents the average score of third grade-students at the beginning of the school year who served as the norm group.

The utility of norm-referenced test information lies in ascertaining how well a particular student, classroom, school, or state compares to others. For example, if I want to know how well my son performed on a reading comprehension test, his national percentile rank score will tell me the percentage of the national norm group that he performed as good as or better than. When evaluating the utility of norm-referenced test information, the recentness of the norms, and the degree to which they are representative of the group they claim to represent (e.g., all fourth graders in the nation) are important factors. If my son's national percentile rank score of 84 were based on norms from 1994, I may be less impressed than if the norms were more recent.

A serious limitation of norm-referenced scores is that in many cases it is less important to know how well a student did relative to others, than it is to know what a student has or has not learned. For this reason, criterion-referenced tests are much more popular today. Rather than reference a student's test score to the performance of other students, criterion-referenced tests compare students' test performance with carefully defined standards of expected performance. Examples of criterion-referenced scores are classifications such as *pass, fail, needs improvement, basic, proficient,* and *advanced.* The information derived from criterion-referenced tests allows one to gauge whether a student mastered specific course material. The standards of *mastery* specified in criterion-referenced testing are typically decided upon by groups of subject matter experts (e.g., experienced and well respected teachers and administrators).

To summarize our discussion of norm- and criterion-referenced tests, it should be clear that norm-referenced tests describe a student's test performance in relation to the performance of one or more specific reference groups of students who took the same test. The group to which a student's performance is compared is called the *norm group.* The statement that Carlos scored at the sixtieth percentile on the ITBS math subtest means that Carlos equaled or outperformed 60% of students in the norm group.

Criterion-referenced tests, on the other hand, describe what a student can and cannot do with respect to a well-defined domain of knowledge or skill. Thus, students' scores are interpreted in terms of *mastery* of the components of this well-defined domain. The statement that Carlos demonstrated mastery of solving algebraic equations, suggests that he attained the knowledge and skill intended in this portion of the school curriculum. In norm-referenced testing, it is critical that the norm group is appropriate for the students tested. In criterion-referenced testing, it is critical that the criterion domain is clearly defined.

What is Reliability? What is Validity?

Reliability and validity are two important concepts that apply to all types of tests. Many people often ask if a test is reliable or if a test is valid, but few people ever ask "what do these concepts mean?" In fact, when people ask me if a test is "reliableandvalid," they often say it as a single word, which leaves me wondering if they realize they are two very different concepts.

Reliability refers to the degree to which test scores are consistent. For example, if you took a test on a Monday and received a score of 80, and then took the same test on Tuesday and received a score of 50, the scores produced by this test are certainly not reliable. Your bathroom scale is reliable. If you weigh yourself, step off the scale, and then weigh yourself a second time, you should get the same reading each time. Such physical measurements are often very reliable. Psychological measurements, such as measuring a teacher candidate's readiness for teaching, are a little trickier. A person's test score could be influenced by the particular sample of questions chosen for the test, how motivated or fatigued the person is on the testing day, distracting test administration conditions, or the previously ingested extra large pastrami sandwich that suddenly causes trouble during the middle of the test. A great deal of statistical theory has been developed to provide indices of the reliability of test scores. These indices typically range from zero to one, with reliabilities of .90 or higher signifying test scores that are likely to be consistent from one test administration to the next. For tests that are used to make pass/fail decisions, the reliability of the passing score is of particular importance.

The reliability of a test score is an important index of test quality. A fundamental aspect of test quality is that the scores derived from the test are reliable. Readers interested in the technical details regarding test score reliability should consult any standard measurement textbook such as Anastasi (1988) or Linn and Gronlund (2000).

Validity is different from reliability. This concept refers to the soundness and appropriateness of the conclusions that are made on the basis of test scores. Examples of questions pertaining to test score validity include "Is this test fair?," "Is this test measuring what it is supposed to measure?," and "Is this test useful for its intended purpose?" Validity refers to all aspects of test fairness. It is a comprehensive concept that asks whether the test measures what it intends to measure and whether the test scores are being used appropriately.

The validity of test scores must always be evaluated with respect to the purpose of testing. For example, the Scholastic Achievement Test (SAT) is designed to help college admissions officers make decisions about who should be admitted to their schools. The validity of SAT scores for this purpose has been supported by studies showing the ability of SAT scores to predict future college grades. However, some people question the utility of using the SAT for a different purpose: to determine whether a student athlete should be eligible to play sports in college. Using test scores for purposes other than what they were originally intended for requires additional validity evidence.

Another way of thinking about validity is the degree to which a test measures what it claims to measure. For educational tests, this aspect of test quality is often described as *content validity*. Content validity refers to the degree to which a test represents the content domains it is designed to measure. When a test is judged to have high content validity, the content of the test is considered to be congruent with the testing purpose and with prevailing notions of the subject matter tested. Given that educational tests are designed to measure specific curricula, the degree to which the tests match curricular objectives is critical. Thus, in educational assessment content validity is a fundamental characteristic of test quality (see Sireci, 1998a, 1998b for further discussion of content validity; for more comprehensive treatment of validity issues in testing see Kane, 1992, Messick, 1989, or Shepard, 1993).

To distinguish between reliability and validity, I often tell the following story. Although many people have trouble losing weight, I can lose 5 pounds in only 3 hours. Furthermore, I can eat whatever I want in this time period. My secret is simple. I weigh myself on my bathroom scale, and then I drive 3 hours to my mother-in-law's house. Upon arrival, I weigh myself on her bathroom scale and, poof!, I'm 5 pounds lighter. I have accomplished this weight loss many times and weighed myself on both scales repeatedly. In all cases, I have found both scales to be highly reliable. Although I hate to admit it, one of these scales is reliable, but probably not valid. It is biased. It systematically underestimates or overestimates my true weight.

Before concluding our discussion of reliability and validity, a few further clarifying words about these concepts are in order. First, reliability and validity do not refer to inherent properties of a test, but rather to properties of test scores, or even more precisely, to the decisions that are made on the basis of test scores. Second, as mentioned earlier, the validity of decisions made on the basis test scores must be evaluated with respect to the purpose of the test. Third, to claim that scores from a test are valid for a particular purpose requires multiple types of evidence—some statistical and some qualitative. Finally, evaluating validity and reliability is an ongoing endeavor. There is not any one study that could validate the use of a test for a particular purpose from now until infinity. Therefore, test validation is comprehensive and continuous.

How Are Passing Scores Set on a Test?

Test takers are ecstatic when they pass a test and upset when they fail. However, unless passing rates for a test are very surprising, the question of *how* the passing score was determined is rarely asked. Setting a passing score on a test is perhaps the most difficult problem in the entire testing enterprise. No matter which method is used, some test takers who are competent will fail, and some who are not yet competent will pass. The goal in setting a passing score is to minimize these two types of errors.

Before describing defensible ways in which passing scores are set on a test, a few words about how passing scores should not be set are in order. For example, it may be tempting to decide upon a passing score that would pass or fail a specific percentage of test takers. Using this logic a score that fails the bottom 30% of test takers could be used to screen out the "worst" candidates for licensure in a profession. However, if all test takers were competent, this procedure would fail 30% of those who are competent. On the other hand, if all test takers were not competent, 70% of those who are incompetent would pass! This type of *norm-referenced* passing score is not defensible for high school graduation, licensure, or certification tests because scores are interpreted with respect to being better or worse than others, rather than with respect to the level of competence of a specific test taker.

Passing scores should also not be set based on arbitrary notions of how many items a student should answer correctly. For example, on the PBS program *The News Hour With Jim Lehrer*, John Silber, former Chair of the Massachusetts Board of Education, exclaimed that the passing scores set on the Massachusetts Teacher Tests corresponded to correctly answering 70% to 75% of the questions. He described this passing standard as a C average. It is hard to know whether the 70%-to-75% standard really corresponds to what most people would consider to be a C. If the test comprised very difficult questions, 70% correct could represent a level of excellence well above a C level. As an example, an unethical person could develop a test comprising only extremely difficult questions to prove the point that teachers were performing poorly. On the other hand, another unethical person could intentionally create a test comprising very easy items to make it appear that teachers are performing extremely well. In this case, 70% correct may represent a very low standard such as what most people would consider to be a D or F. Thus, establishing passing scores based on arbitrary notions of percent correct is indefensible, and is rarely used in practice. The mistake of equating percentage of items answered correctly with school grades should not be made.

In elementary and high school, our teachers decided what constituted a *F* or an *A* and so forth. When the stakes are high, such as in the case of teacher licensure, the judgments of a single person cannot be used to establish a passing score or any other type of test-based standard. The most defensible procedures currently used to set passing scores on tests are done by committee. Experts from a variety of perspectives are brought together to scrutinize all test questions and make judgments regarding the likely performance of competent test takers on each question. These judgments are discussed thoroughly and often statistics summarizing test takers' performance on the items are used to inform the process. The passing scores that are set using this process are often considered to be preliminary. They are sometimes adjusted using statistical analyses that attempt to validate the standard and on the basis of anticipated social and political consequences. A thorough discussion of methods for setting passing scores is beyond the scope of this chapter. However, regardless of the method used, it is critical that the entire process is carefully documented so that the public can judge the appropriateness of the methodology. In fact, clear documentation of the procedures used for setting passing scores is a fundamental requirement stipulated in professional standards for educational and psychological testing.

How Can I Get More Information About a Test?

It is unfortunate that this last question made the list of frequently unasked questions because it is perhaps the most important question a test user or test taker can ask. Tests can be confusing. Sometimes the directions are confusing, sometimes the scores are confusing, and sometimes the content is confusing. Sometimes, the whole process is confusing! Professional standards for testing require test developers to provide documentation to interested parties regarding what the test measures, how the test was developed, how to complete the test, and how to interpret test scores (American Educational Research Association (AERA), American Psychological Association, & National Council on Measurement in Education, 1999). Furthermore, these standards require test developers to provide evidence of the reliability and validity of test scores with respect to the testing purpose. Good test developers are proactive and provide a great deal of technical and non-technical information about their tests. This information can be invaluable to those who want to evaluate the merits of a particular test for a particular purpose. To acquire information about a particular test, start by contacting the test publisher. If you do not know who published the test, ask the person or organization who administered the test.

There are also several reference books available that provide critiques of popular tests, so, ask your local librarian. Examples of such books include the *Mental Measurements Yearbook, Tests in Print,* and *Test Critiques.* The first two books are published by the Buros Center for Testing (www.unl.edu/buros). The third book is published by Test Corporation of America.

A very important source of information for evaluating tests is the *Standards for Educational and Psychological Testing* (AERA et al., 1999). The original version of these standards dates back more than 50 years. The *Standards* stipulate standards of quality in test development, use, interpretation, and evaluation. Given that there is no "policing" organization for the testing industry, these standards have become the authoritative source for gauging how to ensure quality test development and how to evaluate whether a particular test is suited for a particular purpose. They are also useful for determining if specific testing practices are defensible. Anyone interested in challenging the use of a test for a particular purpose will want to be familiar with these standards, as will anyone involved in testing who strives to ensure quality and fairness.

CONCLUSION

This chapter may not have provided complete and satisfactory answers to all the important questions that could be raised about tests, but at least now you know more about the right questions to ask. The next time you receive a score from a test you took, knowing the answers to one or more of these questions may help you better understand the meaning of your performance. Good tests help people make important decisions. Good tests also tend to be accompanied by adequate documentation that provides answers to the important, but often unasked, questions raised above. Understanding fundamental concepts in educational assessment helps us realize the strengths and limitations of such assessments. Educational measurement is an inexact science, but one that is improving steadily. By engaging more people into the test development and test monitoring processes, we can accelerate the process of making our tests more valid and more useful.

REFERENCES

American Educational Research Association, American Psychological Association, & National Council on Measurement in Education. (1999). *Standards for educational and psychological testing.* Washington, DC: American Educational Research Association.

Anastasi, A. (1988). *Psychological testing* (6th ed.). New York: Macmillan.

Kane, M. T. (1992). An argument based approach to validity. *Psychological Bulletin, 112,* 527–535.

Linn, R. L., & Gronlund, N. E. (2000). *Measurement and assessment in teaching* (8th ed.). Upper Saddle River, NJ: Prentice-Hall.

Messick, S. (1989). Validity. In R. Linn (Ed.), *Educational measurement* (3rd ed., pp. 13–100). Washington, DC: American Council on Education.

Shepard, L. A. (1993). Evaluating test validity. *Review of Research in Education, 19,* 405–450.

Sireci, S. G. (1998a). Gathering and analyzing content validity data. *Educational Assessment, 5,* 299–321.

Sireci, S. G. (1998b). The construct of content validity. *Social Indicators Research, 45,* 83–117.

6

Must High Stakes Mean Low Quality? Some Testing Program Implementation Issues

George K. Cunningham
University of Louisville

The beliefs of the public, legislatures, and governors, as well as the rationale behind the No Child Left Behind ACT (NCLB) suggest that the most important purpose of education is increasing student academic achievement. According to this philosophy, the purpose of education is to increase student reading comprehension, skill at performing mathematical computations, knowledge of history, and understanding of science. Academic achievement can be operationally defined as performance on academic achievement tests.

Many education professors, state departments of education staff, and public school administrators, however, may prefer to de-emphasize the importance of academic achievement and its assessment, and focus on other student outcomes, such as the social skills and dispositions of students. The subordination of academic achievement and its assessment has its roots in progressive education and is consistent with a belief that students differ in their capacity to perform academically. Originally, progressive educators attributed these differences to innate characteristics, but now they are more likely to blame them on inherent flaws in our society. Some present-day progressive educators regard standardized tests, which call attention to these differences, as unfair to students from disadvantaged backgrounds.

An examination of the standards promulgated by teacher education organizations such as the National Commission on Teaching and America's Future (NCTAF), the National Council for the Accreditation of Teacher Education (NCATE), the Interstate New Teacher Assessment and Support Consortium (INTASC) gives little indication of a commitment to academic achievement as their highest priority. Instead, they focus on having students learn to get along with others, be sensitive to other cultures, display "high-level thinking" and demonstrate a commitment to the promotion of social justice. *Systematic* instruction in reading, the learning of mathematical algorithms such as the computations associated with long division and the manipulation of fractions may be discouraged, as is the acquisition of the facts associated with science, history, economics, and geography.

Given the large numbers and political leverage of supporters of academic achievement, it would seem that they would have an advantage in this debate, but this is not the case. Those who train teachers, state department of education staff, and local educational leaders are closer to the classroom, exercise enormous influence over what actually happens in schools, and they have political power, too.

Concern about the reluctance of educators to emphasize academic achievement has led to the widespread adoption of standards-based educations reform (SBER), as a way for governors and legislatures to force an achievement emphasis on schools. This means they have defined a set of content standards, adopted an assessment system, set performance standards (cut scores), and implemented an accountability system in which schools, districts, and/or students receive rewards and sanctions depending on their academic achievement. The ultimate in accountability occurs when students are required to pass an exam in order to graduate.

Those state educational leaders who oppose a primary emphasis on academic achievement have responded by broadening and/or changing the purposes of SBER to encompass goals other than the improvement of academic achievement. The problem with this Swiss army knife approach to assessment is that when SBER programs serve conflicting purposes, they are likely to fail at all of them.

Indeed, in some states, the response to SBER has been a demand for opportunity-to-learn standards. This is nice sounding phrase often used to undermine SBER. According to this view, schools should not be held accountable until they receive all of the resources necessary to ensure success. Given the budgetary situation in most states and school districts and the insatiable demand for ever more resources, it is doubtful that any school would ever reach the point where there is consensus that opportunity to learn needs have been satisfied.

The ostensible purpose for SBER is to improve academic performance, but just as taking someone's temperature does not cure a fever, assessing academic achievement does not necessarily improve academic performance. The most important effect of standards is their influence on instruction. If schools respond to poor academic performance by adopting effective instructional methods, SBER can improve academic achievement. But, where instructional leaders do not believe that academic achievement is the most important purpose for schools, they may be less likely to adopt effective strategies for improving academic achievement. This is not an SBER problem; it is an instructional leadership problem.

TYPES OF STANDARDS

Discussions about SBER typically include four types of assessment: standards-referenced, criterion-referenced, norm-referenced, and absolute standards.

Standards-Referenced Assessment

The term, *standards-referenced assessment* refers to tests based on content standards. Because, by definition, all SBER programs utilize standards, labeling their assessments *standards referenced* is a tautology.

Criterion-Referenced Assessment

At one time, the term *criterion-referenced assessment* referred to a specific form of testing—tests that provide information about what each student knows and what each student does not know in terms of mastery of individual instructional objectives—that is, tests used in mastery learning. Mastery learning is a method of instruction in which everything a student is supposed to know is defined precisely using behavioral objectives. Mastery learning instruction is carefully sequenced and students do not move to the next objective until they had mastered previous objectives. Military and medical instruction programs successfully implemented mastery learning, but it never caught on in public schools. Furthermore, much of the content that schools target is not easily described using behavioral objectives. But, although mastery learning techniques in the schools have shrunk in popularity, the use of the term *criterion referenced* to describe tests stuck.

The popularity of the term *criterion referenced* stems from its designation as the opposite of *norm-referenced assessment*, with which it is often contrasted. The term *norm-referenced assessment* seems to carry bad connotations. For some, it suggests relative standards that allow half of students to be designated above average no matter how poor their performance. For others, it is associated with the unpleasant task of categorizing students as winners and losers and guarantees that, no matter how well students perform collectively, someone always has to be on the bottom. As a result, state departments of education, anxious to sell their tests to the public, tend to avoid the term *norm-referenced*. The public seems to like the sound of the term *criterion referenced*, despite uncertainty about its meaning. State departments of education and publishers have been quick to describe their tests as criterion referenced and ignore the fact that the so-named tests have none of the traits formerly associated with criterion-referenced testing.

The final authority on such definitions, the *Standards for Educational and Psychological Testing* (1999; often shortened to *Joint Standards*), define a criterion-referenced test as: "A test that allows its users to make score interpretations in relation to a functional performance level, as distinguished from those interpretations that are made in relation to the performance of others. Examples of criterion-reference interpretations include comparisons to cut scores" (p. 174).

The shift in the definition of *criterion referenced* has allowed state departments of education to describe almost any of their tests as criterion-referenced. In the *Joint Standards* definition, the critical attribute of a criterion-referenced test is the use of a cut-score. Since standards-based education reform (SBER) requires the use of cut-scores and state departments of education are anxious to distance themselves from norm-referenced tests, they prefer to describe their tests as criterion referenced. Ironically, the states using this term often employ the same norm-referenced principles they seem to be rejecting. Furthermore, it is easy to attach a cut-score to a norm-referenced test, which is another common practice. Doing this further obfuscates the distinction between norm- and criterion-referenced tests.

Norm-Referenced Assessment

Historically, measurement specialists had focused on differentiating between norm- and criterion-referenced tests. With the changes in the definition of criterion-referenced testing, this distinction is no longer important. The distinction between tests based on norm-referenced principles and those based on *absolute standards* is far more important because quite different assumptions underlie the two types of assessments. Nevertheless, most statewide tests end up combining the characteristics of both.

A norm-referenced assessment interprets a student's performance by comparing it to typical student performance. Means, standard deviations, and percentile ranks are all norm-referenced measures. Anytime student performance is defined in terms of the average, norm-referenced performance standards are being used. A standard requiring that all students perform "at grade level" in reading is norm-referenced as are the cut-points states set on the various PRAXIS exams. The PRAXIS exam is a test published by the Educational Testing Service, which teachers in most states must pass in order to be certified.

Absolute Standards

Absolute standards interpret student performance by comparing it to predetermined levels of achievement. Comparisons with other students are avoided. Consider the use of absolute standards in a keyboarding class. Suppose the instructor defines adequate keyboarding as a typing rate of 50 words per minute. A student has met the performance standards for the class if he or she types that fast, and has failed if they type slower. It would make no difference whether almost all students met the standard or almost all students did not. There is no expectation, assumption, or need for student performance to be normally distributed.

RECOMMENDATIONS FOR IMPROVING
THE IMPLEMENTATION OF SBER

Although 49 states have adopted SBER as a primary educational reform technique, they have not all chosen the same path. Each state assessment is unique and although the U.S. Department of Education (DOE), through the No Child Left Behind (NCLB) Act, must approve each state's design, it has accepted considerable variation among the states.

One probable cause of the wide variation in state designs is the difference in goals between the legislatures and governors who pass and sign the SBER legislation and the administrators and staff at state departments of education who actually implement it. As described earlier, those in charge of the actual design of the assessments may feel a greater commitment to goals other than increasing academic achievement. This can lead to modifications that render the assessments less effective in increasing academic achievement. For a variety of reasons, they must rely on outside consultants or the test publishers for much of the test design work. There are many psychometric consultants available and they vary greatly in their methodological and philosophical orientation. In providing advice about the structure of assessments, they can find themselves facing conflicts of interest. Their advice can strongly affect the cost and character of an assessment, and their profit margin.

The purpose of the following sections is to provide recommendations about the best practices in those statewide assessments whose primary intended purpose is to increase academic achievement.

Developing Content Standards

Content standards tell us what students are supposed to learn. They usually consist of lists of competencies, objectives, or goals. It is not difficult to compile such lists, but it can be almost impossible to reach consensus about what should be included. The differences of opinion can be as basic as taste, as abstract as ideology, or may involve fundamental philosophical differences about why certain subjects are taught in schools. Those who formulate content standards often find themselves entangled in endless debates about what should be included. What can emerge is a document born in compromise that completely satisfies few and angers many.

The following suggestions are intended to provide recommendations, that, if followed, can lead to the creation of better content standards.

1. Objectives must be written at a reasonable level of specificity. In many states, content standards are written in general, vague terms making it difficult for educators to be sure exactly what they are supposed to teach and for parents to know exactly what their children are supposed to be learning. When the authors of standards go to the opposite extreme and begin specifying in detail exactly what students should know at each grade level they can find themselves trapped. Suddenly, they are expected to write down everything that students are supposed to know and the standards can become impossibly long and detailed. Teachers can justify excluding from instruction anything not precisely specified in such complete standards.

During the 1960s and early 1970s, mastery learning became a popular education innovation. One of the key provisions of this instructional technique is the definition of content using behavioral objectives. Behavioral objectives define what students are supposed to learn in such a way that there is no ambiguity about whether or not the objective has been mastered. This is accomplished by requiring students to display a concrete behavior as an indicator of mastery. Instructional objectives used to define content standards do not need to be written at a behavioral objective level of specificity. This would only be required if scores were reported on an objective-by-objective basis, and few large-scale assessments are so designed.

2. Subject-area specialists must not try to out-do each other in their topical coverage. The usual method of creating content standards is to put content matter specialists in charge. For example, the committee responsible for writing the math content standards might include a specialist in math from the department of education, math teachers from the public schools, school of education faculty, and math professors. All of these specialists have one thing in common. They all believe that math is important and that every educated person needs to have a deep under-standing of the topic. To them, this may be important enough to warrant devoting a larger proportion of the school day to math than is devoted to any other subject. Of course, the members of the language arts committee are likely to feel the same about their subject, as may the science and social studies committees. What this means in practice is that the content standards in each area are written in isolation, with each committee ensuring comprehensive coverage of their own field. This process for writing content standards tends to ignore the limits im-posed by the length of the school day. There is just not enough time to include everything that these different specialists believe is important. Apportioning the time required for different subjects is a zero sum game and more time devoted to one discipline means less time avail-able for others.

A level of decision making above the committees setting standards for each discipline is needed to allocate resources and time to each discipline rationally. The length of the day and the number of days in a year that students will attend school must be considered and the painful task of setting priorities must take place. Because the ensuing battles over turf and proportion of the school day can be difficult, some states skip this stage and accept what each separate committee proposes. This is a mis-take, because content standards constructed in this way will be unrealis-tically lengthy and unlikely to be fully implemented.

3. *An effort should be made to obtain agreement among stakeholders about content standards.* Within communities, schools, and educational insti-tutions, there are strong differences of opinion regarding what should be taught in schools. Historically, local control has been honored, which has permitted a wide diversity of content to be taught and al-lowed decisions about course content to be made at the classroom level. The adoption of content standards shifts decisions about what is taught in schools to the state level. In some disciplines, the controversy is mini-mal, whereas in others there are major differences of opinion. Even those subjects about which there seemed to be consensus in the past have become increasingly contentious. At one time, it was possible to define a continuum of skills and algorithms in math that enjoyed wide-spread acceptance. This consensus disappeared with the controversies engendered by the *Principles and Standards for School Mathematics* first published in 1989 by the National Council of Teachers of Mathematics (NCTM) and more recently revised in 2000. Generally, though, it is eas-ier for educational planners to reach agreement about math and science standards than those for history and literature. It also is easier to reach agreement about what students in the lower grades should be taught than it is for secondary schools.

There is no simple solution to the problems posed by these fundamental differences in what various stakeholders believe are important. The best strategy is to constitute the committees charged with writing content standards in ways that allow a fair representation of the stakeholder groups.

4. Establish a process to determine if the assessment measures the content standards. Once the standards are written and implemented. It is easy for tests to drift in the direction of easily measured content and away from comprehensive assessment of the learning objectives specified in the content standards. Most commercial standardized achievement tests include tables in their appendices, which document the number of items assessing each objective. This is a good practice for states to adopt as well.

5. Write content standards in ways that facilitate the use of item sampling methods. In the process of associating items with instructional objectives from the content standards, test authors often strive to ensure that there is at least one item from each objective. This is not necessary, unless results are to be reported at the instructional objectives level. In order to report results at that level, it would be necessary to include at least ten items for each instructional objective. Because students are typically tested over hundreds of instructional objectives, the resulting test would be impossibly long. A better practice is to select items according to item sampling principles. With this method, items are selected randomly, or as close to randomly as practical, from the domain of all possible items. Not every form of a test needs to include items from each objective. Over time, as more forms of the test are produced, all of the objectives will be assessed. As long as teachers and students do not know the objectives from which items will be selected for a particular form of a test, they will be encouraged to become familiar with the breadth of content covered by the objectives.

Developing Performance Standards

Content standards tell us what students are supposed to know whereas performance standards tell us *how well* students have learned the content standards. There are many difficult decisions to be made in the process of establishing content standards, but once a strategy for describing content has been established, the task itself, though time consuming, is not difficult. It is possible to point out some of the more egregious errors that states make in the standard setting process and to steer the reader away from them and towards practices that seem to work better.

1. Performance standards must balance absolute and norm-referenced criteria. Absolute standards form the philosophical basis for state SBER programs and the tests states use to fulfill the requirements of the federally mandated No Child Left Behind Act (NCLB). NCLB is important because it requires students in Grades 3 to 8 in every state, be tested in both reading and math and it places severe penalties on schools that do not make adequate progress towards having all students proficient in these two areas by 2014.

Philosophically, state tests are based on absolute standards, but in practice they usually have more attributes of a norm-referenced than an absolute standard assessment. State policy makers take this mixed approach because setting cut-points that are independent from typical student performance is exceedingly difficult. For example, it is almost impossible to designate how much science a fifth grade student needs to know without knowing how much the average fifth grader knows. The NCLB Act is designed to promote absolute standards, but leaves it to the individual states to define *proficient*. To prevent states from rigging their system in such a way that all schools are proficient from the start, states must set the cut-points for their tests so that initially, at least 20% of students are below proficient. This is a purely norm-referenced requirement.

When test authors use norm-referenced principles to create tests, they assume that student performance spreads out along a continuum with most students in the middle. The result is the classic normal distribution. If a normal distribution does not emerge during pilot testing, the p-value of items are adjusted to achieve that distribution. A p-value is measure of item difficulty and is simply the percentage of students who got the item correct. The goal is to have items of average difficulty as indicated by midrange p-values. Items that most students get right or get wrong are eliminated because these items do not contribute to variability.

Norm-referenced test developers also want relatively high item-total score correlations. The selection of items with appropriate p-values helps achieve this goal. High item-total correlations are desirable because they lead directly to high coefficient alpha reliability, which is the primary criterion test developers use to evaluate their tests. Test score variability and a normal distribution, key ingredients for acceptable coefficient alpha reliability, are less robust when derived from tests developed using absolute standards. With absolute standards, the goal is to have all students score at the top end of the distribution, which results in a skewed distribution.

The most sophisticated test-development procedures depend heavily on the application of item response theory (IRT). This esoteric set of methodologies is especially useful for large-scale tests because it provides the most efficient way to equate tests from year to year and form to form. IRT can only be used with tests created using norm-referenced principles.

Norm-referenced performance standards require the specification of a cut-score that divides those students who are proficient from those who are not, based on percentages, before the test is administered. The designation of this cut-score depends solely on performance relative to other students. For example, a state could specify a percentile such as the fortieth, as proficient. This would mean that 40% of students would always be below proficient no matter how much performance increased or how much it declined. This is not an appropriate way to set cut-scores if student performance is expected to increase. A system that defines a student's performance based on their rank will never show academic improvement. In such a system, a student can improve relative to other students, but student scores will never reflect an overall increase in student performance. SBER systems are designed to document progress in the percentage of students that have reached the standards of proficiency, which implies a measurement of an absolute level of performance.

Absolute standards are difficult to implement because the definition of proficient performance may depend on the perspective of the person setting the standard. A math teacher is likely to believe that students need to understand math at a level that an English teacher might consider unreasonably high. Because experts from each field are likely to seek high standards for their own subject, failure rates can be high. State educational leaders are willing to accept a high initial failure rate with the expectation that once students and teachers become familiar with these standards, they will begin to work hard, and eventually achieve at the higher levels needed to meet the standards. Unfortunately, this seldom happens quickly and the consequence can be politically unacceptably high failure rates. This can be a particularly difficult problem when states designate proficient performance on the assessment as the primary criterion for determining eligibility for a high school diploma.

2. Panels setting standards should include the important educational stakeholders. Across states, various committees and stakeholders set standards. In some states, it is the state school board; in others, curriculum specialists in the discipline being assessed set the standards. The problem with using curriculum specialists to set standards is a bias in favor of their discipline and a strong, understandable tendency for these experts to believe that students need to perform at a high level in their particular field. For example, scientists believe that all students need to know a lot about science.

The best compromise may be to use a citizen committee made up of various stakeholders to set performance standards. The members of a panel setting standards in a particular subject matter area should include experts in the field, but it should also include nonexperts. As recommended earlier, there needs to a separate committee that monitors the standards set in all disciplines to ensure that they are commensurate.

3. Using a formula, such as the Angoff method, for setting standards, requires caution. The biggest challenge with standards-based assessment is setting the performance standards. In part, the problem stems from the dichotomy between norm and absolute standards. It is possible to set standards from a norm-referenced perspective by simply designating the percent of students that are to pass and to fail. This is a difficult procedure to defend for two reasons. First, no matter how well students perform collectively, the same proportion will always fail. Second, if the overall performance of students is poor, some students will be designated as proficient even if they are clearly not.

Several systems for setting cut-sores based on absolute standards have been proposed and used including the Angoff, Ebel, Jaeger, and Nedelsky procedures (Jaeger, 1989). Of these, Angoff is the most popular. To implement, a panel of qualified judges must first become familiar with the standards and the items planned for use in the assessment. After reaching a consensus about the meaning of the standards in terms of student performance, judges estimate the probability, for each item, that a minimally qualified student would get the correct answer. The responses of the judges are summed across items and totaled to come up with the percent correct needed for a student to be considered to have reached a minimally acceptable level of performance. The standard Angoff format can be modified by giving judges information about student performance in a pilot group and/or permitting the judges to discuss their decisions after receiving this information. The purpose of this modification is to temper the tendency of judges to set standards that are too high. Presumably, once they know how students actually perform, they will be hesitant to set standards that will result in unacceptably high failure rates. This feedback is sometimes labeled *empirical*, but it is more accurately described as norm-referenced. In a second modification intended to make the judging process easier, judges can be presented with a limited number of categories of probabilities in a multiple-choice format, rather than permitting them to use any probability from 1 to 99.

Other methods proposed for setting cut-scores depend more on typical student performance, which makes them more norm- than absolute-standards based. Examples of these are the contrasting-group, Jaeger-Mills, and the CTB Bookmark methods (Green, Trimble, & Lewis, 2003). These three methods can yield quite different results. The Kentucky Department of Education conducted a study to determine how best to set the cut-scores on the state-wide test used in that state. The study compared three different scaling methods, which set quite different cut-scores. The most extreme difference arose in seventh grade reading where the Bookmark method yielded a cut-score that labeled 61% of the students proficient or distinguished, while the contrasting groups method had a 22.7% pass rate, and the Jaeger-Mills, a pass rate of 10.5. The Bookmark method usually sets lower cut-scores, resulting in more proficient students (Green et al., 2003), but in some grades and subjects the contrasting group method sets lower cut-scores. The use of multiple standard setting procedures is expensive and such stark discrepancies can undermine the legitimacy of the process. Kentucky's policy makers selected the method producing the highest pass rates.

In addition to setting lower cut-scores than other methods, the Bookmark method has a further advantage. Most other methods, including the Angoff procedures, are intended for use with the sort of dichotomously scored items found on multiple-choice tests. The Bookmark procedure also can be used with constructed response items that are assigned a range of scores (polytomously scored) rather than scored right or wrong.

4. Set standards with scaled scores, not raw scores or percentages of raw scores correct. The primary responsibility of committees impaneled to set performance standards is the determination of the number of items a student must correctly answer to be considered proficient. Determining that number can be exceedingly difficult for even the most seasoned educators. Even if a panelist has some good ideas about the level of performance to be expected of an eighth grader in social studies, they still must convert that knowledge to a specific number of correct items on a test assessing social studies knowledge.

The percentage of items correctly answered on a test is arbitrary and easily manipulated, however. Psychometrists routinely adjust item difficulty to increase the variability in scores. A test that is too easy or too difficult will have many students with the same score—such a test will have low variability. A test designed to yield a wide range of student scores will be more sensitive to student differences and be more reliable than a test with less variability.

The manipulation of item difficulty is one of the most important norm-referenced test development techniques. Test developers routinely adjust the difficulty of items by changing the distracters. Psychometrists have determined the optimum proportion of correct answers (item difficulty as expressed in p-values) that will maximize reliability. They can compute this optimum proportion of correct answers using a simple formula, which includes the number of items and the number of multiple-choice options. This makes the meaning of the proportion of items correct dependent on item difficulty, which is set at a level that ensures maximum reliability. For these reasons, any interpretation of student performance based solely on the number of items correct will be of dubious value.

Scaled scores have meaning that can transcend the meaning of specific test. Scaled scores are obtained by transforming raw scores onto a common scale. The simplest way to do this is to define student performance in terms of standard scores based on means and standard deviation. In large-scale, statewide tests, item response theory (IRT) is used. IRT makes it possible to equate tests from year to year and form to form so that their meaning remains constant. The scales used with standardized achievement tests such as the Iowa Test of Basic Skills, the SAT9, TerraNova, and Comprehensive Test of Basic Skills as well as academic aptitude tests such as the ACT, SAT, NAEP, and GRE rely on these techniques. The introduction of item response methods and specialized techniques for interpreting tests that include a mixture of multiple-choice and constructed-response item formats have made test scaling increasingly complex and the interpretation of raw scores even more problematic.

Assessment Issues

Some Inherent Advantages of Multiple-Choice Items for Accountability Systems

Throughout the twentieth century, there was a continuing debate about the relative merits of objective and essay test items. The debate has continued into the present century, refined as a debate about the relative merits of the constructed-response (CR) and multiple-choice (MC) item formats. Instead of being framed as an either–or choice, it has more recently become a choice between the exclusive use of MC items or a combination of MC and CR items. Although some states use only MC items, no state currently uses only CR items for high-stakes tests and most states include both item formats. For example, of the 24 states that will have a high school exam in place by 2008, 21 will be using assessments that include CR items in addition to MC items. The need to choose between these item formats is only relevant for large-scale statewide tests. In the classroom, both item types are appropriate and are used along with many other assessment formats. In that setting, the decision about which format or combinations of formats depends on the sort of information for which the teacher has the greatest need.

There is abundant evidence establishing that MC only tests are much more reliable, less expensive and produce and return results more quickly than tests that include both formats. Commenting on the Advanced Placement (AP) tests published by the Educational Testing Service, which uses both formats, Lukhele, Thissen, and Wainer (1993) asserted: "Constructed response items are expensive. They typically require a great deal of time for the examinee to answer, and they cost a lot to score. In the AP testing program it was found that a constructed response test of equivalent reliability to a multiple-choice test takes from 4 to 40 times as long to administer and is typically hundreds of thousands of times more expensive to score" (p. 234).

If the CR format has such disadvantages, it seems reasonable to ask why it is so widely used and to seek to identify the source of the strong pressure in some states to adopt constructed response items. Rodriguez (2003) provided one explanation for the inclusion of CR items:

> Often, CR items are employed because of a belief that they may directly measure some cognitive processes more readily than one or more MC items. Although many argue that this results from careful item writing rather than the inherent characteristics of a given item format, popular notions of authentic and direct assessment have politicized the item-writing profession, particularly in large-scale settings. (p. 164)

In other words, the decision to include CR items can be based more on ideological and political considerations than their value as a measurement tool. Furthermore, the decision to adopt these methods can undermine the support of large-scale statewide assessments because it makes the resulting assessments less reliable and more expensive. Opponents of standards-based reform can then base their case for the elimination of testing and accountability on shortcomings attributable to the constructed response format.

There are four justifications asserted for the use of the CR format that go beyond political and ideological considerations: (1) they can provide information to teachers about what students know and do not know, (2) they can have a positive effect on teacher instructional behaviors, (3) they measure constructs that the MC item format cannot, and (4) they can compensate for the limitations of the MC item format.

1. Useful information for teachers. Constructed response items are useful for communicating what students know and what they do not know. MC items, on the other hand primarily provide information about how students or schools compare. Information about what students know and do not know is quite useful for the classroom teacher, but this useful attribute does not apply to large-scale assessment. Statewide achievement testing usually takes place in the spring. It takes a long time to score CR items. This means that information about the details of student performance would be available the following fall or even later— too late for the classroom teacher to use. By then, he or she will be teaching a new classroom of students. Furthermore, information about how each student performed on specific items cannot be provided if a state intends to reuse the items. Reusing items in later test administrations reduces the need to include some previously administered items on new tests for purposes of equating. State education leaders may also be reluctant to release items if they believe it encourages teaching to the test.

2. A positive effect on teacher instruction. Lukhele et al. (1994) described the case for including CR items as follows:

> Constructed response questions are thought to replicate more faithfully the tasks examinees face in academic and work settings. Thus, there is an indirect benefit of constructed response test formats that has nothing to do with their measurement characteristics. Because large-scale tests are highly visible within the education community, their content may provide cues to teachers about what is important to teach and to students about what is important to learn. If it is known that students will be required to demonstrate competence in problem solving, graphing, verbal expression, essay organization and writing, these skills may be more likely to be emphasized in the classroom. (p. 235)

This is one of the most common justifications for including CR items on statewide achievement tests. It is based on the assertion that it is better to prepare students for CR items than for MC items because, for example, practice in writing seems more beneficial than practice in the sort of recognition tasks associated with MC items. CR items, however, can be written and scored in a number of different ways. Some ways of writing CR items maximize their instructional value and others are intended to increase reliability. CR item format tests can be made more reliable by increasing the number of items they contain or by ensuring that the scoring of the test is objective. Because of the time it takes for a student to answer and for graders to score CR items, increasing the number of items enough, say, to make a CR test as statistically reliable as a typical MC test, would gobble up weeks of class time, produce uncomfortably long delays in the return of test results, and impose enormous financial burden on education budgets. Items can be scored more objectively when they are written in such a way that there is only one clearly correct answer. This results in consistent scoring and agreement among graders because their answers do not engender different interpretations.

CR Items can be scored either analytically or holistically. Analytical scoring includes specifications called rubrics that tell the grader exactly how a student must respond to each part of a question to receive credit. The rubric also may specify the number of points to be awarded according to the quality of the answer. Tests scored analytically tend to be more reliable than those scored holistically. With holistic scoring, the grader makes a judgment based on his or her overall impression of the answer. One advantage to holistic scoring is that it tends to reward effective writing skills. The problem with holistic scoring is that graders tend to disagree about the scoring of student responses.

Linda Mabry (1999) is a supporter of the use of the CR item format, and an outspoken opponent of high-stakes testing. She asserted that the way CR items are currently implemented, with the focus on analytical scoring, rubrics, and an emphasis on grader agreement, renders them ineffective instructionally. Teachers, schools, and even entire school districts have developed strategies for helping students perform better on standardized CR tests. They take advantage of the necessarily mechanical nature of the cursory review of each question by test graders. Mabry described the pernicious effect of rubrics on tests she has evaluated to determine their effect on the development of writing skills. "Compliance with the rubric tended to yield higher scores but produced 'vacuous' writing. Performance was rewarded on the stated criteria only, and those criteria were insufficient to ensure good writing" (p. 678).

3. Capacity of CR items to measure constructs different from those measured by MC items. Factor analytic studies can be used to identify the different constructs assessed by large scale achievement tests. If CR items provide additional information about student performance, such studies should reveal a second robust factor associated with CR item use. Thissen, Wainer, and Wang (1994) found evidence for a CR factor orthogonal to the main MC factor on both Computer Science and Chemistry AP tests. They found that the factor loading for the CR items is usually greater on the general (multiple choice) factor than on the constructed-response factor(s). The loadings of the CR items on the constructed-response factors are small, indicating that the free-response items do not measure something different very well. The MC items also load on the CR factors. Paradoxically, it turns out that MC items measure the CR factors more accurately than CR items. If we want to predict a student's performance on a future CR test, we can actually do this more accurately with MC than with CR items. Measuring something indirectly but precisely yields more accurate prediction than measuring the right thing poorly.

4. Limitations of the MC item format. Unfortunately, the decision to include CR items along with MC items on large-scale statewide tests is sometimes based on misinformation about or distrust of conventional standardized testing. Some of the reasons given for not using multiple-choice items, for example, are as follows:

- They can only measure the recall of facts and isolated pieces of information.
- They cannot assess higher level thinking processes.
- They represent an old-fashion method of assessment that needs to be replaced by more modern assessment techniques.
- They do not provide a fair measure of the achievement of non-Asian minorities and economically deprived students.

None of these assertions, however, can withstand careful analysis. Multiple-choice items can assess facts, dates, names, and isolated ideas, but they also can provide an effective measure of high-level thinking skills. Although they are not appropriate measures of creativity and organizing ability, they can measure virtually any other level of cognitive functioning. The so-called more modern assessment techniques of constructed response items are just the old essay tests that predate multiple-choice items.

Low-income, minority, and ESL students do not perform as well on standardized tests as middle-class nonminority students and most standardized tests employ a multiple-choice item format. This connection has caused critics of standardized tests to assert incorrectly that the item format is the problem. In actuality, the exact opposite is true. The gap between the performance of minority and non-minority is greater for constructed-response than multiple-choice items (Cunningham, 1998). One reason for this is that low-income and minority students do not respond at all to some CR items, and they do this at a much higher rate than nonminorities. Nonresponses are seldom a problem with MC item format tests.

Necessary Statistical Considerations When Both MC and CR Items are Used

Combining Scores.   If a state department of education follows the usual practice and uses both item formats, they must decide how to combine the two. The usual method for combining scores is paradoxical. On one hand, the use of CR items is often justified by their capacity to provide information about student performance that is different from the information provided by MC items. On the other hand, the MC and CR sections of a test can only be combined if they are both measuring the same construct, an attribute referred to as *unidimensionality.* If two sections measuring different constructs are combined, the resulting scale will be less reliable than either of the two scales upon which the combined scale is based. This is because the combined scores will have less variability than the two scores from which they are derived. It is possible to create a test made up of CR items that measures the same construct as a test using MC items measures. For example, a stem equivalent CR test can be constructed using items based on stems from MC items (Rodriguez, 2003). Scores from the two sections can be shown to be measuring the same construct. Even without the use of a stem equivalent approach, the CR items can be written is such a way that they cover the same instructional objectives as MC items and they can be written in such a way that they can be scored objectively. If the CR items emulate MC items, measure the same construct as the MC items, and are constructed so that there is only one correct answer, why not just use the less expensive and more reliable MC items?

When both item types are included in a test, in addition to the question of how to combine them, a further decision about how to weight the two sections must be made. The usual practice is to weight them according to how much time is devoted to each. Wainer and Thissen (1993) demonstrated that when the CR and MC sections of a test are weighted in this way, the resulting overall score will be less reliable than the score obtained from just the MC section because MC items are so much more reliable than CR items. The addition of CR items actually suppresses the reliability of the overall score.

Because it takes longer to answer a CR than an MC item, when equal time is allotted for both, there will be fewer items in the CR section. Because reliability is partially a function of test length, the test section that includes CR items will be less reliable than the one made up of MC items. One solution to differential reliability is to increase the number of CR items so that the reliability of that section is as high as the MC section. Wainer and Thissen (1993) examined a test in chemistry; a subject for which a CR item test can be created that can be analytically scored. They demonstrated that if you increased the number of CR items to the point where that section had reliability equal to that of the MC section, it would need to be 3 hours long as compared to the 75 minutes required for the MC test. It also would cost $30 to score such a test compared with one cent to score the MC section. For a test assessing a less concrete subject like literature or music, scored holistically, 30 hours of CR testing time would be required and the estimated cost to score it would be $100.

Item Difficulty. Item difficulty presents a significant challenge in the implementation of norm-referenced standards-based systems. Even small deviations from the ideal can lead to tests that are either too easy or too hard. It is particularly important when student performance is reported in the form of raw scores or the percentage of raw items correct. If the item difficulty is unstable from year to year, no comparisons across years will be meaningful, and different forms employed in the same year cannot be compared. When multiple-choice items, norm-referenced principles, and item response theory are employed, item difficulty presents few problems. Multiple-choice items can be made easier by choosing distracters that are different from the correct answer or made more difficult by selecting distracters that are similar. The manipulation of the difficulty of multiple-choice items makes it possible for a test author to maximize the variability of scores. For any test, the optimum level of difficulty can be easily determined using a simple formula. Tests with that level of difficulty will yield maximum score variability, which leads to higher reliability. When constructed-response items are used instead of multiple-choice items, there is no way to adjust difficulty other than changing the content of the questions. This characteristic of CR items makes comparing test performance from year to year (test equating) difficult and is another cause of the lower reliability for tests made up of these items.

Content Validity. The most important type of validity associated with large-scale assessments of achievement is content validity. This form of validity refers to the fidelity with which a test can assess instructional objectives. Tests made up of constructed-response items can contain only a limited number of items because each item requires a lengthy response. As a result, tests made up of CR items are usually less construct valid than those that utilize the MC item format because many more items can be included with this latter type of test format.

Conclusions About the Use of CR Items

Lukhele et al. (1994) sum up the case for the exclusive use of MC format items in comparing the CR and MC sections of tests from the Advanced Placement (AP) testing Program of the College Board. This was a good set of tests to examine because the training of their examiners and the sophistication of the scoring methods used with the constructed response items on this test are "state of the art." Whatever defects the study uncovered in the scoring of their constructed response items cannot easily be attributed to flaws in the training of examiners or the methods they employed. The authors conclusions were as follows:

> Overall, the multiple-choice items provide more than twice the information than the constructed response items do. Examining the entire test (and freely applying the Spearman-Brown prophesy formula), we found that a 75-minute multiple-choice tests is as reliable as a 185-minute test built of constructed response questions. Both kinds of items are measuring essentially the same construct, and the constructed response items cost about 300 times more to score. It would appear, based on this limited sample of questions, that there is no good measurement reason for including constructed response items. (p. 240)

> On the basis of the data examined, we are forced to conclude that constructed response items provide less information in more time at greater cost than do multiple-choice items. This conclusion is surely discouraging to those who feel that constructed response items are more authentic and hence, in some sense, more useful than multiple-choice items. It should be. (p. 245)

Be Prepared to Deal With Accommodations and Modifications for Special Education Students

The existence of students with educational disabilities challenges an underlying assumption of some standards-based education reforms—that all students can learn at the same high level. This assumption places considerable responsibility on each state to carefully formulate policies defining the conditions under which students with educational disabilities or students who are English Language Learners (ELL) participate in state assessments.

Federal and state laws, under the umbrella of the 1975, 1991, and finally the 1997 Individual with Disabilities Act (IDEA) include the criteria used to specify the conditions under which students are to be defined as disabled. Section 504, of the Rehabilitation Act signed into law in 1973 states that students with disabilities that "substantially limits one or more major life activities" qualify for a Section 504 plan. The Section 504 rules supplement those included in the more recent IDEA legislation. A multi-disciplinary team of professionals who know the student best, design the student's individual educational plan (IEP) under both IDEA and Section 504 rules. This committee is given different names depending on the state but usually it includes the phrase "admissions and retentions committee" (ARC). The IDEA legislation requires that "children with disabilities be included in general state and district-wide assessments with accommodations where necessary" [612(a)(17)(A)]. The law further requires that ARCs specify the accommodations for individual students with IEPs who are participating in large-scale assessment programs.

The IDEA legislation does not protect a special education student from being tested. Instead, it ensures that they are not denied the opportunity to be tested. For this reason, exempting disabled students is not an option. Even severely disabled students must be included. The IDEA rules require an alternate assessment for students whose disability is so severe that they cannot participate in the regular assessment. Most states have adopted an alternate portfolio for this purpose. For most states, less that one percent of students fit in this category. The use of alternate portfolios for developmentally disabled students is seldom controversial because there is no expectation that these students would graduate from high school.

Accommodations are adjustments in testing procedures that permit disabled students to perform on tests in ways that reflect their true ability. Accommodations should have two characteristics: (1) they should not compromise the construct validity of the test, and (2) the same alteration in the testing procedure given to a nonhandicapped student should not enhance his or her score (Pitoniak & Royer, 2001). Examples of typical accommodations are the provision of more testing time, permitting students to take an exam in a separated area away from other students, the use of signing to provide test administration instructions for hearing impaired students, or the use of Braille for visually impaired students. Scores obtained by students with accommodations are considered equivalent to scores obtained under standard administration procedures, they can become part of school's score, and/or are used to establish eligibility for graduation. Accommodations are intended to give disabled students a fair chance on tests and although the IDEA legislation requires states to include appropriate accommodations, they are not required to include accommodations that compensate for a student's lack of proficiency in what the test is measuring. (For example, a reader on a reading test, having a scribe write down a student's answers to a constructed response question, or permitting the use of a calculator for a math test; Pitoniak & Royer, 2001). These sorts of changes in testing conditions that would alter the underlying meaning of the construct being measured are called *modifications*. The IDEA legislation leaves it to states to distinguish between accommodations and modifications.

When the focus of accountability is on schools and school districts, policies adopted to accommodate educationally disabled students should focus on fairness for the schools being evaluated. These policies should not have the effect of giving an advantage to a school that has a greater or lesser number of students with disabilities. As long as it is the school or district that is held accountable, individual student scores may not seem critically important and many are prone to allow generous accommodations. Parents are happy because their children are given an opportunity for success and are not placed in testing situations where they are likely to fail. Although cut-scores can be adjusted to account for these scores, there is a need to control for the tendency of overzealous educators to over-identify students and use exemptions as a way to increase their school's scores.

Designating the changes in testing conditions to be considered accommodations becomes more difficult when the accountability system is focused on individual students, particularly when the results are used to determine whether a student will be allowed to graduate from high school.

Deciding what are to be considered fair accommodations is most difficult for learning disabled (LD) students. Students in this category make up the majority of students with IEPs. The proportion of the student population classified as LD varies widely across states; in some states, more than ten percent of all students have been given this label. The implementation of high school exit exams has had a dramatic impact on these students. In the past, LD students have been encouraged to follow a course of studies that would permit them to graduate. Many of these students, with the help of teachers and generous accommodations within classrooms have been able to pass a sufficient number of courses to do just that. Some parents of students with learning disabilities have come to view high school graduation as a reasonable expectation.

If generous assistance in test taking is provided to students with learning disabilities to help them pass a state exam, however, parents of other poorly performing students might demand the same. The problem is even more acute because there is no clear distinction between LD and other poorly performing students (Aaron, 1997; Pitoniak & Royer, 2001; Swerling & Sternberg, 1997).

Moreover, the most common accommodation for students with disabilities is the provision of additional time, but state accountability exams are usually not highly speeded and as a result, extra time does not provide much of an advantage.

The NCLB Act focuses on improving the performance of students who historically have not performed well in school and this includes students with learning disabilities. The most important provision of this law is the requirement that the academic progress of such students be monitored separately. Unlike some accountability systems currently employed at the state level, the NCLB Act does not permit the high performance of one segment of students to compensate for other low achieving students. The NCLB policy regarding accommodations is a reiteration of the IDEA rules. As is true of IDEA, the NCLB rules are not intended to protect learning disabled students from being tested. They are intended to ensure not only that they are assessed, but that the results of their assessment are tabulated separately.

State Departments of Education can Provide Clear Explanations for the Public

Both educators and the public deserve to be informed about state SBER programs. As these programs evolve, they can become quite complex and difficult to understand. This makes the task of explaining them difficult. At a minimum, a comprehensive technical manual should be provided. The assessment part of SBER is typically a joint venture between a state department of education and a testing company that produces the actual test. Unfortunately, both parties to the joint venture have strong incentives to minimize disclosure of technical details about their testing program. State departments of education must endure constant attacks by antitesting members of the education community and repeatedly are required to defend their practices. It can be tempting for them to provide a minimum of information as a way of reducing the burden of their defense. The problem with secrecy in such matters is that it can undermine public confidence. Those state education departments that have absorbed the expense and made the effort to divulge as much information as possible have been rewarded by gains in public support.

The test publishing companies that manage statewide achievement tests make up a billion-dollar industry. The bidding process for new and existing contracts has become increasingly competitive. The institutional knowledge of an incumbent contractor gives them a big advantage when they submit proposals for the renewal of their contracts. The value of this knowledge makes test publishers reluctant to release technical details about the testing programs they manage for fear that it would be too useful for competing contractors. For this reason, they may be unenthusiastic about publishing a highly detailed technical manual that could be used by their competitors to win the contracts they currently hold.

One decision about a statewide achievement test that education leaders in a state must make is whether to release used items. There is a reluctance on the part of state educational leaders to do this because when items are released they cannot be reused. Creating new items makes the testing process more expensive. Furthermore, test forms from different years must share some items for the purpose of test equating. In addition to these reasons for not releasing items, there is concern that the release of items will increase the likelihood that teachers will spend too much time "teaching to the test." This is the main reason why the items from the National Assessment for Educational Progress (NAEP) are not released.

Although these may be good reasons for not releasing items, a case can be made for making some items available to the public. In some states there is strong opposition to testing, and a consequent need for state officials to sell the test to the public. One technique opponents use to criticize tests is to claim that the items used are flawed. If they are not released, it will be difficult to convince the public that the items are of high quality. Of course, if the items are not very good, releasing them can be embarrassing. But, if releasing items means that poor items will be identified, this can be seen as a positive aspect of such a policy. There are examples of members of the public identifying items that have been scored incorrectly affecting a large number of students. The identification of the problem allowed it to be fixed.

CONCLUSION

A primary purpose of SBER is to ensure that the educational community recognizes the importance of academic achievement. Even if the governor, the legislature, and the public are committed to having all students reach a high level of academic achievement in conventional academic subjects, some educational leaders may not share this goal, and that difference in aspirations can adversely affect the testing program.

State assessment systems should be both reliable and valid. It is possible to create large-scale tests that meet these criteria without being excessively expensive. State tests tend to go awry when their designers try to make them do too much. State educational decision makers need to recognize the complexity of testing programs. Moreover, they need in-house staff who can design and evaluate the testing program, and monitor the performance of testing contractors. There are right ways of implementing SBER and there are wrong ways. It has been the purpose of this chapter to help the reader distinguish between the two.

REFERENCES

Aaron, P. (1997). The impending demise of the discrepancy formula. *Review of Educational Research, 67*(4), 461–502.

American Educational Research Association, American Psychological Association, & National Council on Measurement in Education. (1999). *Standards for educational and psychological testing.* Washington, DC: American Educational Research Association.

Cunningham, G. K. (1998). *Assessment in the Classroom.* London: Falmer Press

Green, D. R., Trimble, C. S., & Lewis, D. M. (2003), Interpreting the results of three different standard setting procedures. *Educational Measurement: Issues and Practice, 22*(1), 22–35.

Individuals with Disabilities Education Act Amendments of 1997. (1997). 20 U.S.C. 1400, et seq.

Jaeger, R. M. (1989). Certification of student competence. In R. L. Linn (Ed.), *Educational Measurement* (3rd ed., pp. 485–514). New York: MacMillan.

Lukhele R., Thissen, D., & Wainer, H. (1994). On the relative value of multiple-choice, constructed-response, and examinee-selected items on two achievement tests. *Journal of Educational Measurement, 31*(3), 234–250.

Mabry, L. (1999, May). Writing to the rubric: Lingering effects of traditional standardized testing on the direct writing assessment. *Phi Delta Kappan,* 673–679.

Pitoniak, M., & Royer, J. (2001). Testing accommodations for examinees with disabilities: A review of psychometric, legal, and social policy issues. *Review of Educational Research, 71*(1), 53–104.

Rodriguez, M. (2003). Construct equivalence of multiple-choice and construct-response items: A random effects synthesis of correlations. *Journal of Educational Measurement, 40*(2), 163–184.

Swerling, L., & Sternberg, R. (1997). Off track: When poor readers become "learning disabled." Boulder, CO: Westview Press.

Thissen, D., Wainer, H., & Wang, X. (1994). Are tests comprising both multiple-choice and free-response items necessarily less unidimensional than multiple-choice tests? An analysis of two tests. *Journal of Educational Measurement, 31*(2), 113–123.

Wainer, H., & Thissen, D. (1993). Combining multiple-choice and constructed response test scores: Toward a Marxist theory of test construction. *Applied Measurement in Education, 6*(2), 103–118.

7

Whose rules? The Relation Between the "Rules" and "Law" of Testing

Chad W. Buckendahl
Buros Center for Testing, University of Nebraska, Lincoln

Robert Hunt
Caveon Test Security

The testing community generally relies on the *Standards for Educational and Psychological Testing* (AERA, APA, & NCME, 1999) as the arbiter of what is appropriate in test development, psychometric analyses, test administration, score reporting, and test usage.[1] However, because the *Standards* are

---

[1]Other professional organizations have developed standards and guidelines for areas that may not be clearly specified within the Standards. For example, the Society for Industrial and Organizational Psychologists developed the Principles for Validation and Use of Personnel Selection Procedures (2003) that apply specifically to personnel selection testing programs. More recently, the Association of Test Publishers (2001) and the International Test Commission (2003) have been promoting guidelines that focus on the increasingly popular computer-based testing. The Buros Institute for Assessment Consultation and Outreach (BIACO), through their Standards for BIACO Accreditation of Proprietary Testing Programs, focuses on the broader arena of proprietary testing in education, credentialing, and business. Additional agencies such as the National Organization for Competency Assurance (NOCA) through their NCCA Standards for the Accreditation of Certification Programs, and the American National Standards Institute (ANSI) through one of their International Standards Organization (ISO) programs have focused on personnel certification and licensure testing programs. These guidelines represent the collective interpretation of acceptable practice within the profession which gives the courts additional support for their decisions. *(continued)*

professional policies, their influence is generally limited to the self-regulation of testing professionals, lacking an organization or method of redress for aggrieved test users, enforcement authority, or the necessary breadth to anticipate the myriad social issues surrounding the use of tests.

> In short, although the rules and practice of testing professionals provide the framework and tools for sound testing practice, they lack the apparatus necessary for the consideration (and inculcation) of related social issues—typically expressed in legal and political conflicts. To this point, the *Standards* concede that they "… provide more specific guidance on matters of technical adequacy, *matters of values and public policy are crucial to responsible test use.*" (AERA et al., 1999, p. 80, italics added)

In the United States, state and federal legislatures and courts provide many services to support (or restrict) the use of tests for the purposes of licensure, certification, employment selection, as well as the focus of this chapter: educational selection and attainment. Specifically, legislatures and courts provide both an infrastructure that sustains the use of tests for a variety of purposes, and direction to test creators and users regarding test validity and fairness. In recent years, for example, test creators and users have been guided by explicit legal direction regarding test bias (race, gender, disabilities and English-as-a-second-language [ESL]) and validity (relation to employment and curricular requirements).

By their actions, legislatures and courts extend the influence of tests by legitimizing their use for a host of functions—primarily by advancing the use of tests (e.g.; No Child Left Behind), and by providing an authoritative apparatus for the resolution of disputes regarding fairness and validity. The purpose of this chapter is to illustrate the interaction between the *rules* and *law* of testing, beginning with an examination of the role legislatures and courts play in advancing social and professional consensus regarding testing practice, and ending with illustrations of governmental leadership on testing issues.

FAIR TEST CONTENT

Although testing professionals have long supported the goal of test fairness, tests, along with other methods of social and economic differentiation, have been swept along in the tide of egalitarian legal reform originated in the 1950s and 1960s. Prior to these reforms, testing professionals recommended and exercised caution to minimize test bias, but could

---

[1](*continued*) Although it is possible to go beyond their standards and guidelines, the courts have been reticent to stray far from the practices that the professional community has defined in its standards of acceptable practice.

not have anticipated the specificity of legal proscriptions regarding racial, cultural, gender, and disability discrimination.

Perhaps the most significant expression of egalitarian legal reform appeared in the form of the 1964 Civil Rights Act (reauthorized in 1991). Title VII of the Act specifically prohibits discrimination "in all terms and conditions of employment" on the basis of race, color, religion, sex, or national origin. Subsequent legislation such as the Age Discrimination in Employment Act (ADEA) and the Americans with Disabilities Act (ADA) has extended similar protections against discrimination in a variety of settings to age and disability.

Importantly, the jurisdiction of these statutes extends to state education agencies and local education agencies that serve as employment "gatekeepers." For example, because a high school diploma may be used as a criterion for employment or further education, Title VII may apply to high school graduation tests.

In evaluating Title VII challenges to testing programs, courts seek to understand whether a testing program unintentionally discriminates or "adversely impacts" one or more groups protected by the legislation. Adverse impact in testing can arise from a number of sources including biased content, the selection of items, and opportunity to learn (AERA et al., 1999).

In reviewing these unintentional discrimination challenges arising under Title VII, courts typically rely on one of three methods. The first involves an examination of the pass-rates of the members of the protected group (typically females or an ethnic minority) and other examinees (typically males or the ethnic majority); adverse impact is generally regarded to exist if 80% or less of the protected group equals the test performance of other examinees.[2] The second method involves a comparison of the proportions of members of a protected group and other examinees who passed the test (Shoben, 1978). The third method involves a standard deviation analysis wherein mean differences between members of a protected group and other examinees are compared. If these differences are greater than three standard deviations, they are generally regarded as indicative of adverse impact (*Hazelwood School District v. United States*, 1977).

If a court rules that adverse impact exists, the burden shifts to the testing program to demonstrate that the test is "rationally related" to important aspects of the job, curriculum or profession. If a sponsor can satisfy this burden, challengers have a final opportunity to provide evidence that an equivalent, alternative test or method exists that does not result in adverse impact.

The APA, AERA, and NCME candidly concede in their *Standards* that "... fairness is defined in a variety of ways and is not exclusively addressed

---

[2]This method is suggested in the Equal Employment Opportunity Commission (EEOC) Guidelines (1978) and is commonly known as the "four-fifths" rule.

in technical terms; it is subject to different definitions and interpretations in different social and political circumstances," (AERA et al., 1990, p. 80). This admission reveals the organizations' view that law and the legal system are necessary adjuncts to the successful operation of testing programs; they clarify principles articulated by testing professionals, chiefly by specifying concrete social objectives (legislatures), and by providing pragmatic guidance in their application (courts).

FAIRNESS IN TEST ADMINISTRATION

The *Standards* acknowledge that "[a] well designed test is not intrinsically fair or unfair, but the use of the test in a particular circumstance or with particular examinees may be fair or unfair" (AERA et al., 1999) With their long experience in the interpretation and application of the Equal Protection clause of the 14th Amendment, courts have become particularly adept at analyzing the "fundamental fairness" of both the criteria (substance) and procedures used by governments and their agencies to grant or deny individual rights and property.

The idea of "due process" is typically understood in relation to the concepts of "notice," "access," and "hearing"—the building blocks of what the law and courts refer to more specifically as "procedural due process." Each element of procedural due process has a clear and necessary application to testing. Regarding "notice" and "access" for example, the *Standards* provide that "[w]here appropriate, test takers should be provided, in advance, as much information about the test, the testing process, the intended test use, test scoring criteria, test policy ... as is consistent with obtaining valid responses" (AERA, APA, & NCME, 1999, p. 86).

Tests, of course, are both surrounded by processes and are processes in themselves. Because tests are used as tools by which individuals may be denied the right to practice in a chosen profession, secure employment or graduate from high school, evidence that supports the use of these scores for these purposes is critical. In applying the 14th Amendment, courts are also interested in the relationship between the requirements of a test (e.g., minimum proficiency on core content for graduation eligibility) and its purpose (e.g., to differentiate students who have achieved minimum levels of competency from those who have not). This "substantive due process" analysis is concerned, like Title VII, with the validity of tests intended for wide-scale use and their consequences.

Unlike Title VII, however, substantive due process analysis involves more rigorous scrutiny of test requirements and related questions of fairness including "opportunity to learn." In *Debra P. v. Turlington* (1979, 1981, 1983, 1984), 10 African-American high school students challenged the Florida State Student Assessment Test as being unfair because they claimed they had not had an adequate opportunity to master the underlying curriculum. The test was given to the students during their junior year in high school. Students who did not pass the test were placed into programs designed to provide remedial assistance and given the opportunity to retake the exam up to two more times during their senior year. If students did not pass the exam after these additional opportunities to take the exam, they were to be denied eligibility for high school diplomas. In their legal action the students claimed denial of due process because they had not been given adequate in-school preparation for the test and, secondarily that the state was using the test to discriminate against students by race.

The U.S. District Court for the Middle District of Florida initially ruled that the test was being used in a way that potentially disadvantaged minority students due to a historical pattern of unequal educational opportunities. Drawing on prior case law regarding school segregation, the court held that the students did not have the same opportunities to learn the material represented on the test compared to other students. As a result, the courts enjoined the state from using the test for graduation eligibility until 1983 (4 years after the case was filed) when the students would have had the opportunity to learn in an integrated educational system.

This first requirement of due process analysis therefore, is that the students have a right to a reasonable length of time to learn the underlying material prior to being held responsible for it. In *Debra P.*, the court ruled that the appropriate length of time was 4 years, or the equivalent of a high-school career. Courts in other jurisdictions, however, have subsequently ruled that the amount of time varies with circumstances.[3]

The second requirement of substantive due process analysis to emerge from *Debra P.* focuses on the relationship of test content to the underlying curriculum, and is often labeled "opportunity to learn" (OTL).[4] How does a school district or state demonstrate the curricular validity of a test? In *Debra P.*, Florida's Department of Education surveyed the content of classes in four subject areas from a representative sample of Florida schools to sup-

---

[3]For example, the court ruled that a year and a half's notice to handicapped students was inadequate (*Brookhart v. Illinois State Board of Education*, 1983). Another court ruled that adequate notice would be at least two years (*Anderson v. Banks*, 1982).

[4]Phillips (1996) referred to this as evidence of curricular validity. This requirement should not be construed narrowly as requiring instruction on individual items or tasks that might appear on a graduation test, but rather that instruction has occurred in the content domain from which test items or tasks might be sampled on current or future forms of the test. Because a good test represents a sample of the larger content domain of interest, students should have the opportunity to be exposed to instruction in this area before they are held responsible for the material. Any representative sample that is then drawn from that larger content domain should be supported by the curricular evidence that demonstrates that the content on the test is reflected in the curriculum and has been sequenced to allow instruction to occur on this content prior to being tested on it.

port their assertion that the test material was, in fact, covered by both curriculum and instruction.

The evidence presented by the State consisted of an analysis of the content in the curriculum for each district in the state, and the results of a survey sent to all teachers regarding what they taught in their classrooms. A third piece of evidence consisted of reports from on-site, independent audits conducted in each school district for the purpose of validating district reports of the curriculum content and sequencing. The final piece of the State's curricular validity evidence was provided by the results of a student survey—direct testimony regarding whether they had been taught the material that appeared on the test.

For both stakeholders and practitioners, substantiating the curricular validity of a test is obviously nontrivial. Adequate notice under the substantive due process analysis articulated in *Debra P.* requires a reasonable amount of time to implement any necessary curricular changes that may be necessary to give schools and students sufficient time to adequately prepare them for the test. For example, requiring students to demonstrate advanced algebra skills on the graduation test may mean that a district's high school mathematics curriculum may need to be adjusted. It may also necessitate changes at the elementary and middle school levels to prepare students entering high school to master advanced algebra material by the time they are required to demonstrate their skills in this area.

The scope and sequencing of instruction are also of concern. In the example of a district that expects high school graduates to demonstrate some level of advanced algebra skills, without adequate notice, students who are allowed to "opt-out" after prealgebra may be in jeopardy of failing the algebra element of a graduation test. For similar reasons, the sequencing of curriculum is important because students must be exposed to material in a course or grade prior to the point in time they are tested on the material.[5]

OTHER ASPECTS OF TEST DESIGN

In addition to the fairness of tests, the *Standards* articulate other important aspects of test design which the courts, on several occasions, have adopted and reinforced through the application of legal limits. In *GI Forum v. Texas Education Agency* in which high school students sought the suspension of a graduation test on the basis that it was unfair to minority students, for example, the court entertained a number of specific claims about the quality and utility of the psychometric aspects of a testing program.

---

[5]Although not discussed in this chapter, Pitoniak and Royer (2001) provided a summary with relevant citations and case law related to testing examinees with disabilities.

Validity

Of primary importance to a testing program is the usefulness of resulting test scores for their intended (or foreseeable) purpose (i.e., educational attainment, employment selection, etc.; Messick, 1989). For educational tests, this means that the relation of the test content to underlying curriculum is critical. In *GI Forum* the court adopted a professional measure of test validity by examining and upholding the relationship of the graduation test to Texas' curriculum in reading, mathematics, and writing which the State had documented in an associated technical manual (Smisko, Twing, & Denny, 2000).[6] The technical manual, importantly, included content reviews conducted both before and after field testing of the test to allow educators multiple opportunities to examine the test content in relation to the State's curriculum.

A related professional concept of test validity, "curricular validity," or the relationship of test content to the curriculum and instruction provided by an individual school district, received legal recognition in both *Debra P.* and *GI Forum*. In *GI Forum* the court accepted reviews by educators, results from an earlier survey of teachers for the previous graduation test, and the provision of study guides and remedial opportunities as sufficient demonstration of curricular validity.[7]

Additional aspects of test validity reinforced by law include strategies for setting cut-scores (or passing standards) that classify examinees into predefined categories of performance. Courts have generally shown deference to professional processes used to derive cut-scores and the substantive judgments underlying those decisions. In *Tyler v. Vickery* (1975) and *Richardson v. Lamar County Board of Education* (1989), for example, each court ruled that testing programs are responsible for ensuring that professionally acceptable strategies are used to derive cut-scores and also suggested that a rational relationship should exist between the impact of the passing score and the purpose of the test.

---

[6]The content validation strategy recommended by the *Standards* is to document the link between the content that is desired and the content that actually appears in the test or item bank from which tests are developed. This link is generally supported through judgmental reviews by educators who are familiar with the content. These reviews are conducted to ensure that items or tasks that may appear on the test measure content that was deemed important in the curriculum. They are also generally checked to ensure that the correct answer is keyed or a rubric is sufficiently clear to allow for independent raters to evaluate performance.

[7]These interactions among content standards, curriculum, instruction, and testing serve as core elements in the alignment research of Webb (1997). Alignment also shows up frequently in the language of the No Child Left Behind legislation. Thus, practitioners are encouraged to continue to collect, analyze, use, and document the validity evidence from these studies.

Reliability

The concept of test reliability encompasses the dependability of test scores. Within a criterion-referenced setting, however, the stability of scores may be less important than the stability of decisions made about the scores. These related perspectives of reliability both have a goal of reducing the measurement error associated in order to give us greater confidence in using the results. Although there are a number of strategies for estimating score reliability (e.g., parallel forms, test–retest, internal consistency) for objectively scored tests, each bears assumptions that make them more or less attractive in an educational setting.

Most testing programs employ a measure of internal consistency to estimate reliability. Such estimates involve mathematical strategies for examining the relations among the test questions to assess the extent that the questions are related to each other. Values range from 0.0 (reliability is low) to 1.0 (reliability is high).[8] Following the professional practices of the measurement community, the court in *GI Forum* held that the reliability values in the high .80s to low .90s for the Texas graduation test were acceptable (Phillips, 2000).

The discussion of legal issues related to educational testing in this chapter should not be construed as comprehensive review of testing litigation. Numerous cases in credentialing, admissions, and employment have also helped to shape the professional rules of testing. However, we did not want to overwhelm readers with discussions of case law related to testing programs. For additional information about testing litigation that readers could use to further explore this topic, we have provided a summary of cases discussed in this chapter in addition to some of these other cases in Table 7.1. Cases are arranged chronologically and classified by their respective testing application.

CONSIDERATIONS AND RECOMMENDATIONS

As the introduction of this brief chapter intimated, the interaction between the rules and law of testing is more synergistic than competitive: associations of testing professionals articulate best practices which courts tend to adopt and to which they add concrete direction and the authoritative weight of the law.

What, in this environment, can educational testing programs do to protect themselves from the inevitable challenges that high stakes testing programs elicit? The answer seems clear—pay close attention to the *Standards*. In addition, we offer three recommendations that apply primarily to mea-

---

[8]See Anastasi (1996), or similar educational measurement textbooks for a more detailed explanation of reliability.

TABLE 7.1
Influential Cases in Testing Litigation 1970–2000

Case	Testing focus	Year(s)
Bray v. Lee	admissions	1971
Griggs v. Duke Power Company	employment	1971
Board of Regents of State Colleges v. Roth	employment	1972
Larry P. v. Riles	education	1972–1984
Pennsylvania Assn for Retarded Children v. Commonwealth of Pennsylvania	education	1972
Sibley Memorial Hospital v. Wilson	employment	1973
Albermarle Paper Company v. Moody	employment	1975
Tyler v. Vickery	credentialing	1975
Hoffman v. Board of Education of New York City	education	1976–1979
Paul v. Davis	employment	1976
Washington v. Davis	credentialing	1976
Hazelwood School District v. United States	credentialing	1977
United States v. South Carolina	credentialing	1977
Regents of the State of California v. Bakke	admissions	1978
Debra P. v. Turlington	education	1979–1984
Detroit Edison Co. v. National Labor Relations Board	employment	1979
Diana v. California State Board of Education	education	1979
Southeastern Community College v. Davis	education	1979
Woodard v. Virginia Board of Bar Examiners	credentialing	1979
Anderson v. Banks	education	1982
Board of Education of Northport-E. Northport v. Ambach	education	1983
Brookhart v. Illinois State Board of Education	education	1983
Guardian Assn. v. Civil Service Commission of New York	employment	1983
Golden Rule v. Washburn	employment	1984
Haddock v. Board of Dental Examiners	credentialing	1985
Doe v. St. Joseph's Hospital	employment	1986
United States v. LULAC	employment	1986
State of Texas v. Project Principle	credentialing	1987
Richardson v. Lamar County Board of Education	credentialing	1989
Sharif v. New York State Education Department	education	1989
Wards Cove Packing Co. v. Antonio	employment	1989

(continued)

TABLE 7.1   (*continued*)

Case	Testing focus	Year(s)
Hawaii State Department of Education	education	1990
Groves v. Alabama State Board of Education	admissions	1991
Musgrove et al. v. Board of Education for the State of Georgia et al.	credentialing	1991
Pandazides v. Virginia Board of Education	education	1992
Smothers v. Benitez	employment	1992
Association of Mexican-American Educators v. California	credentialing	1993–1996
Maxwell v. Pasadena I.S.D.	education	1994
Allen v. Alabama State Board of Education		
Bartlett v. New York State Board of Law Examiners	credentialing	1997–1998
Price v. National Board of Medical Examiners	admissions	1997
Washington v. Glucksberg	credentialing	1997
Jacobson v. Tillmann	credentialing	1998
GI Forum v. Texas Education Agency	education	2000

surement practitioners. However, consumers can also review these recommendations and ask how well their testing program attends to each.

1. *Develop and maintain a technical manual:* A sound technical manual may include information about the derivation of content specifications, the link to test items/tasks, content and bias review procedures, field test results, form development, form redevelopment, reliability/standard errors, item analyses, standard setting, equating, test administration, test scoring, score reporting, item/task security, item exposure control, re-take policies, and appeal/review policies.

2. *Follow sound psychometric practice:* Within the educational testing arena, sound psychometric practice with respect to the elements described above is defined primarily by the *Standards for Educational and Psychological Testing* (AERA et al., 1999) and address test construction, evaluation, usage, rights and responsibilities of test developers, test takers and test users. When in doubt, courts have tended to rely on the recommended best practices of a profession, so following accepted professional guidelines extends the defensibility of practices to the broader profession.

3. *Utilize psychometric specialists:* Most people consult a medical doctor when they need health-related assistance. Testing programs, too,

should utilize appropriately trained psychometric experts to conduct quality control on the internal processes. Testing programs are also encouraged to conduct an external psychometric evaluation or audit that examines the quality of their program according to both psychometric best practices and legal defensibility criteria. Evidence that a testing program has sought to independently confirm or improve its technical quality provides another layer of protection when defending a challenge (Mehrens & Pophem, 1992).

CONCLUSION

Educational testing programs will continue to be challenged in the courts when a perception exists that they are unfair or being misused. Although time consuming, these challenges to the testing community require that we provide evidence of the soundness of our science to the broader public in a language that it can understand. These activities serve to strengthen the parts of our field to withstand these challenges and expose weaknesses that we may not have addressed in the past due to political or external pressures. The strategies used to defend educational testing programs described in this chapter by no means offer a guarantee that a program will be able to withstand a legal challenge. They are meant, instead, to inform practitioners and consumers of the courts' priorities in their evaluations of these systems.

REFERENCES

AERA, APA, & NCME. (1999). *Standards for educational and psychological testing.* Washington, DC: American Educational Research Association.

Anastasi, A. (1996). Psychological Testing (6th ed.). New York, NY: Macmillan.

Anderson v. Banks, 540 F. Supp. 472 (S.D. Fla. 1981), *reh'g,* 540 F. Supp. 761 (S.D. Ga. 1982).

Association of Mexican-American Educators v. California, 836 F. Supp. 1534 (N.D. Calif. 1993).

Association of Test Publishers. (2001). *Guidelines for computer-based testing.* Washington, DC: Author.

Brookhart v. Illinois State Board of Education, 697 F.2d 179 (7th Cir. 1983).

Buros Institute for Assessment Consultation and Outreach. (2002). *Standards for proprietary testing programs.* Lincoln, NE: Author.

Debra P. v. Turlington, 474 F. Supp. 244 (M.D. Fla. 1979), *aff'd in part, rev'd in part,* 644 F.2d 397 (5th Cir. 1981); *on remand,* 564 F. Supp. 177 (M.D. Fla. 1983), *aff'd,* 730 F.2d 1405 (11th Cir. 1984).

Doe v. St. Joseph's Hospital, 788 F. 2d 411 (7th Cir. 1986).

Equal Employment Opportunity Commission, Civil Service Commission, Department of Labor, and Department of Justice. (1978, August 25). Uniform guidelines on employee selection procedures. *Federal Register, 43,* 38290–38315.

GI Forum et al. v. TEA et al., F.Supp., 1 (W.D. Tex. 2000).

Hazelwood School District v. United States, 97 S. Ct. 2736 (1977).

Mehrens, W. A., & Pophem, W. J. (1992). How to evaluate the legal defensibility of high-stakes tests. *Applied Measurement in Education, 5*(3), 265–283.

Messick, S. (1989). Validity. In R. L. Linn (Ed.), *Educational Measurement* (3rd ed., pp. 13–103). Washington, DC: American Council on Education.

Phillips, S. E. (1996). Legal defensibility of standards: Issues and policy perspectives. *Educational Measurement: Issues and Practices, 15*(2), 5–13, 19.

Phillips, S. E. (2000). GI Forum v. Texas Education Agency: Psychometric evidence. *Applied Measurement in Education, 13*(4), 343–385.

Pitoniak, M. J., & Royer, J. M. (2001). Testing accommodations for examinees with disabilities: A review of psychometric, legal, and social policy issues. *Review of Educational Research, 71*(1), 53–104.

Richardson v. Lamar County Board of Education, 729 F. Supp. 806 (1989).

Shoben, E. (1978). Differential pass-fail rates in employment testing: Statistical proof under Title VII. *Harvard Law Review, 91,* 793–813.

Smisko, A., Twing, J. S., & Denny, P. (2000). The Texas model for content and curricular validity. *Applied Measurement in Education, 13*(4), 333–342.

Society for Industrial and Organizational Psychology. (2003). *Principles for the validation and use of personnel selection procedures.* College Park, MD: Author.

Title VI of the Civil Rights Act of 1964, 42 U.S.C.S. §2000d (1999).

Title VII of the Civil Rights Act of 1964, 42 U.S.C.S. §2000e-2(a)(1) (1999).

Tyler v. Vickery, 517 F.2d 1089, (5th Cir. 1975), *cert. denied,* 426 U.S. 940 (1976).

United States Constitution Amendment XIV, §1.

Webb, N. L. (1997). *Criteria for alignment of expectations and assessments in mathematics and science education.* Madison, WI: National Institute for Science Education and Washington, DC: Council of Chief State School Officers.

8

Teaching For the Test: How and Why Test Preparation Is Appropriate

Linda Crocker
University of Florida

One flashpoint in the incendiary debate over standardized testing in American public schools is the area of test preparation. As noted by Smith, Smith, and DeLisi (2001), "we exist in an era in which student testing and the rigorous standards associated with testing seem to be the educational position of choice amongst politicians. Test scores have become the coin of the realm in education, and with that, concerns about how to get students to do well on tests has risen" (p. 87). Critics of standardized testing often voice at least two types of concern about test preparation:

1. Test preparation requires drilling students on a narrow set of low-level skills covered on the test, ignoring material that would have been covered had the teacher been unfettered by demands of preparing students for the assessment (e.g., Kohn, 2000; Madaus, 1998; Popham, 2003; Smith & Rottenberg, 1991).
2. Instruction aimed at making students skillful test-takers on standardized assessments may be harmful to their educational development and thinking processes (e.g. Hillocks, 2002; Lattimore, 2001; Sacks, 1999).

The focus of this chapter is test preparation in achievement testing and its purportedly harmful effects on students and teachers. The intent is not to argue that educators, and policy makers should dismiss the above concerns, but rather to weigh these concerns realistically against the backdrop of assessment history, research findings, recommended practices for test preparation, and ethical standards of practice already available to mitigate such concerns. The chapter is organized into three major sections. The first section provides a rationale, definition, and historic background for the topic of preparing students for assessment. The second section outlines two broad elements of preparing students for assessment. The final section discusses teacher preparation and professional development in this area.

THE IMPORTANCE OF TEST-TAKING SKILLS

Many teachers view teaching of test-taking skills as a tawdry practice. They may avoid it or undertake instruction geared to preparing students to demonstrate their knowledge in a particular format—multiple choice, essay, and performance assessment—in a shamefaced or clandestine fashion. This unfortunate situation, largely engendered by critics of standardized testing, impedes student performance and harms teacher morale. Yet, more than 20 years ago, McPhail (1981) offered two worthy reasons for teaching test-taking skills: (a) "to improve the validity of test results" (p. 33) and (b) "to provide equal educational, employment, and promotional opportunity" (p. 34) particularly for disadvantaged students who often do not have access to additional educational resources enjoyed by their middle-class cohorts. This rationale remains compelling today.

In the highly mobile twenty-first century, students migrate with their parents across state and national borders, attend colleges thousands of miles from home, and apply for employment and graduate or professional studies in areas where their transcripts and other credentials cannot be measured on a common metric by those making the selection decisions. Standardized tests have become critical tools for decisions regarding college admission, college credits for high school work, graduate or school professional admission, and licensure for many blue-collar and white-collar professions. Put simply, no one becomes a physician, lawyer, teacher, nurse, accountant, electrician, fire-fighter, cosmetologist, or real estate broker without taking a series of tests. Caring, effective teachers should want to prepare their students for these future testing situations.

Furthermore the test-taking skills required by the short-essay or performance assessments, which now accompany the objective-item formats of many standardized assessments, have additional application to many real-world contexts in which individuals encounter demands for spontaneous written communications. Consider, for example, the following requests: "Explain why you have come to the clinic today and describe your symptoms;" "Describe how the accident occurred, and use diagrams, if necessary;" or "Describe your qualifications for the position." The ability to respond to a set of structured questions in a specific format has become a communications skill that is as vital in the repertoire of today's student as rhetoric was to the student of the nineteenth century. It is certainly as appropriate for teachers to impart these skills to students as it is for them to instruct them in other forms of oral and written communication.

DEFINITION OF TERMS

Test preparation, broadly defined, encompasses not only study of content from the domain of knowledge sampled by the assessment, but also practicing the skills that will allow students to demonstrate their knowledge on various types of assessment exercises.

Test-wiseness is commonly considered to be a construct representing an examinee's "capacity to utilize the characteristics and formats of the test and/or test-taking situation to receive a high score" (Millman, Bishop, & Ebel, 1965, p. 707).

Coaching refers to the actions of a teacher or expert in preparing examinees for a particular examination or type of examination.

A *norm-referenced test* is an assessment on which an individual's score is interpreted through comparison to the score distribution of a well-defined norm group who took the test at a given time. In a national norm-referenced achievement test, the exercises are designed and selected to sample content from various curricula used at a nationally representative sample of districts and schools, but the exercises may not systematically represent any particular, local curriculum.

A *criterion referenced test* is an assessment designed to sample specified curricular and/or instructional objectives on which an individual's score is interpreted in relation to a cut score or standard (e.g., a given number of items correctly answered on the current test or on a test form to which scores on the current test are linked).

High stakes assessment is assessment in which significant awards are given or sanctions imposed on individual students, teachers, or schools as result of performance.

HISTORICAL PERSPECTIVE ON TEST PREPARATION

College Admissions Testing. The seeds of test preparation and coaching sprouted first in the area of college admissions testing when Stanley Kaplan in 1946 began to tutor public high school students in Brooklyn for the SAT. Kaplan's approach to test preparation consisted of reviewing available descriptions of the test and asking examinees who previously had taken the test to remember and describe specific test items. He then created practice materials to use in tutoring students who were planning to take the test (Lemann, 1999). Because the SAT was originally conceived as an academic aptitude test, its content and form were deliberately designed not to conform to any one secondary curriculum but to present quantitative and verbal reasoning problems in new contexts. Thus security of the items (which were reused) was necessary to ensure fairness and comparability of examinees' scores. Consequently, coaching programs based primarily on information about test content, obtained through item memorization during live test administrations were controversial and widely regarded as a threat to test score validity (Allalouf & Ben-Shakhar, 1999). In addition, this type of test preparation for college admissions raises issues of fairness and access to opportunity because access to coaching schools, published practice materials, and tutors generally have been limited to those with greater financial resources.

Ultimately the most effective test preparation for the SAT or ACT is a rigorous academic high school curriculum, but experts also recommend that students should be familiar with what to expect in the testing mileau (Schmeisser, 2001). The acquisition of skills such as time management and practice with general item types (e.g., verbal analogies), item formats, and guessing strategies under formula scoring rules (which imposed a penalty for incorrect responses) have been long regarded as legitimate test preparation practices (e.g., Millman & Pauk, 1969). Taking practice tests (consisting of released, nonsecure test items) under time constraints similar to the live testing situation is encouraged to allow examinees to become familiar with item types and formats, test instructions, and test-taking conditions. Topical content areas tested are released so that examinees can review these areas as needed. Research on test preparation for the SAT and GRE has indicated that examinees who engage in such practices on average show some score gain upon retaking the test, but the estimates of the effect sizes vary depending upon the design of the studies and methods of data collection (Linn, 1990; Powers & Rock, 1999). Currently an emerging national trend in admissions and licensure testing is for applicants to receive free access to test preparation and practice materials in electronic formats (e.g., CD-ROMs or interactive websites) upon registration for tests to equalize access to preparation materials.

Advanced Placement Testing

By contrast, a large-scale testing program that generally has generated minimal controversy is the Advanced Placement (AP) program, administered by ETS, in which tests are used for awarding college credit to students on the basis of high school course work. Since the 1950s, a variety of AP high school courses have been created through cooperative efforts of university and secondary education faculty for the purpose of providing junior and senior high school students the opportunity to study introductory level college coursework prior to high school graduation. The course curricula are aligned to standardized assessments, administered at year end or semester end, with substantial stakes for individual students, in the form of college credit for those who receive a prespecified score. Teachers of AP courses plan and deliver instruction in their own ways, but their syllabi are designed to fit the core AP curriculum and they must cover material on schedule to ensure that their students are prepared by the date of the test. AP teachers have access to practice tests and their students generally participate in multiple practice test sessions. The AP assessments, consisting of both multiple choice and constructed response exercises, are developed and scored by ETS, and distributed to universities designated by the student.

More than 70% of the high schools in 23 states offer AP courses; in an additional 11 states, 50% to 69% of the high schools offer such courses; only four states offer AP courses in fewer than 25% of their high schools (Doherty & Skinner, 2003). This popular, long-established instructional and testing program provides a strong counterexample to testing critics' fears. It demonstrates that a prescribed curriculum coupled with an externally administered end-of-course assessment per se does not automatically result in drill-and-practice instruction, avoidance of challenging subject material, or mind-numbing assignments.

Preparation for School Assessment

Until the late 1960s, few states had developed unique statewide achievement testing programs. Many school districts administered norm-referenced standardized test batteries, but results were not compared across districts and often not reported outside of the school building. The notable exceptions were Ohio, Washington, and New York, with only the New York examination meeting the definition of a high-stakes assessment (see Angel, 1968). The New York Regents Scholarship Examination, implemented in the late 1800s, used for the award of the Regents' Diploma and subsequent tuition awards to state universities, was the statewide achievement test with the greatest stakes attached for individual examinees in this era, and was generally recognized has having a significant impact on classroom instruction in New York (Tinkleman, 1966).

But in 1965, the landscape of standardized achievement testing in the United States was altered significantly by new Federal legislation: The Elementary and Secondary Education Act (ESEA). Title I of this act was a specific provision for funding state and local school districts (LEAs) for enhanced education of children from low-income homes. The impact on school testing resulted from a requirement for LEAs to adopt effective procedures for evaluation, including objective, standardized testing, to provide evidence that the programs were improving the learning of poor children. Subsequent amendments to the original ESEA strengthened the teeth of this requirement to bring LEAs into greater conformity in their evaluation efforts. Within 10 years, the vast majority of districts used the norm-referenced model, wherein children were tested on norm-referenced standardized achievement tests and their gains were assessed against the test norm.

As the external monitoring of these programs became more stringent and the number of children enrolled in Title I programs increased (along with the commensurate funding), teachers felt increasing pressure to prepare students for norm-referenced tests so that instructional and support services for delivery of these programs at school and district levels could be maintained. The accuracy of results of district and state norm-referenced achievement testing was called into question sharply by the publication of a report entitled, "Nationally Normed Elementary Achievement Testing in America's Public Schools: How All Fifty States Are Above Average" (Cannell, 1987). This phenomenon of alleged test-score inflation was dubbed the *Lake Wobegon Effect* referring to the fictional Minnesota community in Garrison Keillor's radio monologues where "all the women are strong, all the men are good-looking, and all the children are above average." A variety of explanations were proffered for this finding, including the possibility of overzealous test preparation by classroom teachers and school administrators (Linn, Graue, & Sanders, 1990; Shepard, 1990). Whatever the cause, the credibility of norm-referenced standardized tests as high-stakes measures of school performance was in question.

In the 1970s and 1980s, many states also implemented criterion-referenced state assessment programs to combat critics' charges that norm-referenced tests inevitably created "winners" and "losers" but offered limited information to guide instructional planning (Popham, 1992). Unfortunately, the basis for many of these assessments were objectives based on minimal competencies, so that critics then charged that these assessments caused teachers to focus on relatively low expectations for students (Shortfalls, 1994). By 1994, 45 states had created testing programs for students in K–12 schools, but only a handful had a formal statewide curriculum that would give teachers or students guidance about what to expect and few of these had differentiated benchmarks for desired levels of performance. This led authors of a national study called the New Standards Project to conclude, "We have a history of not training students in the material they will be tested on. Other countries don't hide the tests from the students" (Jennings, 1998, p. 5).

As the twenty-first century arrived, a new accountability movement was afoot under the watchwords of *high and rigorous standards* and *standards-based assessment*. *Standards-based assessment*s are composed of exercises that can be linked to specific content standards in each tested subject (e.g., reading, mathematics, science, etc.) and on which performance standards for accomplishment have been established. *Content standards* are descriptions of what students should know and be able to do in a given subject and are widely available to teachers for use in planning instruction. *Performance standards* are levels of proficiency on the score scale of an assessment, related to specific performance benchmarks. The No Child Left Behind Act of 2001, requiring annual testing of nearly all students in mathematics and reading in Grades 3 through 8 and once in high school using standards-based assessments by 2005–2006 has placed substantial testing and accountability requirements on states (Doherty & Skinner, 2003). This movement has thrust the debate on appropriate test preparation practices to center stage of the ongoing controversy surrounding standardized testing.

PREPARING STUDENTS FOR ASSESSMENT

Teaching "to" the test has a negative connotation among teachers, students, and school administrators. It generally refers to targeting and delivering instruction geared solely at the content or format of a particular test for the express purpose of increasing examinee scores. It implies that improvements in test score performance may not represent corresponding increases in knowledge of the broader universe of content that is sampled by the test specifications and test items.

Teaching for assessment, as used in this chapter, has a broader connotation. It refers to teaching students the broader content domain represented by the curricular standards, not simply to that subset of content sampled by the items on a single test form. Four essential elements of teaching for the assessment include (a) a challenging core curriculum, (b) comprehensive instruction in that curriculum, (c) developing students' test-taking skills, and (d) adherence to ethical guidelines regarding preparation of students for assessment. The next sections of this chapter address these elements.

Curriculum Alignment Versus Measurement Driven Instruction

One of the greatest fears of testing opponents is that with high-stakes assessments, teachers will be shackled to teaching content that is easily tested in restricted formats, and forced to subvert their professional judgment and restrict their efforts to covering only that content likely to appear on high-stakes tests at the expense of more comprehensive student learning. This latter view has given rise to such phrases as *curricular reductionism, measure-*

ment-driven curriculum. Many accountability advocates, however, are comfortable with the notion that standardized achievement tests, particularly those tied to state-developed curricular standards, legitimately should play a vital role in shaping curricular and instructional practice. As one district level assessment expert noted, "Often you will hear teachers complain that they have to teach something because it is on the test. If a test is the only reason that students are taught concepts such as graphing data, writing hypotheses, genres in literature, or the Pythagorean theorem, then thank goodness for tests!" (see Wilson, 2002, p. 17). Their comfort arises from the notion of curricular alignment and its distinction from measurement-driven instruction. Most accountability advocates would view curriculum alignment as desirable, but would view measurement driven instruction as abdication of professional responsibility.

Curricular alignment is the process of selecting or developing an assessment to ensure that test objectives and exercises are representative of the content domain defined by a prescribed curriculum or set of objectives. It also refers to systematic adaptation of a classroom curriculum to include specific content objectives covered on an assessment. By contrast, *measurement-driven instruction* emphasizes specific content or processes solely because that material is likely to be included on a particular assessment, while de-emphasizing other important aspects of the curriculum that are untested. Unfortunately in practice, the boundary between beneficial curriculum alignment and detrimental measurement-driven instruction is often ambiguous (see Koretz, McCaffrey, & Hamilton, 2001).

Classroom Instructional Practices

It is noteworthy that, despite the great concerns about measurement driven instruction, after reviewing empirical research literature, both Mehrens (1998) and Cizek (2002) found relatively sparse evidence to support the claims of negative consequences of classroom teachers' test preparation on student learning. However, when Stecher (2002) also found "little evidence about the extent of negative coaching," he suggested this may be due "in part because it is so difficult to detect" (p. 95). He maintained that mounting evidence of score inflation suggests widespread curricular alignment and coaching practices with potential negative consequences.

A continuum of approaches to test preparation, offered by Smith et al., (2001) is useful to classroom teachers in differentiating curriculum alignment from measurement-driven instruction. The first four stages of this continuum are as follows:

1. Teach ... without paying attention to the standardized test and hope that the students' abilities will show through on the assessment.

2. Spend most of your time in instruction as you normally do, but spend some time going over item formats to be found on the assessment so that students will be familiar with these formats ....
3. Analyze the content of the assessment, make certain that you cover the content in your regular instructional program, then work on item format and test-taking skills as well.
4. Analyze the content of the assessment and restructure your instructional program around that content exclusively. Then in addition engage in Item 3 above. (pp. 90–91)

Approach 1 illustrates teaching without test preparation and without curricular alignment. Approach 2 illustrates instruction without curricular alignment, but with some attention to test-taking skills. Approach 4 crosses the line toward measurement-driven instruction. Approach 3 describes a reasonable balance of instruction with curricular alignment and instruction in test-taking skills, especially there is a concerted effort to teach subject-matter knowledge and test-taking skills that will have broad utility to the students beyond this immediate examination situation. Two important caveats of Approach 3 are that (a) the assessment represents a good sample of the core curriculum, and (b) the core curriculum is worthy and important.

Developing Test-Taking Skills

A taxonomy of elements of test-taking skills, developed by Millman et al. (1965) includes the following categories: time-using strategies, error-avoidance strategies, guessing strategies (that make use of student's partial knowledge), and deductive reasoning strategies. Most well-designed interventions aimed at developing student test-taking skills involve learning and practice activities in all of these categories.

Research on Test Preparation.   In the 1980s, research on the effectiveness of test preparation strategies for school achievement tests flourished. A substantial meta-analysis, of the effects of 30 controlled studies on coaching for achievement tests, revealed that test preparation programs generally had positive impact on test scores, raising student scores on average by approximately one-quarter standard deviation. Furthermore, the greatest effects were achieved by longer programs that incorporated more opportunities to practice and that were designed to improve broad cognitive skills (Bangert-Drowns, Kulik, & Kulik, 1983). Even young children can benefit from appropriate instruction in test-taking strategies (Sarnacki, 1979; Scruggs, White, & Bonnur, 1986). For example, Callenbach (1973) devised a treatment requiring second graders to listen to oral directions over an extended period of time, understand the directions, ask for clarification if confused, and mark an answer booklet according to directions, which resulted in a positive effect of nearly one quarter of a standard deviation for students receiving the instruction.

Elements of Effective Test Preparation. Test preparation and good teaching can go hand in hand. Development of good test-taking skills is not a frenzied activity to be tackled just prior to administration of a major assessment, but rather a year-long activity to be incorporated into classroom instruction throughout the year for greatest effectiveness. An compilation of illustrative suggestions for test preparation from a sampling of sources is provided (Brown, 1982; Campanile, 1981; Crocker & Hombo, 1997; McPhail, 1981; Mehrens, Popham, & Ryan, 1998; Millman & Pauk, 1969; Smith et al., 2001; Wilson, 2002):

1. Always demonstrate a positive attitude in talking with students and parents about tests;
2. Build concentration endurance in test-like conditions over the course of a year, working from shorter to longer tests until students can work for the length of test standardized test period without becoming fatigued or distracted;
3. Practice listening to and reading instructions similar to those used on standardized tests, working sample items, and asking questions if they do not understand the directions;
4. Occasionally use separate answer sheets that require bubbling or circling the correct response.
5. Review responses to practice tests and explain why incorrect answers are incorrect;
6. Provide students with practice on timed tests and teach them how to be self-monitoring in using their time wisely;
7. Model good problem-solving strategies when demonstrating how to approach test items;
8. Talk through the problems to help students learn how to determine what question the item is really asking;
9. Encourage students to explain how they arrived at correct answers;
10. Teach students different ways that questions can be posed (e.g., inclusion of irrelevant information, backward thinking);
11. Provide practice with a variety of item formats;
12. Vary item difficulty to expose students to challenging items. This gives them practice in continuing to work through a test even if they encounter items that they cannot answer.
13. Have students practice systematic strategies for choosing one best answer for multiple-choice items (e.g., eliminate obviously incorrect responses and compare remaining responses. Select response that most

closely addresses the question, not simply a response that contains true information that is irrelevant to the question.)

14. Have students practice in reviewing their item responses and deciding when response change is indicated;

15. Grade homework and classwork diagnostically, being on the lookout for individual student response patterns that should be corrected before testing. For example, does Sarah frequently miscopy numbers in setting up math problems? Does James not label his diagrams? Does Marty only complete the first step of a two-stage problem? Does Sue often focus on irrelevant information in the paragraph?

16. Teach students to check on the reasonableness of answers to math problems. If possible, the numeric solution should be inserted into a sentence to answer the question (e.g., "Mary washed _____ cars.") to see if it makes sense.

17. Build students' test-taking vocabulary, using terms that they are likely to encounter on tests in various disciplines. For example, in eighth-grade mathematics, students should be able to read and comprehend terms such as *digit, numeral, quotient, remainder, direction, fraction, decimal, sum, difference, estimate,* and *multiply.* Do not assume that students will recognize a word in print, simply because they recognize its meaning orally. For example, many high school students hear and understand the word *genre* in English class, but fail to recognize it in print.

18. Give students practice on various types of tasks that test exercises may present. For example, some math problems require the student to specify only the correct operation, others require solving the problems, and still others require identification of an error in a solution. Even simple variations such as vertical or linear set-ups of computational problems should be practiced.

19. Teach students the types of phrases commonly used in reading items that require inferences or conclusions from reading passages rather than simply factual information, so that they do not spend valuable time reading and rereading trying to locate an answer which is implied but not specifically stated.

20. For performance assessment items, explain how score rubrics are used to award points and provide students with examples of responses to practice items that would generate full, partial, or no credit. Help students learn to evaluate their own responses.

Upon reviewing this list of recommended practices, four points seem obvious. First, development of good test-taking skills is not limited to low-level content or basic cognitive processes. These generic skills are as applicable in elementary mathematics as they are in AP calculus or twelfth grade English.

Second, students who develop good testing skills also acquire a repertoire of problem-solving skills that will enhance study habits and future learning. Third, good test-taking skills are not a "bag of tricks" enabling students who know nothing about the content domain to achieve high scores. Rather, these skills allow students to demonstrate what they know (or do not know) about the material without interfering "noise" in the scores resulting from lack of familiarity with the assessment format. Finally, instruction in test-taking skills should be grounded in content, offering practice and reinforcement in application of newly acquired content knowledge.

Ethical Test Preparation Strategies

Even as research was emerging to document that some teachers were engaged in inappropriate test preparation practices (Herman & Golan, 1993; Smith & Rottenberg, 1991), measurement experts focused attention on criteria for evaluating the propriety of test preparation strategies. For example, Mehrens and Kaminski (1989) proposed a well-known continuum for the appropriateness of various test preparation practices in terms of their contribution to validity of test score interpretations. The most appropriate practices enhance student knowledge of subject matter while improving their test performance (e.g., using estimation skills in mathematics to check on the accuracy of a solution). Acceptable practices are those designed to help students improve scores using test-taking skills (e.g., practice with a variety of item formats and budgeting time). Activities at the inappropriate end of the continuum are designed to improve student scores on a particular test with no increase in generalizable knowledge or skill (e.g., practice on a test form that closely parallels the form to be given or practice on items that will appear on the test form to be used.)

From these efforts, four broad criteria have emerged which are widely used by measurement professionals in judging the appropriateness of test preparation activities:

1. Academic ethics: Test preparation should be consistent with the ethical canons of the education profession, dealing with cheating, misrepresentation, and respect for intellectual property or work of others (Popham, 1991);
2. Validity: Test preparation should improve validity of test scores by allowing only students who have knowledge or partial knowledge of content being tested in an exercise to display that knowledge (AERA, APA, & NCME, 1999);
3. Transferability: Test preparation should provide student with skills that have applicability to a broad range of testing situations (Mehrens et al., 1998; Popham, 1992);

4. Educational value: test preparation that leads to improvement in student scores should simultaneously increase student mastery of the content domain tested (AERA et al., 1999; Popham, 1991; Reeves, 2001).

Test preparation activities that meet these criteria will be worthwhile, effective, and improve both student learning and assessment quality.

PREPARING TEACHERS WHO CAN PREPARE STUDENTS FOR ASSESSMENT

CRITICS of testing seem convinced that, given the high stakes now attached to some assessments, teachers will abandon their professional responsibilities to teach a balanced curriculum in preference for a narrowly focused measurement-driven approach to instruction. No doubt, there are cases in which this has occurred. For example, in a survey of more than 2,000 teachers in one state, 25% reported such questionable practices as directly teaching vocabulary words and 10% reported teaching items that would appear on the current year's test (Nolen, Haladyna, & Haas, 1992). However, many widely advocated educational practices (e.g., cooperative learning, phonemic awareness, whole-language instruction, or use of calculators) have been implemented by some teachers in ineffective, or even counterproductive, ways. Such events, do not lead to a clamor to abandon these instructional innovations, but rather to calls for emphasizing them more in teacher education and professional development programs. Logically, then should we not urge that teachers need more preparation in how to appropriately prepare their students for assessment?

What should teacher preservice and inservice professional development programs include to prepare teachers who can teach for standardized tests in effective, legitimate ways? Teachers must be armed with appropriate knowledge, attitudes, skills, and ethical values about test preparation or their efforts may actually undermine student test performance. Crocker (2003) suggested five areas of assessment training that should be addressed in teacher preservice education or inservice professional development and identified specific instructional activities for teacher preparation in each area. Incorporating these areas and activities into teacher preparation could result in teachers who: (a) are well-informed about assessment history and the current movement; (b) display positive attitudes toward assessment of student learning; (c) demonstrate competence in integrating effective test preparation learning activities into day-to-day instruction in content areas; (d) can readily discriminate between ethical and unethical test preparation activities; and (e) are prepared to collaborate as professional partners in large-scale test development and validation activities, such as item review, standard setting, and score-reporting tryouts.

CONCLUSION

In the current accountability movement, policy makers have established strong expectations that teachers will provide instruction linked to state-wide core curricula and that students will approach the accompanying assessments armed with both content knowledge and skills to succeed on those assessments. Critics of testing have charged that instruction linked to preparation for assessment must be mind-numbing and antithetical to higher order thinking. The literature reviewed in this chapter offers substantial hope that these fears are exaggerated. Teaching students from a curriculum that has been aligned with challenging content standards and helping them develop test-taking skills is good instructional practice that can be offered in ways that are both ethical and pedagogically appropriate. We should not assume, however, that beginning teachers emerge from typical professional preparation programs with sufficient information or practice in these areas or even attitudes that are amenable to these practices. Gaps in teacher knowledge about appropriate methods of curricular alignment and ethical test preparation practices can, and will, lead to instructional lapses that will further fuel criticisms of assessment. The goal of having classroom teachers who are competent and enthusiastic about preparing students for assessment will be realized only if teacher educators can be convinced of its value. This means that continued investigation of the benefits (and negative side effects) of test preparation is needed. In the battle for the hearts and minds of teachers and those who prepare teachers, it should be research, not simply rhetoric, that carries the day.

REFERENCES

Allalouf, A., & Ben-Shakhar, G. (1998). The effect of coaching on the predictive validity of scholastic aptitude test. *Journal of Educational Measurement, 35,* 31–47.

American Educational Research Association (AERA), American Psychological Association (APA), & National Council on Measurement in Education (NCME). (1999). *Standards for educational and psychological testing.* Washington DC: Author.

Angel, J. L. (1968). National, state, and other external testing programs. *Review of Educational Research, 38,* 85–91.

Bangert-Drowns, R. L., Kulik, J. A., & Kulik, C. C. (1983). Effects of coaching programs on achievement test performance. *Review of Educational Research, 53,* 571–586.

Brown, D. (1982, February). Increasing test-wiseness in children. *Elementary School Guidance and Counseling,* 180–185.

Callenbach, C. (1973). The effects of instruction and practice in content-independent test-taking techniques upon the standardized reading test scores of selected second grade students. *Journal of Educational Measurement, 10,* 25–30.

Campanile, P. (1981, March). Evening up the score. *Instructor,* 58–59.

Cannell, J. J. (1987). *Nationally normed elementary achievement testing in America's schools: How all fifty states are above the national average.* Daniels, WV: Friends for Education.

Cizek, G. J. (2002). More unintended consequences of high-stakes testing. *Educational Measurement: Issues & Practice, 20*(4), 19–27.

Crocker, L. (2003). Teaching for the test: Validity, fairness, and moral action. *Educational Measurement: Issues and Practice, 3,* 5–10.

Crocker, L., & Hombo, C. (1997). Teaching test-taking skills. *The Education Advisor, 1*(8), 1–5.

Doherty, K. M., & Skinner, R. A. (2003, January 9). State of the states. *Education Week, 22*(17), 75–103.

Herman, J. L., & Golan, S. (1993). The effects of standardized testing on teachers and schools. *Educational Measurement: Issues and Practice, 12*(4), 20–25, 41.

Hillocks, G., Jr. (2002). *The testing trap.* NY: Teachers College, Columbia University.

Jennings, J. F. (1998). *Why national standards and tests?* Thousand Oaks: Sage.

Kohn, A. (2000, September 27). Standardized testing and its victims: Inconvenient facts and inevitable consequences. *Education Week, 60,* 46.

Koretz, D., McCaffrey, D., & Hamilton, L. (2001). Toward a framework for validating gains under high-stakes conditions. *CSE Technical Report 551.* Los Angeles: National Center for Research on Evaluation, Standards and Student Testing.

Lattimore, R. (2001). The wrath of high stakes tests. *Urban Review, 33*(1), 57–67.

Lemann, N. (1999). *The big test.* New York: Farrar, Strauss and Giroux.

Linn, R. L. (1990). Admissions testing: Recommended uses, validity, differential prediction, and coaching. *Applied Measurement in Education, 3,* 297–318.

Linn, R. L., Graue, M. E., & Sanders, N. M. (1990). Comparing state and district test results to national norms: The validity of the claims that "everyone is above average." *Educational Measurement: Issues and Practice, 9*(3), 5–14.

Madaus, G. (1998). The distortion of teaching and testing: High-stakes testing and instruction. *Peabody Journal of Education, 65,* 29–46.

McPhail, I. P. (1981, October). Why teach test-wiseness? *Journal of Reading,* 32–37.

Mehrens, W. A. (1998). Consequences of assessment: What is the evidence? *Educational Policy Analysis Archives, 6*(13), 1–16.

Mehrens, W. A., & Kaminski, J. (1989). Methods for improving standardized test scores: Fruitful, fruitless, or fraudulent? *Educational Measurement: Issues and Practice, 8*(1), 14–22.

Mehrens, W. A., Popham, W. J., & Ryan, J. M. (1998). How to prepare students for performance assessments. *Educational Measurement: Issues & Practice, 17*(1), 18–22.

Millman, J., Bishop, C. H., & Ebel, R. L. (1965). An analysis of test wiseness. *Educational and Psychological Measurement, 25,* 707–726.

Millman, J., & Pauk, W. (1969). *How to take tests.* New York: McGraw Hill.

Nolan, S. B., Haladyna, T. M., & Haas, N. S. (1992). Uses and abuses of achievement test scores. *Education Measurement: Issues & Practice, 11,* 9–15.

Popham, W. J. (1991). Appropriateness of teachers' test-preparation practices. *Educational Measurement: Issues and Practice, 10,*12–15.

Popham, W. J. (1992). A tale of two test-specification strategies. *Educational Measurement: Issues & Practice, 11*(2), 16–17, 22.

Popham, W. J. (2003). Seeking redemption for our psychometric sins. *Educational Measurement: Issues and Practice, 22*(1) 45–48.

Powers, D. E., & Rock, D. A. (1999). Effects of coaching on SAT I: Reasoning test scores. *Journal of Educational Measurement, 36*, 93–118.

Reeves, D. B. (2001). Standards make a difference: The influence of standards on classroom assessment. *NASSP Bulletin, 85*, 5–12.

Sacks, P. (1999). *Standardized minds.* Cambridge, MA: Perseus.

Sarnacki, R. E. (1979). An examination of test wiseness in the cognitive domain. *Review of Educational Research, 49*, 252–279.

Schmeiser, C. B. (2001). Promoting a healthy environment for college admissions testing. *NASSP Bulletin, 85*, 27–36.

Scruggs, T. E., White, K. P., & Bonnur, K. (1986). Teaching test-taking skills to elementary grade students: A meta-analysis, *The Elementary School Journal, 87*, 69–82.

Shepard, L. A. (1990). Inflated test score gains: Is the problem old norms or teaching to the test? *Educational Measurement: Issues and Practice, 9*(3), 15–22.

Shortfalls in 1980s reform: Refocused educational strategies on the results of schooling. (1994, July). *R&D Preview*, p. 6.

Smith, M. L., & Rottenberg, C. (1991). Unintended consequences of external testing in elementary schools. *Educational Measurement: Issues & Practices, 10*(4), 7–11.

Smith, J. K., Smith, L. F., & DeLisi, R. (2001). *Natural classroom assessment.* Thousand Oaks, CA: Corwin.

Stecher, B. M. (2002). Consequences of large-scale, high-stakes testing on school and classroom practice. In L. S. Hamilton, B. M. Stecher, & S. P. Klein, (Eds.), *Making sense of test-based accountability in education.* Santa Monica: Rand.

Tinkleman, S. N. (1966). *Regents Examination in New York State after 100 years.* Albany: University of the State of New York, State Department of Education.

Wilson, L. W. (2002). *Better instruction through assessment.* Larchmont, NY: Eye on Education.

9

Doesn't Everybody Know That 70% is Passing?

Barbara S. Plake

Buros Center for Testing, University of Nebraska Lincoln

Standardized tests are used for many purposes. In high-stakes testing, test results are often used for making critically important decisions about people. Such decisions include which students are eligible for high school graduation, which applicants pass a licensure test, and who, among qualified applicants, will receive scholarships or other awards and prizes. In order to make these decisions, typically one or more score values are identified from the possible test scores to be the "passing score" or "cutscore." To most members of the public, the methods for determining these score values are a mystery. Many people believe that the often-used passing score from their educational experiences is the appropriate value for these purposes. For some, the familiar 70% of the total score points seems the appropriate passing score to use for these tests.

The purpose of this chapter is to describe several methods that can be used to set passing scores on tests. The chapter also presents strengths and weaknesses of these methods. It is hoped that the reader will gain an understanding of the principles and issues that need to be considered when setting passing scores on tests. Likewise, it is hoped that the reader will come to understand why using the "70% right" as the passing score is not an appropriate strategy for setting passing scores on high-stakes tests.

STANDARD SETTING METHODS

Setting passing scores, or cutscores, is often referred to as *standard setting*. This is because, by determining the passing score, the "standard" is set for the performance needed to pass the test. Standard-setting methods are often differentiated by whether they focus on the test takers (the examinee population) or on the test questions. Methods are presented that illustrate both of these approaches.

Examinee-Focused Methods

Two different examinee focused methods are discussed. The first method includes strategies whereby examinees are assigned to performance categories by someone who is qualified to judge their performance. The second method uses the score distribution on the test to make examinee classifications.

When using the first of these methods, people who know the examinees well (e.g., their teachers) are asked to classify them into performance categories. These performance categories could be simply *qualified to pass* or *not qualified to pass*, or more complex, such as *Basic*, *Proficient* and *Advanced*. When people make these classifications, they do not know how the examinee did on the test. After examinees are classified into the performance categories, the test score that best separates the classification categories is determined.

These examinee focused methods have substantial appeal due to their strong mathematical basis and because they are based on how examinees actually did on the test. However, there are also substantial limitations to the utility of these approaches. First, it is necessary that the examinees be classified into the performance categories by some person. In some applications (especially in education where these classification decisions are made for students by their teacher), the person making the classification decisions may have considerable information about the skill levels of the examinees. Even under these conditions, teachers are often not very accurate in making performance classifications for their students, even when they have been working with their students for nearly a full academic year (Impara & Plake, 1998). Students who are classified by their teachers in the lowest performance category, for example, sometimes perform very well on the test, even exceeding the average performance of students who were classified by their teachers into the *Advanced* performance category. Likewise, students who have been classified into the most advanced performance categories will sometimes do very poorly on the test, with test scores that are below the average score on the test by the students classified into the lowest performance category. Because of these problems with classifications into performance categories, there is often less certainty about the appropriate values for the cutscores from these methods.

Even more challenging is the use of these examinee-based methods in licensure and certification testing. Most often, the skills of the examinees are not well known prior to their taking the test. In fact, it is the purpose of the test to learn if these examinees have the needed skills to pass the test. The fact that the skills of the examinees are not known in advance of the test limits the usefulness of examinee-based methods for determining the cutscores in licensure and certification testing.

The second general approach to setting cutscores using examinee performance data are *norm-based methods*. When using norm-based methods, the scores from the current examinee are summarized, calculating the average (or mean) of the set of scores and some measure of how spread out across the score range the test scores fall (variability). In some applications, the cutscore is set at the mean of the score distribution or the mean plus or minus a measure of score variability (standard deviation). Setting the passing score above the mean (say one standard deviation above the mean) would (in a bell-shaped score distribution) pass about 15% of the examinees; likewise, setting the passing score one standard deviation below the mean would fail about 15% of the examinees.

In other applications of norm-based methods, a quota system is used such that examinees are selected starting with the highest scoring examinee until all the available slots are filled. Thus the "passing score" is the score obtained by the lowest scoring examinee among those selected to fill the quota.

The rationale for using this approach is that some people feel this is a fair method for setting the passing score because it adjusts the expectation for passing based on how well examinees did on the test. This is similar to "grading on the curve" that many people have experienced in their educational programs. There are serious problems with these norm-based approaches, however. These problems are especially severe in licensure and certification settings. In those settings, it is necessary that persons who pass the test have the requisite skills and competencies to function effectively (and safely). If the passing score is based on how the group of examinees performed on the test, there is little assurance that passing examinees will be qualified. This is because all we know is that the passing examinees did "better" than those who did not. It could be the case that none of the examinees have the skills needed to perform on the job, but that there were some who were better skilled than others who took the test. However, they may still not be qualified to perform in the designated profession. Another concern is the continuity of standards across examinee groups. It is often the case in licensure and certification testing, that examinees who take the test at different times of the year have different overall skill levels. The test administration that coincides most closely with the end of the training or educational program often has the highest number of examinees and typically they are the most skilled. Later administrations often include examinees who did not pass an earlier administration and who have not as recently completed their training. Therefore, the skill levels of the examinees who score at or above the mean on the first administration will likely be higher than the skill levels of the examinees who score at or above the mean on subsequent administrations. However, if the passing score was set after each administration, less able examinees would likely pass the examination if they took it at a different test administration. This is not only unfair to the examinees (who may pass or fail not only as a function of their skill levels but also based on the skill levels of the examinees who also took the test at the same test administration) but also risky for the public who will not know whether or not the person they are using in a profession has been warranted to have the needed skill levels to competently function in that profession.

Test-Based Methods

Test-based methods for setting passing scores consider the questions that comprise the test. In a limited way, the "70% correct" method could be considered a test-based method because it is based on the total number of questions in the test. However, this isn't really a test-based method because the content of the questions is not taken into account. The problem with the 70% correct approach is that it does not reflect the difficulty of the questions in the test. It is possible to construct a test where achieving 70% correct would be trivial and not indicate that the needed level of performance on the content has been reached. Likewise, a very difficult test could be developed so that hardly anyone, regardless of their skill level, could pass the test. Therefore, only knowing that a certain percentage of the total number of test questions has been answered correctly does not assure that the skill levels of examinees who pass the test are at the required levels for passing the test.

Before discussing test-based methods, it is necessary to know more about the kinds of questions that comprise the test. Many licensure and certification tests are composed of multiple-choice test questions. These questions (sometimes called *items*) have a question and then several (often four) answer choices from which the examinee selects the right or best answer. Some licensure tests have as few as 30 to 50 questions whereas others have nearly 800. Multiple-choice test questions are often favored by licensure and certification boards because they are quick and easy to score and, with careful test construction efforts, can cover a broad range of content in a reasonable length of testing time. Other tests have questions that ask the examinee to write an answer, not select an answer from a set list (e.g., with multiple choice questions).

Sometimes these types of questions are called *constructed-response* questions because the examinee is required to construct a response. Some licensure and certification agencies find these kinds of questions appealing because they are more directly related, in some situations, to the actual work that is required by the occupation or profession. These types of questions also are frequently seen in educational testing for several reasons. First, some educational outcomes are not well measured by multiple-choice questions. Writing skills are a good example. Multiple-choice questions could measure whether an examinee knows grammatical rules or whether they can select a more compelling argument in a persuasive essay, but they are not good measures of whether the examinee can write a persuasive argument that uses good grammar. Second, some examinees are better able to demonstrate their skill levels through constructed response questions than with multiple-choice questions. Therefore, if a high-stakes decision were based on examinee test performance (e.g., high school eligibility or licensing a dentist), it may be desirable to allow the examinee different ways to demonstrate his or her levels of skill and competency.

A limitation of these kinds of questions is the additional time they require, both for administration and for scoring. Because they take longer for an examinee to complete, less content can be covered than in the same amount of time for a multiple-choice test administration. Further, at least until recently, these constructed response questions needed to be scored by human raters who had been trained to accurately score the examinee responses. This has two ramifications: more cost is incurred for the scoring and more time is needed to complete the scoring. Recently, computer systems have been developed to score answers to some types of constructed response questions. At least one high-stakes testing program is using one human scorer and a computerized scoring system. Both methods are used for each essay, with rules on how to reconcile any score differences between the computerized score and the score provided by the human rater.

There is another type of question that sometimes appears in licensure, called *performance tasks*. These kinds of tasks are also sometimes used in educational settings, especially in the sciences. With performance tasks, examinees are asked to perform a task that is similar to what they would be asked to do in the profession. For example, dentists must demonstrate their skills on actual patients. Sometimes simulations (using actors or mannequins) are used instead of having unlicensed persons work with human subjects in some medical fields.

The methods used for setting passing scores will vary based on the type of questions and tasks that comprise the test. In every case, however, a panel of experts is convened (called *subject matter experts*, or SMEs). Their task is to work with the test content in determining the recommended minimum passing score for the test, or in some situations, the multiple cutscores for making performance classifications for examinees (e.g., *Basic*, *Proficient*, and *Advanced*).

Multiple-Choice Questions

Until recently, most of the tests that were used in standard setting contained only multiple-choice questions. The reasons for this were mostly because of the ability to obtain a lot of information about the examinees' skill levels in a limited amount of time. The ease and accuracy of scoring were also a consideration in the popularity of the multiple-choice test question in high-stakes testing. Two frequently used standard setting methods for multiple-choice questions are described in this chapter.

Angoff Method.   The most prevalent method for setting cutscores on multiple-choice tests for making pass–fail decisions is the Angoff method (1971). Using this method, SMEs are asked to conceptualize an examinee who is just barely qualified to function in the profession (called the *minimally competent candidate*, or MCC). Then, for each item in the test, the SMEs are asked to estimate the probability that a randomly selected MCC would be able to correctly answer the item. The SMEs work independently when making these predictions. Once these predictions have been completed, the probabilities assigned to the items in the test are added together for each SME. Therefore, each SME will have an estimate of the minimum passing score for the test. These estimates are then averaged across the SMEs to determine the overall minimum passing score. Because the SMEs will vary in their individual estimates of the minimum passing score, it is possible to also compute the variability in their minimum passing score estimates. The smaller the variability, the more cohesive the SMEs are in their estimates of the minimum passing score. Sometimes this variability is used to adjust the minimum passing score to be either higher or lower than the average value.

In most applications of the Angoff standard-setting method, more than one set of estimates is obtained from the SMEs. The first set (described previously) is often called *Round 1*. After Round 1, SMEs are typically given additional information. For example, they may be told the groups' Round 1 minimum passing score value and the range so they can learn about the level of cohesion of the panel at this point. Sometimes they will be told their individual estimate of the minimum passing score (typically privately so that their minimum passing score estimate isn't revealed to the full panel). In addition, it is common for the SMEs to be told how recent examinees performed on the test. This may include the proportion of examinees who answered each item correctly (a measure of the item's difficulty) and the consequences of using the panel's Round 1 minimum passing score on the passing rate. The sharing of examinee performance information is somewhat controversial. However, it is often the case that SMEs need performance information as a reality check. SMEs may be somewhat removed from the skill level of the MCC and believe that MCCs are, as a group, more able than is reasonable. An individual SME, for example, may think that an item is easy, and that the probability that a MCC will answer the item correctly is .80. However, if the SME sees that only 30% of the total examinee group was able to correctly answer the question, then that SME may decide that he or she was being unrealistic in his or her first, Round 1 estimate. If data is given to the SMEs, then it is customary to conduct a second round of ratings, called *Round 2*. The minimum passing scores are then calculated using the Round 2 data in a manner identical to that for the Round 1 estimates. Again, panel's variability may be used to adjust the final recommended minimum passing score.

There have been many modifications to the Angoff method, so many in fact that there isn't a single, standard set of procedures that define the Angoff standard setting method. Variations include whether or not performance data is provided between rounds, whether there is more than one round, whether SMEs may discuss their ratings, and how the performance estimates are made by the SMEs. Another difference in the application of the Angoff method is in the definitions for the skill levels for the MCC. Obviously, if an SME is to estimate the probability that a randomly selected MCC will be able to answer the item correctly, the SME must have a clear understanding of the skills and competencies of the MCC. Depending on the leaders of the standard setting effort, more or less time may be devoted to defining and characterizing the skills and competencies of the MCCs.

Because the task posed to the SMEs is cognitively complex, some researchers have questioned whether the Angoff method is truly viable as a standard setting method. One of the variations to the Angoff method, called the *Yes/No Method* (Impara & Plake, 1997) attempts to reduce the cognitive demand by asking SMEs to keep in mind a typical MCC and to estimate whether that MCC would answer the item correctly. Research has shown that the Yes/No Method, using only Round 1, gives results consistently similar to the Angoff methods using two rounds. Therefore, the Yes/No Method does not rely on probability estimates by the SME, reduces the need for controversial performance data between rounds, and could stop after only one round, reducing the overall time needed to conduct the standard setting effort.

Bookmark Method.   Another standard-setting method that is used with multiple-choice questions (and also with mixed formats that include multiple-choice and constructed-response question) is called the *Bookmark*

Method (Mitzel, Lewis, Patz, & Green, 2001). In order to conduct this method, the test questions have to be assembled into a special booklet with one item per page and organized in ascending order of difficulty (easiest to hardest). SMEs are given a booklet and asked to page through the booklet until they encounter the first item that they believe that the MCC would have less than, for example, a 67% chance of answering correctly. They place their bookmark on the page prior to that item in the booklet. The number of items that precedes the location of the bookmark represents an individual SME's estimate of the minimum passing score. The percent level (here shown as 67%; values other than 67% are sometimes used) is called the *response probability* (RP). Individual SME's estimates of the minimum passing score are shared with the group, usually graphically. After discussion, SMEs reconsider their initial bookmark location. This usually continues through multiple rounds, with SME's minimum passing score estimates shared after each round. Typically there is large diversity in minimum passing score estimates after Round 1, but the group often reaches a small variability in minimum passing score estimates following the second or third round.

Currently, the Bookmark Method is used most often in educational settings where multiple cutscores are established. Sometimes the cutpoints are for *Basic*, *Proficient*, and *Advanced* categories of student performance. The method has appeal because of its task simplicity for the SMEs. In general, SMEs find the method easier to apply than the Angoff Method (even with the Yes/No variation). Cutscores are often similar across these two methods (Buckendahl, Smith, Impara, & Plake, 2002). The method requires more work in preparation of the standard setting effort because the test booklets need to be assembled with one item per page ordered in ascending difficulty. This may require weeks of preparation and some additional costs.

Constructed-Response Questions

As stated previously, constructed-response questions ask the examinee to prepare a response to a question. This could be solving a problem in mathematics, preparing a cognitive map for a reading passage, or presenting a critical reasoning essay on a current events topic. What is common across these tasks is that the examinee cannot select an answer but rather must construct one. In addition to providing more direct measures of some important skills that are not well measured by multiple-choice questions, it is unlikely that the examinee could correctly answer the questions by guessing. Another distinguishing feature of constructed-response questions is that they typically are worth more than one point. There is often a scoring rubric or scoring system used to determine the number of points an examinee's answer will receive for each test question.

There are several methods for setting standards on constructed-response tests. One method, called *Angoff Extension* (Hambleton & Plake, 1995) asks the SMEs to estimate the total number of points that the MCC is likely to earn out of the total available for that test question. The calculation of the minimum passing score is similar to that for the Angoff method, except that the total number of points awarded to each question is added to calculate the minimum passing score estimate for each SME. As with the Angoff method, multiple rounds are usually conducted with some performance data shared with the SMEs between rounds.

Another method used with constructed response questions is called the *Analytical Judgment* (AJ) method (Plake & Hambleton, 2000). For this method, SMEs read examples of examinee responses and assign them into multiple performance categories. For example, if the purpose is to set one cutscore (say, for *Passing*), the categories would be *Clearly Failing, Failing, Nearly Passing, Just Barely Passing, Passing,* and *Clearly Passing.* Usually a total of 50 examinee responses are collected for each constructed-response question, containing examples of low, middle, and high performance. Scores on the examples are not shown to the SMEs. After the SMEs have made their initial categorizations of the example papers into these multiple-performance categories, the examples that are assigned to the *Nearly Passing* and *Just Barely Passing* categories are identified. The scores on these examples are averaged and the average score is used as the recommended minimum passing score. Again, the variability of scores that were assigned to these two performance categories may be used to adjust the minimum passing score. An advantage of this method is that actual examinee responses are used in the standard-setting effort. A disadvantage of the method is that it considers the examinees' test responses question by question, without an overall consideration of the examinees' test performance. A variation of this method, called the *Integrated Judgment Method* (Jaeger & Mills, 2001) has SMEs consider the questions individually and then collectively in making only one overall test classification decision into the above multiple categories.

Other methods exist for use with constructed response questions but they are generally consistent with the two approaches identified above. Standard-setting methods for performance tasks are typically variations on the ones identified for constructed response questions. More information about these and other standard setting methods can be found in Cizek's (2001) book, *Setting Performance Standards: Concepts, Methods, and Perspectives.*

CONCLUSION

Tests are used for a variety of purposes. In some cases, test scores help to identify if an examinee has learned material taught in school, whether special services are needed to improve the student's level of knowledge, or whether a student has talent for certain kinds of programs. Many of these uses of tests could be considered low stakes because there are often other ways the information can be obtained and decisions made based on the test results can more be changed fairly easily. Other uses of test results are considered high stakes because the decisions that are made, in some cases, have more serious consequences for the examinee. If an examinee fails to pass a licensure test, for example, he or she will be denied the opportunity to practice in an occupation or profession for which he or she may have committed substantial time and resources preparing. Further, any salary that would have been available for practicing in the occupation will not be available to a person who does not pass the licensure test. Many times promotions or other rewards are available for persons who pass a certification examination; these resources and honors would be denied to a person who does not pass the examination. In many states, students must pass tests in reading and mathematics in order to be eligible to graduate from high school. Not passing the high school competency tests has serious consequences for these high school students.

Because these decisions are based on test performance, the score value for passing the test must be determined. This chapter presents several methods that are used to identify reasonable and defensible score values for making these important decisions. Typically, a standard-setting procedure is used to identify recommended values for these cutscores. The final decision about the value of the cutscore is a policy decision that should be made by the governing agency, such as the school board for high school graduation tests or the agency that has authority over the profession. For most licensure tests in the United States, states have the legal authority for governing access to these occupations and professions. Thus, legislative bodies in most cases have the authority to set passing scores on licensure tests. Professional organizations generally have the authority for setting passing scores on certification tests. Often these governing agencies are not trained in testing and in particular do not understand the need for conducting standard setting studies to learn what should be considered reasonable values for passing scores on these tests. The passing rule of 70% (or any other percent value) correct is often written into state legislation. One goal of this chapter is to educate the public on issues related to setting cutscores so that future governing agencies will be better informed about appropriate and fair methods for setting cutscores on these tests.

High-stakes testing serves an important purpose. It is desired to certify that the examinee does have the requisite skills and competencies needed to graduate from school programs, practice in an occupation or profession, or receive elevated status within a profession. These tests serve the public by certifying that students are learning needed skills through their high school programs and that the persons they seek for professional services have demonstrated levels of competency. If the passing scores on these tests are not set appropriately there is no assurance that these outcomes will be achieved. High school students who deserve to graduate may be denied a diploma and persons who have the needed skills may be denied the opportunity to practice in their chosen occupation or profession. Possibly even worse, students who have not learned what was intended in their educational programs may be given high school diplomas and persons who are not qualified will be allowed to practice in their chosen occupation or profession on an unsuspecting public. Therefore, it is critically important that sound methods are used when determining these cutscores. The standard setting methods presented in this chapter are some of the ways that fair, appropriate, and defensible cutscores can be set.

REFERENCES

Angoff, W. H. (1971). Scales, norms, and equivalent scores. In R. L. Thorndike (Ed.), *Educational measurement* (2nd ed., pp. 508–600). Washington, DC: American Council on Education.

Buckendahl, C. W., Smith, R. W., Impara, J. C., & Plake, B. S. (2002). A comparison of Angoff and Bookmark standard setting methods. *Journal of Educational Measurement, 39,* 253–263.

Cizek, G. J. (Ed.). (2001). *Setting performance standards: concepts, methods, and perspectives.* Mahwah, NJ: Lawrence Erlbaum Associates.

Hambleton, R. K., & Plake, B. S. (1995). Extended Angoff procedure to set standards on complex performance assessments. *Applied Measurement in Education, 8,* 41–56.

Impara, J. C., & Plake, B. S. (1997). Standard setting: An alternative approach. *Journal of Educational Measurement, 34,* 353–336.

Impara, J. C., & Plake, B. S. (1998). Teachers' ability to estimate item difficulty: A test of the assumptions in the Angoff standard setting method. *Journal of Educational Measurement, 35,* 69–81.

Jaeger, R. M., & Mills, C. N. (2001). An integrated judgment procedure for setting standards on complex, large-scale assessments. In G. J. Cizek (Ed.), *Setting performance standards: concepts, methods, and perspectives.* Mahwah, NJ: Lawrence Erlbaum Associates.

Mitzel, H. O., Lewis, D. M., Patz, R. J., & Green, D. R. (2001). The bookmark procedure: Psychological perspectives. In G. J. Cizek (Ed.), *Setting performance standards: concepts, methods, and perspectives* (pp. 249–281). Mahwah, NJ: Lawrence Erlbaum Associates.

Plake, B. S., & Hambleton, R. K. (2000). A standard setting method for use with complex performance assessments: Categorical assignments of student work. *Educational Assessment, 6,* 197–215.

10

The Testing Industry, Ethnic Minorities, and Individuals With Disabilities

Kurt F. Geisinger

The University of St. Thomas, Houston

The use of testing in educational, clinical, and industrial settings has undoubtedly benefited the vast majority of organizations as well as society at large, as evidenced by chapters throughout this book. Considerable documentation supports the notion that decisions aided by information from valid psychological measures, in combination with other information used to make such decisions, are more likely to yield both correct and additional efficient judgments.

Nevertheless, long-standing, persistent complaints (Cronbach, 1975) about the use of psychological and educational tests have continued, have frequently been voiced in print media from books to daily newspaper articles (e.g., Gould, 1981; Haney, 1981; Haney, Madavs, & Lyons, 1993; Hanson, 1993; Hoffman, 1962; Kohn, 2000; Sacks, 1999), in both the professional literature and the public press, and have led to scrutiny by governmental and professional groups. Further, some critiques have been aimed primarily against specific tests, most specifically those that are *high-stakes* measures, such as tests for entry to higher educational programs or for graduation from educational programs, especially high school. Many complaints have been lodged against the SAT (e.g., Lemann, 1999; Owen & Doerr, 1999) and, in somewhat less frequent circumstances, against the largest testing company in the

United States, the Educational Testing Service (e.g., A. Nairn, & Associates, 1980). Intelligence and other tests of general mental ability have certainly been the most frequently criticized psychological constructs (e.g., Kamin, 1974), although even tests used in making psychodiagnostic decisions in psychiatric settings have not been immune from criticism (Dawes, 1994). (Psychologists use the term *construct* hypothetically to represent what the public might call a *characteristic*.) General mental-ability tests, similar to tests of intelligence, have been subjected to intensive scrutiny by the National Research Council (Wigdor & Garner, 1982). Certain employment tests used in industry to hire employees have also engendered significant concern and debate (Hardigan & Wigdor, 1989).

It is not, however, a goal of this chapter to enumerate all the various factors identified in criticisms of testing, all of which have varying degrees of truth and falseness. Rather, it shall focus on the persistent complaints regarding the effect of testing on particular groups in our society. To be certain, most of the groups about whom complaints have been associated are those underserved and generally underprivileged in our society: ethic minority groups, especially African Americans, Hispanic Americans, and Native Americans (Samuda, 1975); language minorities, including recent immigrants and those in foreign countries (Hamayan & Damico, 1991); women[1]; and those with disabilities.

These criticisms include:

- tests, even tests of academic achievement, measure middle-class (mostly White) culture, values, and knowledge;
- examples and test material selections are selected that favor men, Whites, and privileged groups;
- language used on tests favors those whose home language is English and, further ...
- arcane and difficult vocabulary is accentuated to aid those who have advantaged, English-speaking home environments;
- test formats (especially multiple choice and other objective testing forms [see Gifford & O'Connor, 1992]) hinder the performance of some groups, primarily women and members of minority groups (see, e.g., Williams, 1970, 1971);
- testing generally is detrimental to the educational process;
- testing is too prevalent and stakes in the schools and in employment settings are too high (i.e., the consequences of not performing well on tests is too severe and sometimes too permanent); and

[1]This chapter does not deal with issues specific to the fairness of tests for women. The interested reader is referred to Willingham and Cole (1997), a book written when both authors were officers at Educational Testing Service.

- the timing and the manner in which a test is administered required by test standardization procedures favor those without disabilities (e.g., Geisinger, 1994b) and those whose primary language is not English.

These criticisms, of course, occur in a milieu where efforts to increase quality and to increase diversity sometimes seem at odds (Gardner, 1961; Jenifer, 1984).

TEST BIAS AND TEST FAIRNESS

The testing industry has responded in many ways to these complaints. One of the primary areas of focus has been the consideration of test bias. Some authors consider test bias and test fairness to be opposites; others describe them as fundamentally different. Schmeiser (1992) differentiated test bias as a characteristic of a test and test fairness as a manner in which scores are used, for example. In this chapter, however, test bias and test fairness are simply opposites. Numerous models and methods have been devised to discern whether tests are biased. Generally, these procedures look at scores earned by members of different societal groups to determine whether scoring is comparable from the perspective of validity. That is, they attempt to establish whether test scores are equally valid for members of underserved groups relative to the majority group. It is interesting that psychometricians who were employees of organizations that develop, sponsor and use tests developed many of the procedures used to identify whether test scores are fair or biased. This fact should not be surprising as such individuals have been charged to make their tests as fair and valid as possible. Anne Cleary (1968; Cleary et al., 1975), for example, who was then an employee of the College Board, performed some of the earliest work. Her model of test bias, based upon predictive validity[2] and regression, remains the predominant model some 35 years after it was initially developed. Other models were advanced by Nancy Cole (1973, 1981) who was later president of Educational Testing Service; Darlington (1971), a university professor; and Nancy Peterson and Mel Novick (1976), both of whom were then employed by the American College Testing Program. Flaugher (1978), another Educational Testing Service researcher, summarized the various models effectively. This topic is one that test publishers took seriously.

---

[2]A test is valid generally if it does what it is supposed to do. Tests used in college admissions are normally supposed to predict the scholastic behavior (e.g., grades) of potential college students—the people taking the tests. To the extent that a test is able to predict academic behavior accurately, it is considered valid for that purpose. Because there are several different kinds of validity, that is, ways that tests can be evaluated formally, this type of validity is called *predictive validity*.

ITEM BIAS/DIFFERENTIAL ITEM FUNCTIONING

Although the models and techniques alluded to previously relate to entire tests and the review of such tests, testing specialists have also attempted to identify individual test questions or items that are biased within what might be otherwise fair tests. If such test items can be identified, they can be removed as components of tests. Further, if specific types of questions could be identified as biased, then they too could be avoided when possible during the construction of future tests. Such procedures have been developed and were known in the early 1980s as *item bias detection methods*. More recently, they have been identified using a more neutral name, as indices of *differential item functioning* (or dif). These techniques led to considerable research in the 1980s and the 1990s (see Angoff, 1982; Berk, 1982; Holland & Wainer, 1993; Scheuneman, 1982; Tittle, 1982). Most professional test publishers now pre-test all items prior to their operational use and evaluate these items for validity and fairness as well as their appropriateness in other respects. When items indicate differential effects on specific societal groups, they are generally not included in the actual tests that are used operationally. Berk's (1982) volume on test bias includes statements by a number of the larger test publishers describing how they then used such procedures to "de-bias" the tests that they publish. Statements from many of the largest test publishers—California Test Bureau/McGraw-Hill, Riverside Press, The Psychological Corporation, Science Research Associates, The American College Testing Program, and the Educational Testing Service—were included in that volume. In describing their procedures publicly, they were espousing standards of fairness to which they were committed. Most test publishers also agreed to abide by the Code of Fair Testing Practices in Education[3], which further provided fairness standards to which they needed to be committed.

In the past decade, two groups have been particularly the focus of complaints about testing: those with disabilities and language minorities. Issues concerning the testing of each group are considered in the following discussion. Both groups present complications not seen generally, for example, in the testing of women and English-speaking minority group members. It is difficult to administer many tests using standard test administration procedures in a meaningful manner to those with disabilities and to members of groups whose dominant language is not English.

---

[3]The Code of Fair Testing Practices is a document that was developed by professionals such as psychologists and counselors, some of whom worked for test publishers. It set out appropriate practices that professional testing companies could and generally do utilize to keep tests valid, fair, and of value to testing clients.

TESTING MEMBERS OF LANGUAGE
MINORITY GROUPS

When a test is offered only in English, this situation may represent a significant problem for someone whose English is not at the level that the test developer expected. Consideration of the special concerns of this group is accentuated by rapid increases in the size of certain language minority populations (especially many Hispanic and some Asian groups; see Eyde, 1992, or Geisinger, 2002). Sometimes, tests must be translated (Geisinger, 1994a) and at other times one must also administer a test of English competence and to interpret the score on the measure of interest in light of the person's performance on the measure of English language ability (Sandoval & Duran, 1998).

TESTING THOSE WITH DISABILITIES

The test-taking problems of those who are language minority group members may be similar to those of those with disabilities in some cases. Those with disabilities and their advocates have documented serious complaints about test use, too, especially in high-stakes situations. Some issues related to proper test administration are particularly sharp. In other venues (Geisinger, 1994b, 2002) I have shown that, with the passage of the Rehabilitation Act of 1973 and the Americans with Disabilities Act of 1990, testing companies are charged to avoid inappropriate practices when testing those with disabilities.

Initially, the primary complaint concerned test administration procedures and formats. Historically, in the training of psychologists and other testing professionals, test administration procedures have rightly been stressed as invariant. This invariance has been seen by some as necessary for each administration to be comparable to that of the test standardization sample, and to one other.

Such invariance simply is illogical for many individuals with disabilities and has led to complaints. (Consider testing an ability to interpret a graph or to recognize colors for an individual who is completely visually disabled.) A number of changes to tests are needed to assess the performance of people with a wide range of disabilities, disabilities that differ both in their nature and in their extent. Primary among the changes that are needed for individuals with many different types of disabilities are changes to the timing of the test; more time is generally needed for many individuals with disabilities.

To their credit, the major testing companies were remarkably swift in making such accommodated test administrations available and they have undertaken some research on the appropriateness of accommodated test administrations. Nevertheless, too little research has been conducted that investigates the validity of scores produced by individuals with disabilities under test administration conditions accommodated to their needs. Willingham and his associates (1988) at the Educational Testing Service studied tests for admission to college (the SAT) and to graduate study (the Graduate Record Examination, or GRE) and, in large measure, found that the accommodated test administrations provide substantial validity. In the period immediately after the passage of the Rehabilitation Act of 1973, tests were administered using accommodations (as described later in this chapter). Until about 2002, the results of most tests taken with an accommodation in high-stakes educational situations were identified as different. In general, the scores were marked with an asterisk, or "flag," indicating that they were not administered in the standard fashion.

During the 1990s, however, a number of testing companies decided to flag only those scores emanating from one type of test accommodation: that of extra time in the test administration (Geisinger et al., 2002). The use of the flag was controversial; even the professional testing standards (American Educational Research Association, American Psychological Association & National Council on Measurement in Education, 1999) acknowledge this controversy. For example, the *Standards* state:

> The inclusion of a flag on a test score where an accommodation for a disability was provided may conflict with legal and social goals promoting fairness of individuals with disabilities .... Further, reporting practices that use asterisks or other, non-specific symbols to indicate that a test's administration has been modified provide little useful information to test users. (p. 108)[4]

Extra time remains the most common form of accommodation by large measure because they have learning disabilities.[5] Around 2000, the Educational Testing Service stopped the practice of "flagging" test scores; this decision was a brave and decisive one taken by the then new president of the company, Kurt Landgraf, in response to a lawsuit filed by Disability Rights Advocates, of Oakland, California. This decision applied to those tests owned by the company, namely the Graduate Record Examination, the Graduate Management Admissions Test and some other examinations. (The SAT, used for college admissions, is developed and administered by the Educational Testing Service, but owned by the College Board.) Subsequent to the settled court case with the Educational Testing Service, the College Board, under the leadership of its relatively new president, Gaston

---

[4]It may be noted that the *Standards* makes a similar reference to the treatment of individuals who are linguistically diverse (see p. 95).

[5]The definition of *learning disabilities* is a complex matter, far beyond the scope of this chapter. However, the central characteristic of students and others with learning disabilities is that their tested ability is higher than their actual performance in school.

Caperton, also changed its policy and stopped flagging scores of individuals with disabilities. Almost immediately after the College Board made this decision, the American College Testing Program, too, changed its policy and stopped flagging the scores of students with disabilities who took the test with extra time.

It is clear that the diversity of our society—one of the United States of America's greatest strengths—has presented certain complications for the testing industry. Let us turn now to review how it has historically dealt with such diversity.

TESTING IN A DIVERSE SOCIETY

It is not obvious how to use test results such as scores when they earned by taking tests that differ in meaningful ways from how such tests are normally administered and scored (as described in the test manuals written by the test publisher to be employed by professional test users). In the following, some of the assessment adaptations and accommodations[6] for those whose dominant language is not English and for those with disabilities are described; in many instances in which language differences are at issue, cultural factors are as well. Before talking about these types of accommodations, however, some information regarding the traditional wisdom concerning fairness in testing needs clarification.

The Traditional Wisdom

The traditional conception of how test publishers attempt to build and use fair assessments might be described with the following six statements.

1. In test construction, groups who are diverse and representative of the entire population should write, review, and evaluate the assessment instruments.

2. Assessments should be pre-tested with groups that are broadly inclusive and fully representative. Comments regarding the instruments should be solicited from those taking the assessments.

3. Components of the test need to be checked to insure that no differential item functioning, or item bias, is present (e.g., Holland & Wainer, 1993). Differential item functioning is found when one component, typically a test item, is differentially more difficult for one group than for other groups. In general, items may differ in their difficulty across groups, but only if the differences in item performance parallel that

---

[6]The term, *test accommodation* is generally used with a test is changed for someone with a disability. Changes that are made for members of language minorities, such as when a test is translated, are known as test adaptations.

found in the test as a whole. Test components should be developed in a manner that is mindful of the diversity of the group taking the test. If a section is not likely to be taken in a meaningful manner by those whose English is not strong or who have disabilities, a discussion centered upon the validity of the test scores resulting from the test should evaluate the necessity of the inclusion of the section. If it is included, then consideration should be given as to how to assess those unable to meaningfully complete this component of the test. It is also sometimes useful to employ panels of individuals representing various segments of society to review test materials for potentially biasing or stereotyping content.

4. Norms must also be considered. Norms help those using test scores to interpret the scores. A typical set of norms, for example, lets a test user know, for every possible test score, what percentage of the entire population earned scores in that range and below. To develop such norm tables, considerable data collection is required, often in the form of pretesting. Samples used for pretesting must be inclusive and representative. Some of the worst examples of test construction have occurred because the norms for given tests were not developed with norms appropriate for their actual use. Two examples will make this point.

The *Peabody Picture Vocabulary Test* (Dunn, 1959) was developed as an individually administered test of intelligence by a special education professor at Vanderbilt University in Nashville, TN. The test consists of pictures that are presented by an examiner four at a time. The examiner then reads a word and the test taker points to the picture that corresponds best to the word; it is, then, a pictorial test of vocabulary, with vocabulary being a strong correlate of intelligence. The original norm sample for this instrument was limited to Whites residing in Nashville, most of whom were children of university professors. Although a second form of the examination remedied this deficiency with respect to norms (Dunn & Dunn, 1981), it was not before serious damage was done. Because experts believed that the test would be relatively culture neutral, it was selected as the primary instrument for the evaluation of Project Head Start a federally funded preschool program designed to improve the academic achievement of underprivileged students. Problems occurred because the Peabody Test's norms were used with populations for which they should not have been used. This use of inappropriate norms led to negative and unwarranted evaluations of the Head Start program.

The *Nebraska Test of Learning Aptitude* (NTLA) provides a second example of norm misuse. Originally called the *Hiskey-Nebraska Test of Learning Aptitude* after its author (Hiskey, 1966), the test "is an individually administered test designed to assess the learning aptitude of deaf and hearing individuals" (Salvia & Ysseldyke, 1991, p. 201). Although it was originally published in 1941 as an instrument for the assessment of individuals with hearing impairments, it was not until 1957 that norms first became available. Those norms were based solely on the testing of individuals without hearing impairments, and it was not until 1966 that norms for those with hearing impairments became available. Clearly, such an instrument would have had limited interpretability until both sets of norms were available. Any use of the examination before 1959, or before 1966 with the hearing impaired, would have produced results absent information that most would consider essential for proper interpretation.

5. We evaluate measures against standards of reliability and validity (see Anastasi & Urbina, 1997). To insure that test scores are stable (e.g., over time) and provide us with the information we seek for the explicit purpose in which the scores are to be used. The extent to which measures are reliable and valid is for psychologists an empirical question, one that needs to be established before tests are subjected to widespread use, just as medicines are analyzed by the Food and Drug Administration (FDA) before widespread use. In our studies of reliability and validity, at a minimum, we must include members of all legally protected (and, preferably, underserved) groups with whom a test will be used.

6. We also need to check the overall fairness of measures for all relevant groups. This statement has multiple implications. For example, in the use of an achievement examination such as a high school graduation test, we need to be certain that members of different groups have equal access to the instruction upon which the test is based. For tests that are used to make predictions, such as the SATs, we need to assess whether the predictions that are made are in fact fair for all groups. The development of the methodology to make these determinations was developed by Cleary and others, as previously noted, and is generally available.

That is what I term the *traditional wisdom* for the fair construction of tests would be applied when considering a diverse test-taking group. Let us now consider the particular situation of testing those whose dominant language is not English.

Language Differences

The testing of individuals whose dominant language or only language is not English in the United States has a long and varied history. Geisinger (2000), after Thorndike and Lohman (1990), demonstrated how the developers of the first group intelligence test for the military were concerned about the testing of those who could not fairly be tested in English.[7] Evaluations of the use of the Army Alpha and Army Beta indicate that the tests achieved widespread success. Unfortunately, the history of testing is not always so rosy. Kamin (1974), for example, documented how English language tests of intelligence were administered to potential immigrants on Ellis Island, with visa decisions often based upon the score one achieved. Conclusions were made about the relative native intelligence of different immigrant groups using these data, and published. No account seems to have been taken of the circumstances compelling different individuals from different countries to come to this country, the different proportions of individuals knowing English from each immigrant group, or the relative similarity, if any, between the languages of their home countries and English.

Pennock-Roman (1990, 1992) studied the relationships between scores from English language and Spanish language tests of academic aptitude on one hand and the later academic performance of Hispanic students in an English language academic environment. These studies are limited by a methodological problem, however. Most of the Spanish-speaking students desirous of studying at American universities have relatively good English; in fact, all of the students in her studies had spent at least 2 years in a U.S. high school. So, her findings are not surprising. Whereas the future academic performance of Hispanic students is not predicted with English language measures quite as accurately as that of English-speaking students, the difference in predictability is slight. In general, the future academic performance of Hispanic students tends to be overpredicted relative to English-speaking students with the same test scores.

Pennock-Roman also analyzed data on the performance of foreign students applying to study in the United States, however. These results indicate the clear existence of an English language proficiency effect on test performance. "The degree to which an aptitude test reflects talent in bilingual examinees varies according to the examinee's proficiency in the language of the test, the degree of difficulty of verbal content of the test, and the specificity of the test vocabulary to a subject domain familiar to examinees" (Pennock-Roman, 1992, p. 127). Furthermore, she stated, "it is plain that test scores underestimate cognitive abilities for bilinguals with low levels of English proficiency ... the academic potential of students with low levels of English proficiency is substantially reduced by verbal tests" (p. 128).

---

[7]The authors of the Army Beta built it to be a test that employed no use of English. Most of the problems were based on figures and the manipulation of figures. Instructions for taking the test were presented in pantomime.

Considering the education of non-English language dominant students studying in English in the United States, Pennock-Roman believed that English language aptitude tests work effectively in predicting success in academic work when the students' language skills in English are strong. Tests in the dominant language—not in English—are preferred when English skills are not strong. She advocated using measures of English language proficiency to determine a student's ability to use the English language. Measures of English language proficiency are themselves moderately related to academic success for bilinguals, but the relation only exists for those whose English language ability is not high. She believed that the use of Spanish language tests for those whose English is weak is a promising alternative that should be explored for those student applicants who are Spanish dominant. Furthermore, measures of language proficiency should be used in conjunction with more traditional admissions measures whenever an individual is a bilingual.

Unfortunately, there are not many tests developed in more than one language. So, tests must be translated and adapted. (The translation and adaptation of psychological measures has been addressed [Geisinger, 1994a].) Commonly, tests are developed in English first and then translated. In traditional wisdom (e.g., Butcher & Pancheri, 1976), a test is translated from the original language to that of a target language. Then, to assess the fidelity of the translation, it is translated back to the original language by individuals blind to the original test version. The original version is then compared to the double translated version for meaning. If the meaning has changed, the translation lacks fidelity.

This technique is known as *back translation*. This technique has been used in the translation of many tests, often with resultant difficulties. In fact, until recently, this approach was preferred to others. However, when test developers know that their work will be evaluated through back translation, they may use wording that ensures that the phraseology of the back translation will converge upon the original. When this occurs, the target language version of the assessment is frequently less than optimal.

Newer methods of test translation incorporate the use of culturally sensitive translators who not only translate the assessment device linguistically, but from a cultural perspective as well. Idioms, for example, do not translate well. Rather than rely on literal translations, it is better to hire culturally sensitive translators who can evoke comparable rather than literally parallel content for test questions. Culturally sensitive changes, however, may alter the nature of the questions. As a check, however, it is appropriate to evaluate the work of the translators with a panel of others who are knowledgeable about the content covered by the assessment, fluent both in the original and target languages, and thoroughly experienced in the two cultures.

Americans should also be sensitive to the number and variety of non-American cultures. Although it may be possible to employ a single assessment instrument for the vast majority of Americans, the same Spanish language instrument may not be equally appropriate for those from Spain, Mexico, Puerto Rico, or from other countries in Latin America. Both the cultures and the language differ in significant and meaningful ways across these regions.

Assessing Individuals With Disabilities

The past 20 years of legislation relating to individuals with disabilities have attempted to safeguard their rights. According to Section 504 of the Rehabilitation Act of 1973, tests used in admissions decisions in higher education that are administered to individuals with disabilities must be validated, and test scores must reflect whatever the test was intended to measure—rather than any disabilities extraneous to the subject matter. The Americans with Disabilities Act of 1990 (PL 101-336), known as ADA, underscores and extends those rights.

Under ADA, a disability is defined as:

1. a physical or mental impairment that substantially limits one or more life activities,
2. documentation of such an impairment, or
3. being regarded as having such an impairment whether or not the impairment substantially limits major life activities.

Testing research has generally classified individuals with disabilities into one of four categories: those with visual impairments, those with hearing impairments, those with physical handicaps, and those with learning disabilities. There are different types of testing accommodations associated with each of these disabilities, although many different disabilities may receive the same accommodation.

Under ADA, individuals with disabilities must have tests administered to them with reasonable and appropriate accommodations. The number of types of reasonable test accommodations devised for persons with every variety of disability is itself almost overwhelming. Further, we can multiply that number by the almost infinite variation in degrees of disability, thereby producing a staggering number of potential departures from the standard test administration format. Thus, although the uniform administration of tests has generally limited sources of variation in test performance to individual differences among test takers, there are now new sources of variation arising from differences in test administration as well. With individually administered tests, for example, test givers may adapt an assessment to the specific needs and abilities of the test taker. In large-scale, group administered standardized testing situations, a number of discrete modifications are likely to be offered regularly, but individually developed accommodations may not be available.

Standardized admissions tests in higher education for applicants with disabilities is perhaps the only type of testing that has been researched seriously with regard to the impact of accommodations (see, e.g., Willingham et al., 1988). The general objective of any modified test administration is to: "provide a test that eliminates, insofar as possible, sources of difficulty that are irrelevant to the skills and knowledge being measured" (p. 3).

A large variety of accommodations in testing format can be provided. Some accommodations are made in a group format; others are individualized, even for tests that are generally group administered. Test forms are provided in regular (standard) format, or with improved (or high resolution) type, large type, braille, or on audio-cassette. Time limits can be enforced, extended, or waived altogether. Test takers may be offered extra rest pauses, a reader, a recorder, a sign-language interpreter, a tape recorder to register answers, convenient test-taking locations and testing times, or other accommodations as needed to meet their particular requirements. Accessibility to the test site is a basic requirement for individuals with many kinds of disabilities. In extreme circumstances, changes in the abilities addressed and content covered in an examination may be required (Geisinger, 1994b).

Obviously, such accommodated measures must be researched with regard to what additional pre-test analyses are needed, whether scores earned on such adapted measures are comparable to those earned under more traditional administrations, and whether the scores that come from adaptations of assessment devices continue to be stable and meaningful. Conclusions to date, with few exceptions, indicate that scores earned under nonstandard test administrations are relatively comparable to those earned when the test is administered under standardized testing conditions. One exception may arise from extending time limits for those with learning disabilities, which may inflate scores and may slightly reduce the validity of scores. A considerable amount of research is being performed on this specific topic currently, including attempts to identify an optimal, but limited time extension that would increase the validity of the examinations and reduce score inflation. It is also possible that some disingenuous individuals may receive the designation of learning disabled simply to receive extra time for high stakes tests. Such a factor could also have the effect of raising scores and lowering the validity of the test to an extent.

Some accommodations clearly change the meaning of test content. Consider test questions that rely on students' ability to interpret graphs. How can such questions be meaningfully "translated" for a person with a visual disability? Similarly, if a reading passage from a test is read to a individual with a visual disability, and then questions about that passage are read to the examinee, is the test still a measure of reading ability? And how do we know that experiences that are common for those without physical or mental disabilities remain common for those with such disabilities?

The difficulty of research to answer such questions is easy to imagine, but it is made still more difficult by the very small numbers of individuals who take examinations with these accommodations. Over a 3-year period, for example, the use of the Graduate Record Examination was studied with regard to those with visual disabilities. Although approximately 60,000 individuals took the examination under standard conditions, only 151 took the large-type, extended time administration—not enough for meaningful comparisons to be made. Those 151 students, moreover, were applicants for graduate study in more than three dozen academic disciplines, making research still more difficult. Accumulating sample sizes large enough for statistical analysis could require a wait of many years, or may not even be possible in the case of the more uncommon disabilities or tests. Until such time, we must use our best judgment both in the manner in which we test individuals with disabilities and in which we interpret the results of such assessments. In some cases, we may need, instead or in addition, to test the so-called "compensatory skills" that those with disabilities use to help offset a disability. In other cases, we must talk with those individuals with disabilities and the persons who work closely with them, such as special education teachers, to determine more specifically how they confront academic challenges and to build tests accordingly.

CONCLUSION

I noted in 2000 (Geisinger, 2000) that the history of testing indicates that necessity begets innovation. A conclusion of some historians of psychology is that that those involved in testing are primarily concerned with differences among individuals. That is why psychologists are concerned about uniformity or standardization in the administration of tests. The conflict between psychologists' understandable desire to standardize test administration and the diverse requirements for fairly testing those who are not English language dominant and those with disabilities is apparent. Test publishers have been active in moving the testing profession in this direction. To facilitate this effort toward accommodating accommodations, we should continue to be vigilant and listen critically to those making complaints to evaluate whether we need to change and improve our processes and procedures.

REFERENCES

American Educational Research Association, American Psychological Association & National Council on Measurement in Education. (1999). *Standards for educa-*

tional and psychological testing. Washington, DC: American Educational Research Association.

Anastasi, A., & Urbina, S. (1997). *Psychological testing* (7th ed.). New York: Prentice Hall.

Angoff, W. H. (1982). Use of difficulty and discrimination indices for detecting item bias. In R. A. Berk (Ed.), *Handbook for detecting test bias* (pp. 96–116). Baltimore: Johns Hopkins.

Berk, R. A. (Ed.). (1982). *Handbook for detecting test bias.* Baltimore: Johns Hopkins.

Butcher, J. N., & Pancheri, P. (1976). *A handbook of cross-national MMPI research.* Minneapolis, MN: University of Minnesota Press.

Cleary, T. A. (1968). Prediction of grades of Negro and White students in integrated colleges. *Journal of Educational Measurement, 5,* 115–124.

Cleary, T. A., Humphreys, L. G., Kendrick, S. A., & Wesman, A. (1975). Educational uses of tests with disadvantaged students. *American Psychologist, 30,* 15–41.

Cole, N. S. (1973). Bias in selection. *Journal of Educational Measurement, 10,* 237–255.

Cole, N. S. (1981). Bias in testing. *American Psychologist, 36,* 1067–1077.

Cronbach, L. J. (1975). Five decades of public controversy over mental testing. *American Psychologist, 30,* 1–14.

Darlington, R. L. (1971). Another look at "culture fairness." *Journal of Educational Measurement, 8,* 71–82.

Dawes, R. M. (1994). *House of cards: Psychology and psychotherapy built on myth.* New York: The Free Press.

Dunn, L. M. (1959). *Peabody Picture Vocabulary Test.* Minneapolis, MN: American Guidance Service.

Dunn, L. M., & Dunn, L. M. (1981). *Peabody Picture Vocabulary Test-Revised.* Circle Pines, MN: American Guidance Service.

Eyde, D. (1992). Introduction to the testing of Hispanics in industry and research. In K. F. Geisinger (Ed.), *The psychological testing of Hispanics* (pp. 167–172). Washington, DC: American Psychological Association.

Flaugher, R. L. (1978). The many definitions of test bias. *American Psychologist, 33,* 671–679.

Gardner, J. W. (1961). *Excellence: Can we be equal and excellent too?* New York: Harper.

Geisinger, K. F. (1994a). Cross-cultural normative assessment: Translation and adaptation issues influencing the normative interpretation of assessment instruments. *Psychological Assessment, 6,* 304–312.

Geisinger, K. F. (1994b). Psychometric issues in testing students with disabilities. *Applied Measurement in Education, 7*(2), 121–140.

Geisinger, K. F. (2000). Psychological testing at the end of the millennium: A brief historical review. *Professional Psychology: Issues and Practice, 31,* 117–118.

Geisinger, K. F. (2002). Testing members of an increasingly diverse society. In J. F. Carlson & B. B. Waterman (Eds.), *Social and personality assessment of school-aged children: Developing interventions for educational and clinical use* (pp. 346–364). Boston: Allyn & Bacon.

Geisinger, K. F., Boodoo, G., & Noble, J. P. (2002). The psychometrics of testing individuals with disabilities. In R. B. Ekstrom & D. K. Smith (Eds.), *Assessing individuals with disabilities in educational, employment and counseling settings* (pp. 33–42). Washington, DC: American Psychological Association.

Gifford, B. R., & O'Connor, M. C. (Eds.). (1992). *Changing assessments: Alternative views of aptitude, achievement and instruction.* Boston: Kluwer.

Gould, S. J. (1981). *The mismeasure of man.* New York: W. W. Norton.

Hamayan, E. V., & Damico, J. S. (Eds.). (1991). *Limiting bias in the assessment of bilingual students.* Austin, TX: Pro-Ed.

Haney, W. (1981). Validity, vaudeville, and values: A short history of social concerns over standardized testing. *American Psychologist, 36,* 1021–1034.

Haney, W., Madaus, G. F., & Lyons, G. (1993). *The fractured marketplace for standardized testing.* Boston: Kluwer.

Hanson, F. A. (1993). *Testing, testing: Social consequences of the examined life.* Berkeley, CA: University of California Press.

Hartigan, J. A., & Wigdor, A. (Eds.). (1989). *Fairness in employment testing: Validity generalization, minority issues and the General Aptitude Test Battery.* Washington, DC: National Academy Press.

Hiskey, M. S. (1966). *Hiskey-Nebraska Test of Learning Aptitude.* Lincoln, NE: Union College Press.

Hoffman, B. (1962). *The tyranny of testing.* New York: Crowell-Collier.

Holland, P. W., & Wainer, H. (Eds.). (1993). *Differential item functioning.* Hillsdale, NJ: Lawrence Erlbaum Associates.

Jenifer, F. G. (1984). How test results affect college admissions of minorities. In C. W. Davis (Ed.), *The uses and misuses of tests* (pp. 91–105). San Francisco: Jossey-Bass.

Kamin, L. J. (1974). *The science and politics of I.Q.* Hillsdale, NJ: Lawrence Erlbaum Associates.

Kohn, A. (2000). *The case against standardized testing: Raising the scores, ruining the schools.* Portsmouth, NH: Heinemann.

Lemann, N. (1999). *The big test: The secret history of the American meritocracy.* New York: Farrar, Straus and Giroux.

Nairn, A., & Associates. (1980). *The reign of ETS: The corporation that makes up minds.* Washington, DC: Learning Research Project.

Owen, D., & Doerr, M. (1999). *None of the above: The truth behind the SATs.* New York: Rowman & Littlefield.

Pennock-Roman, M. (1990). *Test validity and language background: A study of Hispanic American students at six universities.* New York: The College Board.

Pennock-Roman, M. (1992). Interpreting test performance in selective admissions for Hispanic students. In K. F. Geisinger (Ed.), *The Psychological Testing of Hispanics* (pp. 99–135). Washington, DC: American Psychological Association.

Petersen, N. S., & Novick, M. L. (1976). An evaluation of some models for culture-fair selection. *Journal of Educational Measurement, 13,* 3–29.

Sacks, P. (1999). *Standardized minds: The high price of America's testing culture and what we can do to change it.* Cambridge, MA: Perseus.

Salvia, J., & Ysseldyke, J. E. (1991). *Assessment* (5th ed.). Boston: Houghton Mifflin Co.

Samuda, R. J. (1975). *Psychological testing of American minorities.* New York: Dodd, Mead & Co.

Sandoval, J., & Duran, R. P. (1998). Language. In J. Sandoval, C. L. Frisby, K. F. Geisinger, J. D. Scheuneman, & J. R. Grenier (Eds.), *Test interpretation and diversity:*

Achieving equity in assessment (pp. 181–212). Washington, DC: American Psychological Association.

Schmeiser, C. B. (1992). Reactions to technical and social issues in testing Hispanics. In K. F. Geisinger (Ed.), *The psychological testing of Hispanics* (pp. 79–85). Washington, DC: American Psychological Association.

Scheuneman, J. D. (1982). A posteriori analysis of biased items. In R. A. Berk (Ed.), *Handbook for detecting test bias* (pp. 180–198). Baltimore: Johns Hopkins.

Thorndike, R. M., & Lohman, D. F. (1990). *A century of ability testing*. Chicago: Riverside.

Tittle, C. K. (1982). Use of judgmental methods in item bias studies. In R. A. Berk (Ed.), *Handbook for detecting test bias* (pp. 31–63). Baltimore: Johns Hopkins.

Wigdor, A., & Garner, W. R. (Eds.). (1982). *Ability testing: Uses, consequences, and controversies* (Vols. I & II). Washington, DC: National Academy Press.

Williams, R. L. (1970). Danger: Testing and dehumanizing Black children. *Clinical Child Psychology Newsletter, 9*, 5–6.

Williams, R. L. (1971). Abuses and misuses in testing Black children. *Counseling Psychologist, 2*, 62–77.

Willingham, W. W., & Cole, N. S. (1997). *Gender and fair assessment*. Mahwah, NJ: Lawrence Erlbaum Associates.

Willingham, W. W., Ragosta, M., Bennett, R. E., Braun, H., Rock, D. A., & Powers, D. E. (Eds.). (1988). *Testing handicapped people*. Needham Heights, MA: Allyn & Bacon.

11

A School Accountability Case Study: California API Awards and the *Orange County Register* Margin of Error Folly

David Rogosa
Stanford University

This school accountability episode has the following timeline.

August 2002. The *Orange County Register* (*OCRegister*; Orange County, California), after months of preparation, launches a week-long series of attack pieces against the state of California school accountability system, which offered rewards for improvements in the Academic Performance Index (API). The main assertions by the *Orange County Register* to be examined in this case study:

> California's $1 billion school-testing system is so riddled with flaws that the state has no idea whether one third of the schools receiving cash awards actually earned the money (8/11/02)

> the Register's findings, which showed about one-third of the award-winners gains were within the error margin making it impossible to tell if the school really improved (8/16/02)

> That error rate means that of the $67.3 million the state plans to give to schools as rewards this year 35 percent is slated for schools where improvement had little or no statistical significance. (8/11/02)

These claims by the newspaper garnered considerable press attention and serious governmental concern (*OCRegister*, 8/14/02). For this series, the *Orange County Register* received from the Education Writers Association the 2002 National Award for Education Reporting in the Investigative Reporting category. Obviously, if these claims were at all correct, the California school accountability system would not be credible or defensible.

The *OCRegister* reporters repeatedly cite the advice and contributions to their analysis by Richard Hill, Center for Assessment (e.g., Hill, 2001). Additional experts cited include Thomas Kane of UCLA.

September 2002. David Rogosa (9/9/02) distributed "Commentaries on the *Orange County Register* Series" (Rogosa, 2002a) on the California Department of Education (CDE) Web site demonstrating that instead of the 1/3 or 35% claimed by the *OCRegister*, the correct answers were 2% of schools, 1% of funds. The lead from (Rogosa, 2002a): "The *Orange County Register* analysis (8/11–8/16/02) of the California API awards is so riddled with statistical blunders and misstatements that credibility should not be given to their numerical assertions" (p. 1).

In addition, Rogosa (2002b) addressed the Education Writers Association Meetings on September 5, 2002 including a panel discussion with the *OCRegister* reporters.

October 2002. Unabashed, the *OCRegister* reporters repeated their assertions and stress the importance of the *margin of error*:

> in the first three years, the state handed out about $1 billion in awards and money for remedial programs based on API scores that sometimes fell within the margin of error, so it was unclear if the school really improved or dropped. (10/17/02)

September 2003. The *OCRegister* assertions receive national exposure by Malcolm Gladwell in the *New Yorker* (9/15/2003):

> But the average margin of error on the A.P.I. is something like twenty points, and for a small school it can be as much as fifty points. In a recent investigation, the *Orange County Register* concluded that, as a result, about a third of the money given out by the state might have been awarded to schools that simply got lucky.

The major lesson demonstrated in this chapter is that the *OCRegister* use of the *margin of error*, which they defined as 1.96 times the standard error of the school score, represents a serious misunderstanding of basic material from introductory statistics courses. Regrettably, the statistical blunders involved in the *OCRegister* margin of error calculations also arise in slightly different contexts in many state accountability plans for *No Child Left Behind* (CCSSO, 2002). More broadly, the calculations mustered to refute the *OCRegister* claims also provide useful approaches and tools for understanding the properties of accountability systems.

CALIFORNIA API AWARD PROGRAMS
AND THE *OCREGISTER* CALCULATIONS

The California Academic Performance Index (API) is a weighted index of student national percentile ranks on the Stanford 9 battery, producing a possible range for school (or subgroup) scores of 200 to 1,000 (see Appendix A for computational details). To provide some calibration of the scale it's useful to note that a school with about one half of its students above the national fiftieth percentile on the tests will have an API score around 650; also, a one percentile point improvement by each student on each test translates into a 8 to 10 point improvement in the school API (Rogosa, 2000). Data analysis for student and school progress in the California testing programs is provided in Rogosa (2003).

The focus of the *OCRegister* series, and thus this analysis, is the California Governor's Performance Awards (GPA). For most schools (schools below API 800) the API growth target for GPA awards is an arithmetic form of 5% toward the interim state goal of API 800. To receive a GPA award, targets for the numerically significant subgroups in the school must also be met (see Appendix A). The dollar awards to schools and teachers for 1999–2000 API improvement totaled $227 million from GPA (plus another $350 million from the Schoolsite Employee Performance Bonus program to GPA schools); for 2000–2001 API improvement GPA awards totaled $144 million (disbursed in 2 fiscal years).

OCRegister Calculations

The margin of error tallies that produce the claimed one third or 35% start out by counting the schools receiving GPA awards for 1999–2000 and for 2000–2001. The calculation that best matches the *OCRegister* description frames the calculation in terms of year-to-year improvement in the school API. The *OCRegister* margin of error for improvement is given as: 1.3*1.96*(standard error for that school's API score). Tag a school with the designation "state has no idea if it really improved or earned the money" whenever the school's second year API score does not exceed the first year API score by more than this margin of error. The proportion of GPA award schools in 1999–2000 and 2000–2001 passing that criteria for is (3357 + 1895)/(4526 + 3200) = .68; i.e., 32% of the GPA award schools fail these criteria.

Appendix A considers three related versions of the margin of error calculations, all of which produce numbers reasonably consistent with the *OCRegister* claims. As all the margin of error calculations are seen to be statistically unsound, the exact form doesn't much matter. The following sections demonstrate how the *OCRegister* application of the margin of error produces such misleading results, a folly which can be summarized as piling might-have's upon could-be's and counting all those as certainties.

THE MARGIN OF ERROR FOLLY: IF IT COULD BE, IT IS

The margin of error, the main *OCRegister* tool for analysis of the California API awards, is shown to have no value and to lead to preposterous results. A series of examples show California schools with year-to-year improvement in the API falling within this margin of error (and therefore no real improvement according to *OCRegister*) also having probability .98 and larger that true change is greater than 0.

Blood Pressure Parable

As a lead-in to API data demonstrations, consider an artificial setting, using diastolic blood pressure (DBP) for hypertension diagnosis. Like educational standards, standards for blood pressure diagnosis are subject to revision (Brody, 2003). The example uses part of the hypertension standard: DBP, 90 or higher. For this statistical demonstration consider the distribution of DBP for adult males to be represented as normally distributed with mean 82, standard deviation 11.5, which would indicate about 25% of DPB at or above 90. (Hypertension diagnoses can also be based on elevated systolic pressure, leading to a hypertension rate of 1/3 or more.) Also, for purposes of this example assume DPB has measurement uncertainty indicated by standard error of measurement of 6.12 (due to time of day, patient factors, etc.) Consequently, the margin of error for DPB is taken to be 12.

A patient is measured to have DPB = 101. The margin of error logic indicates that the physician has "no idea" whether the patient is indeed hypertensive (as by the margin of error a reading of 101 is indistinguishable from 89). To the contrary, this single DPB measurement does provide information, and the statistical question is: What does a DPB reading of 101 indicate about hypertension status? That is, calculate the conditional probability that true DBP is at least 90 given a DPB measurement of 101. As shown in Appendix B, this probability is .912. That is, the probability is better than 9 out of 10, or odds of 10 to 1, that the true DPB is at least 90. Figure 11.1 provides a depiction of this example. Does the application of the margin of error appear to promote good health (or good educational policy)?

California School Examples:
Margin of Error Versus Actual Probability Calculations

In the API context, the disconnect between the margin of error logic and any reasonable probability statement is even larger than that seen in the Blood

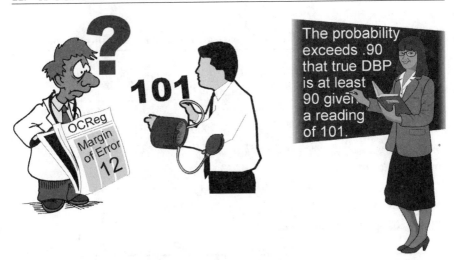

FIG. 11.1. Nonverbal depiction of blood pressure parable. Man (center) has diastolic blood pressure reading 101. Doctor (left) heeding the *Orange County Register* margin of error "has no idea" of whether the man is hypertensive. Statistician (right) explains the probability is greater than .9 that the patient's perfectly measured DBP is at least 90.

Pressure Parable. Three school examples, all telling the same story, are displayed in Table 11.1. Bottom line: Application of the *OCRegister* margin of error to API scores produces nonsense.

School Example 1. The *OCRegister* hypothetical elementary school (from *OCRegister* 8/11/02, "API's error margin leaves a lot to chance") has API score 620 in year 2000 implying a growth target of 9 points. The growth target is surpassed by the 640 score in year 2001. However the *OCRegister* margin of error for improvement is 21.2, exceeding the observed improvement. The *OCRegister* piece, by Ronald Campbell, poses the question "How do you know if the score really increased?" His answer is that the margin of error for improvement (here 21.2 points) indicates "how much the score could have risen by chance alone." His conclusion is "Bottom line: Chance, not improved academics, might be behind that 20 point increase."

Anything "might" or "could" happen; probability calculations (formally or informally) are useful to quantify the "mights" and "coulds" of life. The relevant calculations (see Appendix B), using this *OCRegister* hypothetical school data and the actual California 2000–2001 Elementary school data, are that P{true change ≤ 0 | observed data} = .0189 and P{true change < 9 | observed data} = .125. The probability exceeds .98 that the

TABLE 11.1
Three School Examples: Probability Calculations for API Improvement

	School Example 1		School Example 2		School Example 3	
	yr1	*yr2*	*yr1*	*yr2*	*yr1*	*yr2*
API	620	640	685	701	616	647
n	900	900	900	1002	349	355
se(API)	8.32	8.32	7.5	6.95	14.2	13.2
margin of error						
API	16.3	16.3	14.7	13.6	27.8	25.9
Improvement	21.2		18.4		34.9	
**P{true change ≤ 0	observed data}**						
	.0189		.0341		.00798	

true change is positive for this school (and the odds are 7 to 1 that the true improvement meets the growth target of 9 points).

But according to the *OCRegister*, because the 20-point improvement does not exceed their 21.2 margin of error, this hypothetical school would be a school for which it's impossible to tell if the school really improved. Most importantly, this school would be included in the *OCRegister* tally (approximately 35% total) of schools for which the state has no idea of whether they really improved. In effect, the *OCRegister* would regard this school as having probability 1 (i.e. certainty) of no real change. What this amounts to is rounding the .0189 probability up to 1.0 (in effect multiplying the actual probability by more than a factor of 50). Pile on enough "might haves" upon "could be's" and then count all of those as certainties, and it's not hard to obtain a dramatically inflated number such as the 1/3 or 35% trumpeted by the *OCRegister*.

School Example 2.   This California middle school (CDS code 19644516057616) for years 2000–2001 was chosen for similarity to the *OCRegister* hypothetical school in Example 1. This schools has 3 significant subgroups, Socioeconomically Disadvantaged (SD), Hispanic, and White and received a GPA award of $44,404 for year 2000 to 2001 improvement. The year-to-year improvement of 16 points for the school (see Table 11.1) is 10 points higher than the growth target of 6 points, but still less than the margin of error for improvement calculated to be 18.4 points.

Again the probability that true (real) change is positive is very large, greater than .96, although the school's improvement is less than the stated margin of error and, therefore, not real according to the *OCRegister*. The *OCRegister* calculation for the award programs counts this school as one for which "it's impossible to tell if the school really improved (OCR, 8/16/02)" and includes this school in the tally that yields their 35% figure; in effect the *OCRegister* is taking the small probability .0386 and rounding it up to 1.0. Also note that the P{true change < 6 | observed data} = .133 and thus the odds are better than 6 to 1 that this school's true change met its growth target of 6.

School Example 3. This elementary school (CDS code 19647336018253) for years 1999–2000 has two significant subgroups, Socioeconomically Disadvantaged (SD) and Hispanic, and this school received a GPA award of $40,262 for year 1999 to 2000 improvement. The year-to-year improvement of 31 points for the school is 22 points above the growth target of 9 points, but still less than the margin of error for improvement, calculated to be 34.9 points.

The probability is .992 that the true improvement is greater than 0. Yet, because the observed improvement of 31 points is less than the margin of error for improvement of 34.9, according to the *OCRegister* we are to have "no idea" whether this school actually improved and this school is included in the 35% tally. In effect *OCRegister* rounds .008 up to 1.0 in their tabulation of "impossible to tell" schools. Moreover, P{true change < 9 | observed data} = .0386 and thus the odds are 25 to 1 that the true improvement exceeded the year 2000 growth target.

The intent of these examples is to expunge the margin of error from any discourse about the California API awards or any other educational assessment or accountability program. Understanding the accuracy (statistical properties) of all aspects of an assessment program is essential; botching the important task of understanding accuracy must be avoided in both policy research work and press reporting.

AGGREGATE RESULTS FROM THE SCHOOL PROBABILITY CALCULATIONS

The statistician would calculate for each of the GPA award schools the quantity: P{true improvement ≤ 0 | data}. This empirical Bayes calculation is described in some detail in Appendix B. The calculation is carried out separately by school type (elementary, middle, high) and by award cycle (1999–2000, 2000–2001) because improvement differs over school type and between year-to-year comparisons. The California Data set used here had 4,545 GPA award schools out of 6,630 in 1999–2000 and 3,167 award schools out of 6,570 in 2000–2001. The aggregate results of this collection of six analyses are shown in Table 11.2.

TABLE 11.2
Probability Calculations: No Real Improvement for Schools Given Awards

Award Cycle	School type		
	Elementary	Middle	High
1999–2000	.0098	.0199	.0277
	35.0	12.67	8.95
	(3585/4717)	(637/1100)	(323/813)
2000–2001	.0296	.0304	.0448
	74.53	14.21	7.94
	(2522/4667)	(468/1100)	(177/803)

Note. Each cell contains: the average probability of no improvement for GPA award schools, the expected number of schools having no real improvement and given GPA award, and (number of GPA awards / number of schools).

The expected number of schools in each cell (schools having no real improvement and given GPA award) is simply the sum of the probabilities of all the schools (or the mean probability times the number of GPA award schools). The 1.25% result for 1999–2000 award cycle is obtained from $(35 + 12.67 + 8.95)/4545 = 0.01246$ and the 3% result for 2000–2001 is obtained from $(74.53 + 14.21 + 7.94)/3167 = 0.03053$. The cumulative 2% of schools is $(35 + 12.67 + 8.95 + 74.53 + 14.21 + 7.94)/(4545 + 3167) = 0.01988$.

The total funds associated with the P{true improvement ≤ 0 | data} calculations are closer to 1% of the award monies than to the overall 2% of schools. Two factors make the expected amount of funds relatively smaller than the expected number of schools; GPA awards in the 1999–2000 cycle were about twice as large as the awards in the 2000–2001 cycle, and because these funds are per student, the small schools which tend to have the higher false-positive probabilities receive less total funds.

Most GPA award schools have very large calculated values of P{true change > 0 | observed data}. As displayed in Appendix B (Table 11B.3), for the 4,545 elementary school GPA award winners in 1999–2000, the median value of P{true change > 0 | observed data} was .9988, more than 75% of the schools had probabilities greater than .99, and more than 90% of these schools had probabilities greater than .97. Yet the OCRegister applied their margin of error to assert "no idea" of whether many of the schools really improved. Moreover, results for the probability that true change exceeded the growth target, P{true change $>$ growth target | observed data}, further refute the OCRegister claims. For elementary schools, the median probability for those schools receiving GPA awards is .9926 for 1999–2000 and .951 for 2000–2001. Percentiles for the distributions of these probabilities are given in Appendix B, Table 11B.3.

HOW A HIGH SCHOOL STUDENT COULD HAVE SET THE *ORANGE COUNTY REGISTER* STRAIGHT

The fable of "The High School Intern and the API Dollars" is used to demonstrate a simple plausibility check on the *OCRegister* claims, one that yields results remarkably close to the more complex probability calculations. This discussion also introduces a familiar framework for discussing and evaluating properties of accountability systems.

Medical Diagnostic Test Context

The statistical approach to the accuracy of award programs follows standard ideas from medical diagnostic and screening tests. The accuracy of the award programs is expressed in terms of false positive and false negative events, which are depicted in the chart in Table 11.3. Commonly accepted medical tests have less than perfect accuracy. For example, prostate cancer screening (PSA) produces considerable false positives and in tuberculosis screening, false negatives (sending an infected patient into the general population) are of considerable concern. In the context of API awards, false positives describe events where statistical variability alone (no real improvement) produces award eligibility. False negatives describe events for which award status is denied due to statistical variability in the scores, despite a (stated) level of underlying ("real") improvement.

The common derived quantities from Table 11.3 are *sensitivity*, $a/(a + c)$, which determines the proportion of false-negative results, and *specificity*, $d/(b + d)$ which determines the proportion of false-positive results. Note especially that the *OCRegister* quantity of interest, P{no real improvement | award} $= b/(a + b)$, which would be termed $1 -$ predictive value positive.

TABLE 11.3
2 × 2 Diagnostic Accuracy Table With Joint Probabilities a,b,c,d

	Good Real Improvement	*No Real Improvement*
GPA Award	True positive	False positive
	(a)	(b)
No GPA Award	False negative	True negative
	(c)	(d)

The High School Intern and the API $$$

The short version of this fable is expressed in the equation:

Smart High School Statistics Student + Publicly Available Information
= Correct Answer

The setting for the fable is California, July 2002. A newspaper preparing a series on the API has a summer intern who has recently completed a high school statistics course. The intern is asked by supervisors: "Do you think our finding is reasonable that a third or more of the GPA award schools made no real improvement? That is, can you confirm the statement P{no real improvement | GPA award} > .3"

The high school statistics student makes the following presentation to the newspaper's reporters:

In my class we learned about false positives and false negatives, for disease diagnosis and stuff [see Table 11.3]. To get the information I needed for the API, I did the following:

a. From reports on the CDE Web site I can get P{award | no improvement} for two examples, a typical elementary school with a .1 probability, and a typical high school with a .01 probability. Middle schools will be in between elementary and high, and since there are more elementary schools, that probability might average out over California schools to .07 or .08.

b. But P{award | no improvement} is not the probability I was asked about. From my statistics course, I know a little about conditional probability; namely that P{no improvement | award} = P{award | no improvement}*P{no improvement}/P{award}.

c. From newspapers or CDE site I see that the GPA award rate for 1999–2000 was just about 2/3, which is my P{award}.

d. From reports on the CDE Web site [Rogosa, 2001a,b], I can get the observed distribution of year-to-year change in the API, and I calculate that proportion of schools with observed improvement less than or equal to 0 (which overstates proportion no true improvement) is approximately .1.

So now I can plug into my conditional probability formula and get a *guesstimate* for the 1999–2000 GPA awards that P{no real improvement | GPA award} is approximately .07*.1/.67 = .01 . For 2000–2001 awards, less awards were given, and the CDE reports (Rogosa, 2001b) tell me that at least twice as many schools showed no improvement compared to 1999–2000. Combine those factors, and for 2000–2001 I can compute that P{no real improvement | GPA award} is at least .03. The two results average out to an overall .02. As 1/50 is a whole lot less than 1/3, I can't confirm the reporters' story.

APPLYING MARGIN OF ERROR
TO AWARD QUALIFICATION

Using their margin of error the *OCRegister* claimed that in 35% of schools statistical uncertainty is too great to justify an award; although that head-line is seen to be far off the mark, it does serve to suggest a constructive ex-ercise of considering the properties of alternative award rules. A legitimate award, indicated by the *OCRegister* logic and rhetoric, would be given if and only if the school exceeded the growth target by the margin of error; then the award would not be due to chance and not subject to *OCRegister* criticism. In his justified protest of the *OCRegister* series, Haertel (2002) stated "your reporting suggests that only schools that exceeded their target by 20 points should get rewards." Properties of such an award system can be examined, and some examples are examined here.

For example, suppose a more stringent GPA award rule withheld awards from those schools that are currently eligible but do not exceed their school API targets by at least 20 points. Another alternative award rule would (conservatively) apply that school 20 point surcharge also to the subgroups. Table 11.4 provides probability calculations on the properties of these amended award rules (in the rightmost columns) to illustrate the tradeoffs between false positives and false negatives for a typical elemen-tary school (upper portion) and typical high school (lower portion).

Explaining the structure of Table 11.4 requires introduction of some new quantities. The award probabilities, both for the existing CDE GPA rules and for the margin of error modifications, are expressed as a function of the Incrementation (rows). This representation of school improvement has two forms: Integer Incrementation (Ik) and Partial Incrementation (Pk). In Inte-ger Incrementation (Ik) every student increases k percentile points on each test. Partial Incrementation (Pk) provides an intermediate improvement between the levels of the Integer Incrementation. For Grades 2 through 8, each student increases k percentile points on Math and $k - 1$ on the other three tests (Reading, Language, Spelling), and for Grades 9 through 11 each student increases k percentile points on Math and Reading and $k - 1$ percen-tile points on the other three tests (Language, Science, Social Science). In Table 11.4 the form of incrementation (*Ik*, *Pk*, $k = 0, \ldots 6$) is shown in the Incrementation column, and the school API score resulting from the incrementation is given in the API column (note: *Base* is *I0*). (In Section 2 of Rogosa, 2000, these forms of incrementation, and their consequences for API scores, are covered in detail; Rogosa, 2002c, did the CDE GPA award calculations for these two schools.)

The calculation of probability of award for a specific incrementation is done by bootstrap resampling because subgroups overlap with each other

TABLE 11.4
Comparing Award Rules: Probabilities of Award Eligibility

Elementary School Example. CDS 19643376011951
$n = 350$, CA Rank = 5, API = 613, growth target = 9, s.e.(API) = 13.7,
Significant Subgroups: SD, Hispanic, White

Incrementation (Real Improvement)	API	CDE GPA P{API&Subgr> Target}	Applying OCRegister MOE	
			P{API–20& Subgr>Target}	P{API–20& Subgr–20> Target}
P0	610	0.0655	0.0080	0.0028
Base (I0)	613	0.1002	0.0169	0.0036
P1	615	0.1275	0.0234	0.0054
I1	621	0.2446	0.0597	0.0196
P2	624	0.3111	0.0849	0.0309
I2	630	0.4590	0.1857	0.0774
P3	634	0.5321	0.2602	0.1180
I3	640	0.6515	0.3995	0.1963
P4	642	0.7136	0.4766	0.2588
I4	647	0.7927	0.5992	0.3639
P5	651	0.8639	0.7105	0.4752
I5	658	0.9299	0.8566	0.6345
P6	661	0.9564	0.9017	0.7275
I6	668	0.9832	0.9665	0.8647

High School Example CDS 15635291530708
$n = 1115$, CA Rank = 5, API = 609, growth target = 10, s.e.(API) = 7.8,
Significant Subgroups: SD, African American, Hispanic, White

Incrementation (Real Improvement)	API	CDE GPA P{API&Subgr> Target}	Applying OCRegister MOE	
			P{API–20& Subgr>Target}	P{API–20& Subgr–20>Target}
P0	605	0.0015	0.0000	0.0000
Base (I0)	609	0.0097	0.0002	0.0000
P1	613	0.0307	0.0002	0.0000
I1	618	0.1457	0.0025	0.0000
P2	622	0.2700	0.0145	0.0002
I2	626	0.4480	0.0525	0.0052
P3	629	0.5737	0.1047	0.0150
I3	634	0.7207	0.2432	0.0512

| Incrementation | | CDE GPA | Applying OCRegister MOE | |
(Real Improvement)	API	P{API&Subgr> Target}	P{API–20& Subgr>Target}	P{API–20& Subgr–20>Target}
P4	638	0.8717	0.4515	0.1532
I4	644	0.9555	0.7725	0.3917
P5	648	0.9792	0.8825	0.5647
I5	653	0.9935	0.9690	0.7792
P6	655	0.9932	0.9830	0.8152
I6	662	0.9982	0.9987	0.9405

(i.e., SD subgroup) and with the full school. The calculation starts with the actual 1999 data for the school. First increase all student scores according to the incrementation protocol; then resampling (e.g. 10,000 bootstrap resamples) is used to estimate the probability of award for that specified true improvement (e.g. *no improvement, moderate improvement, large improvement*). These calculations address: What is the probability of award for a specified true improvement?

The *Base (I0)* row provides information about false positives: the probability of achieving award status due to statistical variability alone (no real improvement). Applying a margin of error adjustment to the award criteria does markedly lower that (already often small) probability. But because most schools are making good improvement (c.f. Rogosa, 2003, for documentation of the continuing improvement in California student performance) the consequences of nonzero false-positive probabilities are minimal.

The middle school in Example 2 from the Margin of Error Folly section provides an additional note on false positives. For this school the probability that statistical variability alone producing an award, P{GPA award | no real improvement}, is .077. To illustrate the role of the subgroups criteria (and the minimal information about awards from just the standard error of the school API), note that this probability would be .226 if awards were based solely on the school API, without the additional subgroup criteria.

The marked consequences of adding the margin of error adjustments to the award criteria are seen from considering false negatives. For calibration, consider the *P3* row to indicate *moderate* real improvement (incrementation corresponding to about 20 API points) and the *I4* row to indicate "stronger" real improvement (incrementation corresponding to over 30 API points). For the moderate improvement scenario the false negative probabilities are a little less than .5 under the existing GPA award but soar under the margin of error adjustments to as high as .985 using subgroups and even to .90 just applying the adjustment to the school score. For strong improvement (I4), the false negative probabilities are small for GPA: .05 for the high school and .2 for the elementary school. These probabilities increase by .2 if the school margin of error adjustment is applied and exceed .6 if the adjustment is also applied to the subgroups.

One important issue relating to false negatives is the claim that "small schools [have] an advantage in winning awards" (OCR, 8/11/02, c.f. OCR, 8/12/02). The fallacy of a small school advantage (also claimed by Kane & Staiger, 2002) lies in the neglect of false negatives. A small school having made no real improvement has statistical variability as its friend, in that a false-positive result may occur more often than for a large school. But a small school that has made substantial real improvement (which so far has been the more likely event) has statistical uncertainty as its foe, in that a false-negative result may occur more often than for a large school. An imperfect illustration using Table 11.2 compares the elementary school example ($n = 350$) versus the high school example ($n = 1115$). For true improvement 29 points the false-negative probability P{no award | strong real improvement} is more than twice as large for the smaller school, .13 versus .29. (c.f., Rogosa, 2002d, demonstrations of even larger differences in false negatives between the two school sizes from cleaner comparisons between elementary schools of similar subgroup configuration.)

The short summary is that false positives in GPA awards can be lowered further by more stringent rules, but the cost is a large increase in false negatives (i.e. lower probability of award for a school that really improved). If false positives aren't much of a problem (which is the case if most schools are making good improvement), then measures to reduce those further constitute an unwise policy option.

REFERENCES

Brody, J. E. (2003, August 12). 'Normal' blood pressure: Health watchdogs are resetting the risk. *New York Times.*

Carlin, B. P., & Louis, T. A. (2000). *Bayes and empirical Bayes methods for data analysis* (2nd ed.). New York: Chapman & Hall.

Council Of Chief State School Officers (2002). Making valid and reliable decisions in determining adequate yearly progress. A paper in the series: implementing the state accountability system requirements under the No Child Left Behind Act of 2001. ASR-CAS Joint Study Group on Adequate Yearly Progress, Scott Marion and Carole White, Co-Chairs. Retrieved from http://www.ccsso.org/content/pdfs/AYPpaper.pdf

Haertel, E. H. (2002, August 18). State test program among most reliable in nation [Letter to Editor]. *Orange County Register.*

Hill, R. (2001, February). The reliability of California's API. Center for Assessment. Retrieved 11/10/03 from www.nciea.org

Gladwell, M. (2003, September 15). Making the grade. *The New Yorker*.

Kane, T. J., & Staiger, D. O. (2002). Volatility in school test scores: Implications for test-based accountability systems. In D. Ravitch (Ed.), *Brookings papers on education policy, 2002* (pp. 235–269). Washington, DC: Brookings Institution.

Lehman, E. L., & Casella, G. (1998). *Theory of point estimation* (2nd ed.). New York: Springer-Verlag.

Morris, C. N. (1983). Parametric empirical Bayes inference: theory and applications. *Journal of the American Statistical Association, 78*, 47–55.

The Orange County Register. August 2002 series available from http://www.ocregister.com/features/api/text_version/index.shtml :

Sunday August 11, 2002: Test scores unreliable: Error margin means state can't precisely measure how schools are doing, but the cash still flows. By Keith Sharon, Sarah Tully Tapia, & Ronald Campbell.

API's error margin leaves a lot to chance: Mathematical imprecision could lead to inaccurate interpretations. By Ronald Campbell.

Monday August 12, 2002: Rules hurt diverse schools: Groupings create more hurdles than chances for educators in the hunt for state money. By Keith Sharon, Sarah Tully Tapia, & Ronald Campbell.

Wednesday August 14, 2002: Lawmakers urge changes in school testing law: Flaws uncovered in Register probe prompt calls for reform, but governor's office defends system. By Keith Sharon, Maria Sacchetti, Sarah Tully Tapia, & Kimberly Kindy

Friday August 16, 2002: State testing expert says API margin of error is insignificant Leader who helped design index calls it as accurate as possible. By Sarah Tully Tapia & Keith Sharon.

Thursday, October 17, 2002: State will not cite error margin in API scores: Missing data on results to be released today would reveal numbers' precision, By Keith Sharon & Sarah Tully.

Rogosa, D. R. (2000). *Interpretive notes for the Academic Performance Index*. Retrieved April 1, 2004 from California Department of Education, Policy and Evaluation Division Web site: http://www.cde.ca.gov/ta/ac/ap/researchreports.htm

Rogosa, D. R. (2001a). *Year 2000 update: Interpretive notes for the Academic Performance Index*. Retrieved April 1, 2004 from California Department of Education, Policy and Evaluation Division Web site: http://www.cde.ca.gov/ta/ac/ap/researchreports.htm

Rogosa, D. R. (2001b). *Year 2001 growth update: Interpretive notes for the Academic Performance Index*. Retrieved April 1, 2004 from California Department of Education, Policy and Evaluation Division Web site: http://www.cde.ca.gov/ta/ac/ap/researchreports.htm

Rogosa, D. R. (2002a). *Commentaries on the Orange County Register Series: What's the magnitude of false positives in GPA award programs? and application of OCR "margin of error" to API award programs*. Retrieved April 1, 2004 from California Department of Education, Policy and Evaluation Division Web site: http://www.cde.ca.gov/ta/ac/ap/researchreports.htm

Rogosa, D. R. (2002b, July 15). *Accuracy Is Important, in Testing Programs and in Reporting*. Education Writers Association Meetings (Is School Reform Working in California?), Stanford California.

Rogosa, D. R. (2002c). *Plan and preview for API accuracy reports*. Retrieved April 1, 2004 from California Department of Education, Policy and Evaluation Division Web site: http://www.cde.ca.gov/ta/ac/ap/researchreports.htm

Rogosa, D. R. (2002d). *Irrelevance of reliability coefficients to accountability systems: Statistical disconnect in Kane-Staiger "Volatility in school test scores" CRESST deliverable*. Retrieved October 2002 from Stanford University Web site: http://www-stat.stanford.edu/~rag/api/kscresst.pdf

Rogosa, D. R. (2002e). *Accuracy of API Index and school base report elements*. Retrieved December 1, 2002 from California Department of Education, Policy and Evaluation Division Web site: http://www.cde.ca.gov/ta/ac/ap/researchreports.htm

Rogosa, D. R. (2002f). *Year 2000 update: Accuracy of API index and school base report elements*. Retrieved December 1, 2002, from California Department of Education, Policy and Evaluation Division Web site: http://www.cde.ca.gov/ta/ac/ap/researchreports.htm

Rogosa, D. R. (2003). *Four-peat: Data analysis results from uncharacteristic continuity in California student testing programs*. Retrieved September 1, 2003, from California Department of Education, Policy and Evaluation Division Web site: http://www.cde.ca.gov/ta/ac/ap/researchreports.htm

APPENDIX A:
COMPUTATIONAL DETAILS FOR CALIFORNIA
API INDEX, GPA AWARDS, AND *OCREGISTER*
MARGIN OF ERROR

To compute the API, start with a Stanford 9 test and transform the national percentile rank into quintiles: 1–19, 20–39, 40–59, 60–79, 80–99. The quintiles are assigned values 200, 500, 700, 875, 1000; an individual's API score on a single test is the value for the attained quintile. For any collection of students, the API component score for a single test (e.g. Reading) is the average, over the individuals, of these values (any missing test scores are imputed by the mean of the group). The resulting scores are combined across tests; API scores in Grades 2 through 8 are a combination of Math (.4), Reading (.3), Language (.15), and Spelling (.15) whereas API scores in Grades 9 through 11 are a combination of Math (.2), Reading (.2), Language (.2), Science (.2) and Social Science (.2).

The school API growth target for GPA awards is a rounded version of $40 - API/20$, an arithmetic form of 5% toward the interim state goal of API 800 (for schools below API 800). For example, the school-wide yearly growth target for a school with a 600 API is 10 points. The API target is simply the previous year API plus the growth target. To receive a GPA award, targets for the numerically significant subgroups in the school must also be met; for subgroups the growth target is 4/5 of the school-wide improvement target. In addition, for the 2000–2001 award cycle minimum growth targets of 5 points for the school and 4 points for subgroups were imposed.

OCREGISTER CALCULATIONS

For completeness, consider the variants of the tallies based on the margin of error that indicate the claimed 1/3 or 35% numbers.

Version 1

Set the requirement to be 20 points (the *OCRegister* mean margin of error) above the API GPA award target. Then the proportion of GPA award schools passing (combining 1999–2000, 2000–2001 award cycles) is $(3263 + 1785)/(4526 + 3200) = .653$.

Version 2

Almost equivalently, do the calculation school-by-school, using the criteria 1.96*(standard error for that school's API score) above the API target. Then the proportion of GPA award schools passing is $(3230 + 1726)/(4526 + 3200) = .641$.

Version 3

Framing the calculation in terms of improvement rather than moving past the API school target for GPA award, then the requirement would be 1.3*1.96*(standard error for that school's API score) above the previous year API, and the proportion of GPA award schools passing is (3357 + 1895)/(4526 + 3200) = .68.

APPENDIX B:
TECHNICAL DETAILS FOR PROBABILITY CALCULATIONS

POSTERIOR DISTRIBUTION FOR GAUSSIAN VARIABLES

The basic statistical facts for what is termed the normal/normal model can be found in Carlin and Louis (2000, sec. 1.5.1, eqs. 1.6, 1.7 and sec. 3.3.1) and Lehman and Casella, (1998, sec. 4.2). The likelihood specification (following notation in Morris, 1983) is that $Y_i \mid \theta_i \sim N(\theta_i, V_i)$, a Gaussian distribution with mean θ_i and variance V_i for units (e.g., schools) $i = 1, \ldots, k$. Specifying the (prior) distribution of θ over units as $\theta_i \mid \mu \sim N(\mu, A)$ yields the distribution of the unknown parameter given the data:

$$\theta_i \mid y_i \sim N(B\mu + (1 - B)y_i , (1 - B)V_i), \qquad (1)$$
$$\text{where } B = V_i /(V_i + A).$$

Blood Pressure Example

The DPB example serves to illustrate the simplest form of calculations based on Equation 1. In this example θ_i is the perfectly measured DBP for individual i, and for the DPB measurement $V_i = (6.12)^2$. The prior distribution of true DPB in the adult male population has $\mu = 82$, $A = (11.5)^2$. Consequently, $B = .221$, and for the DBP observation of 101, the posterior distribution is $N(96.8, 29.21)$ and $P\{\text{true DPB} > 89.5 \mid DBP = 101\} = .9117$.

DETAILS ON THE THREE SCHOOL EXAMPLES

Start with the quantities in Table 11.1: standard errors and margins of error. For school Example 1, the *OCRegister* hypothetical school, the margin of error for the yearly API is stated to be 16.3 (OCR 8/11/02), implying that the standard error of the school API, se(API), is 8.32 (= 16.3/1.96). To obtain the *OCRegister* margin of error for year-to-year improvement, the method

TABLE 11B.1
Probability Calculations for School Examples
With Alternative Calculations of V_i

	P{true change ≤ 0	observed data}		
	overlap	*OCR 1.3*	*independence*
Ex1	.0049	.0189	.0259
Ex2	.0105	.0341	.0449
Ex3	.0025	.0080	.0104
	P{true change < target	observed data}		
	overlap	*OCR 1.3*	*independence*
Ex1	.0768	.125	.1404
Ex2	.0777	.1328	.1511
Ex3	.0207	.0386	.0445

(credited to Richard Hill) is to multiply the yearly margin of error by 1.3 to obtain 21.2 (1.3*16.3 = 21.2). For the California schools in Examples 2 and 3, the se(API) values for each year, $se(API_1)$ and $se(API_2)$, are obtained for each school each year from bootstrap calculations described in Rogosa (2002e, 2002f). The margin of error values shown for each of the school scores are simply $1.96*se(API_j)$. The margin of error for improvement is calculated as $1.3*1.96*[(se(API_1)^2 + se(API_2)^2)/2]^{\frac{1}{2}}$.

For the probability calculations shown for each school example, the parameterization is in terms of year-to-year improvement; thus for school i y_i is the observed Year 1, Year 2 improvement, θ_i is the true improvement and V_i is the (error) variance for improvement. The prior distributions are calculated separately by school-type and award cycle, from the improvement data over all schools (see *Calculation for Table 11B.2*). Special attention needs to be given to the calculation of the V_i; in Table 11B.1 results for the posterior probabilities are shown for three versions of V_i, described by the column headings: overlap, OCR 1.3, and independence.

The probabilities reported in the text and Table 11.1 are taken from the column labeled OCR 1.3. For this column $V_i = 1.69*[(se(API_1)^2 + se(API_2)^2)/2]$, following the *OCRegister* method of multiplying se(API) by 1.3 to obtain standard error of improvement. The independence column, using $V_i = [(se(API_1)^2 + se(API_2)^2)]$ has larger mistake probabilities than in OCR 1.3, and represents an upper bound for these calculations. The column labeled overlap takes into account the within-school correlation between Year 1 and Year 2 scores and the partial overlap of student populations (e.g.

Grades 2–6) in Year 1 and Year 2. Setting the score correlation at .75 and the proportion of students present both years at 2/3 would indicate $V_i \approx [(se(API_1)^2 + se(API_2)^2)/2]$. This quantity is used in the column labeled overlap, in which the mistake probabilities are the smallest.

CALCULATIONS FOR TABLE 11.2

The prior distributions used for the school examples and the Table 11.2 results are calculated separately by schooltype and award cycle, using API data from all California schools. Values of μ and A for the prior distributions are calculated from the improvement data over all schools. The value used for μ is the mean improvement, and the value of A is the variance of observed improvement corrected for the error variance in the API scores. Table 11B.2 shows those prior distributions in the form NormalDistribution [mean, sd].

The values in Table 11.2 accumulate the P{true improvement ≤ 0 | data} computed for each school, using the independence calculation for V_i. This upper bound for the mistake probabilities overstates the error rate for awards in a manner most favorable to the *OCRegister* claims, and the school examples above would indicate these are a factor of four larger than probabilities computed with the partial overlap specification.

Data Description for Calculated Probabilities

Two probabilities are calculated for each GPA award school at each award cycle: no improvement and failure to meet growth target. Over the collection of schools, distributions of these probabilities have extreme shapes, with only a relatively few schools having sizeable probabilities. Percentiles of these distributions (expressed in parts per thousand) are given in Table 11B.3. As with Table 11.2 quantities, these probabilities use the independence assumption in calculation of variance improvement, therefore representing an upper bound.

TABLE 11B.2
Distributions for True API Year 1–Year 2 Improvement

	Elementary	Middle	High
1999–2000	[38.23, 22.67]	[21.58, 18.82]	[15.19, 18.95]
2000–2001	[20.94, 22.15]	[12.88, 19.25]	[2.388, 18.12]

TABLE 11B.3
Percentiles of School Distributions for Probability Calculations

		10	20	30	40	50	60	70	80	90
		percentiles of 1000*P{true change ≤ 0	observed data}								
Elem	1999–2000	.0013	.022	.131	.436	1.19	2.68	5.84	12.5	29.9
	2000–2001	.025	.413	1.91	5.22	10.9	19.1	32.0	51.8	93.8
Middle	1999–2000	.0008	.022	.226	.813	2.44	5.44	14.6	31.4	65.5
	2000–2001	.0029	.196	1.16	3.08	7.48	13.8	27.9	49.9	102
High	1999–2000	.00003	.0002	.038	.352	2.20	6.37	14.7	36.0	94.6
	2000–2001	.024	.334	1.64	4.54	11.8	23.8	46.0	83.3	148
		percentiles of 1000*P{true change < growth target	observed data}								
Elem	1999–2000	.039	.383	1.35	3.60	7.43	14.8	26.6	47.7	88.8
	2000–2001	.811	4.98	15.5	29.8	49.5	73.6	113	170	242
Middle	1999–2000	.089	.839	2.96	8.43	22.1	42.3	76	119	197
	2000–2001	.582	5.53	17.6	39.1	63.9	96.6	15.5	212	327
High	1999–2000	.032	.305	2.71	10.5	27.8	54.0	114	187	243
	2000–2001	.583	5.53	17.6	39.1	63.9	96.6	15.5	212	327

ACKNOWLEDGMENTS

Preparation of this chapter was supported under the Educational Research and Development Centers Program, PR/Award Number R305B960002, as administered by the Institute of Education Sciences, U.S. Department of Education.

The findings and opinions expressed in this report do not reflect the positions or policies of the National Institute on Student Achievement, Curriculum, and Assessment, the Institute of Education Sciences, or the U.S. Department of Education.

12

Leave No Standardized Test Behind

Mary Lyn Bourque
Mid-Atlantic Psychometric Services Inc.

INTRODUCTION

On January 8, 2002, President George W. Bush signed into law the most recent reauthorization of the Elementary and Secondary Act (ESEA), a landmark piece of legislation designed to catapult student achievement in the twenty-first century through the requirements of No Child Left Behind (P.L. 107-110). This chapter examines the background of this legislated educational reform that has testing and accountability at its fulcrum; examines some specific requirements of the law; explores the possible positive impact on related school and district policies; and finally provides a few real-time examples of initial impact of the law in various states.

EDUCATIONAL REFORM AND TESTING IN THE 1990s

To unravel the historical and sociopolitical events that have contributed to the current reform effort would be more than this chapter could discuss in the limited amount of space. Suffice it to say that federal concern about educational reform had its beginnings in the late 1950s with the federal funding of science and foreign languages after the launch of Sputnik by the Russians, and was followed by the legislative agenda of Lyndon B. Johnson in the mid 1960s. The Johnson administration was successful in mounting a

227

battle for academically challenged and economically disadvantaged children. The passage of the first ESEA legislation in 1965 was testimony to this country's concern for the low-performing segment of the school-age population who did not fare well in school. However, several administrations of recent memory have tried to turn up the heat on educational reform that would impact the full school-age population using testing, accountability, and other approaches to prod improvements at the state and local levels.

In the late 1980s, the first Bush administration was concerned enough about poor academic performance in the schools to call together the nation's governors in Charlottesville to craft a set of national education goals (National Governors Association, 1991). The initial six priority areas included school readiness; school graduation rates exceeding 90%; competency over challenging subject matter in nine academic areas; the challenge to be first in the world in math and science by the year 2000; adult literacy; and drug-free and violence-free schools. The main thrust of this effort was to put in place a set of agreed-to national goals that all states could invest in, and then encourage districts, schools, teachers, students, and parents to strive to reach the goals. The America 2000 plan, as it was called, included a federally sponsored voluntary national test, the American Achievement Tests (AAT), as well as content standards as part of the total package. The AAT was to be administered in Grades 4, 8, and 12, in five subject areas.

The proposed reform program also spawned several legislated panels including the National Goals Panel and the National Council on Education Testing and Standards, charged with monitoring progress toward achieving the goals, and the testing and standards component of the plan. The content frameworks of the American Achievement Tests would reflect world-class standards and would be developed under the auspices of the U.S. Department of Education (USDOE). Between 1991 and 1992, USDOE awarded a series of grants to develop "New World Standards" in five of the nine academic goal areas, including English, mathematics, science, history, and geography (Education Week, 1991; Miller, 1991).

Despite the best efforts of the Bush administration and the work of a politically savvy Secretary of Education in Lamar Alexander, the America 2000 legislation languished on Capitol Hill until 1994, when the six national goals and two additional goals on parental involvement and teacher preparation were codified in the 1994 Goals 2000 legislation (P.L. 103-227). However, the American Achievement Test component of the original plan never saw the light of day. The perception of a national curriculum and a national test to match loomed large in its failure.

The Clinton administration, which followed, made new efforts to pick up the banner of education reform using some of the same tools of previous administrations. Under Clinton and then-secretary of Education Richard Riley, contracts were awarded by the U.S. Department of Education to various professional organizations to develop national standards, viewed as precursors to any future national assessments. Content standards were developed in English, U.S. history, mathematics, science, civics, and the arts.

In 1997, during the state of the union address to Congress, Clinton announced his intentions to develop and implement a Voluntary National Test (VNT). The purpose of this test was to report to the American public on the academic achievement of individual students, schools, districts, and states. Initially the tests would be limited to Grade-4 reading and Grade-8 mathematics. As in the case of the AAT, the VNT languished on Capitol Hill for want of full authorization and funding by Congress and was abandoned after 15 million dollars and 2½ years of development effort. Again, the fear of a national curriculum loomed large along with the concern that federalizing the content of what is taught and measured in schools would be abandoning the constitutionally protected rights and responsibilities of the states.

Educational Reform and the Sociopolitical Milieu at the Turn of the Century

The country had been struggling with educational reform for almost four decades by the time George W. Bush came to office. Starting with the Great Society programs of the Johnson administration, suffering the national embarrassment of *A Nation at Risk* two decades later (National Commission on Excellence in Education, 1983), and intensifying the debate with the false starts of the 1990s (National Goals Panel, 1993), this nation had made many attempts to respond to low student achievement, particularly among minorities and the poor. The futility of these efforts over several decades spawned a determination to "make a difference" and prepared the fertile ground for the quick passage of NCLB, less than 1 year after President Bush took office. By early 2000, the nation's lawmakers had finally developed the political will to hold the educational establishment accountable for its actions (or inaction). It is interesting to note that not since 1954 had both houses of Congress and the White House been under the control of the Republican Party. For readers who may be interested, Wong (1998) provided a detailed look at the symbiotic relation between political institutions and educational policy, particularly focusing on the 1990s and the deinstitutionalization of the U.S. Congress as new (Republican) members take over leadership roles in the House and Senate in the 103rd Congress.

The Clinton effort, along with the earlier efforts of Presidents Bush and Reagan, from all accounts ostensibly failed, except in one way. Those earlier efforts paved the way for the Bush administration's No Child Left Behind Act of 2001 (NCLB). A hard lesson was learned through those earlier initiatives of education reform during the 1980s and 1990s. Still clinging to the principles that "what is measured gets taught" and that accountability is the *sine qua non* of systemic reform, the current legislation seems to be on a route unlike any other reform effort of the last four decades.

THE BUSH EXPERIENCE IN TEXAS
COMES TO WASHINGTON

The Bush plan had a dress rehearsal in Texas before making its debut in Washington. Although the Texas testing program, the TAAS (Texas Assessment of Academic Skills), was initiated before George W. Bush took over the Governor's office in 1995, Governor Bush supported the program and took full advantage of the good press that accompanied its much-touted results for Texas students.

The TAAS program, initiated in 1990, was administered in reading and mathematics in Grades 3 through 8, and Grade 10 as an exit examination from high school. In addition, a writing test was administered at Grades 4, 8, and 10, along with science and social studies tests in Grade 8. The phase-in was completed by 1994, and until 2003 remained relatively unchanged in character. A new assessment program in Texas (called the Texas Assessment of Knowledge and Skills [TAKS]) was phased in during the 2002–2003 academic year.

The goals of the TAAS program were to improve student learning, to narrow the performance gaps among major demographic groups, and to press toward accountability by rewarding schools and teachers that could demonstrate gains in student achievement scores. However, there are varying opinions on how well the TAAS actually achieved those goals. Some research supports the results reported from the Texas program (Grissmer, Flanagan, Kawata, & Williamson, 2000), whereas other research claims the Texas results may be misleading (Klein, Hamilton, McCaffrey, & Stecher, 2000), or even fraudulent, calling it "the myth of the Texas miracle" (Haney, 2000).

Notwithstanding, NCLB has many similarities to the TAAS program. NCLB will be phased in over a period of several years and requires annual testing in Grades 3 to 8 in mathematics and reading or language arts, and by the academic year 2005–2006, in science. Most importantly, it flows out of a similar accountability philosophy. Schools will be held accountable for their results measured by student achievement on tests aligned with state curricula. The crafters of the NCLB legislation understood well the nuances of the TAAS program, its strengths and weaknesses, and attempted to build into the federal legislation the positive assets of the Texas program, while correcting for the negative ones.

LEGISLATIVE BACKGROUND
TO NO CHILD LEFT BEHIND

The road to the passage of NCLB (P.L. 107-110) was long and winding, although traveled upon, with what some in Washington DC would call, meteoric speed. The earlier version of the Elementary and Secondary Education Act (ESEA) reauthorized in 1994 included a number of accountability requirements, including the adoption of state standards, state assessments that measured student progress toward those standards, and a state accountability system. Prior to the passage of NCLB 7 years later only 15 states had achieved full compliance with the 1994 law, while another 4 states and Puerto Rico were operating under a timeline waiver on their compliance agreement with the Department of Education, and timeline waivers were pending for an additional four states (Education Week, 2001). Although less than one half the states had met the requirements of the 1994 law, none had suffered the loss of any federal monies. Draft versions of NCLB contained many of the same provisions as the 1994 law.

The groundwork for passage of NCLB had been laid during the 106th Congress in the heated debates over the ESEA reauthorization. Some in Congress wanted school vouchers to be part of the picture; some wanted block grants for the states with no strings attached; some wanted rewards and sanctions for teachers and schools not meeting the accountability measures, particularly academic progress for students. In the end, resolution was achieved through a *quid pro quo*, more control for the states in terms of how they used the federal dollars and how much flexibility they had in federal programs, in return for the provisions of NCLB. The final bill contained several contentious components including annual testing, adequate yearly progress (AYP) for student achievement along with sanctions for those who do not meet AYP, report cards for states and districts, professional competency requirements for teachers, a program called *Reading First*, and a new role for the National Assessment of Educational Progress (NAEP). The bill passed the Senate 87-10, and the House by a margin of 381-41 (Robelen, 2001).

Principle Requirements of P.L. 107-110: NCLB

This section will describe in detail the major components of the law intended to drive both the educational reform of public education and student academic improvements. Although it is not possible to include in this brief *exposé* all the arguments of the law and the Department of Education regulations published in December 2002, the author will try to cover the most salient issues as they pertain to the testing and accountability requirements. As in any piece of legislation, clarity sometimes remains elusive.

And so it devolves upon the regulatory process to shed light on Congressional intent. This analysis will draw on both documents for its elaboration (P.L. 107-110, Sec. 1111; Title 1, 2002).

Annual Testing

Clearly the most burdensome and resource-intensive aspect of NCLB is the annual testing requirement. Under the 1994 ESEA legislation, states must administer annual testing in mathematics and reading or language arts in Grade clusters, 3 through 5, 6 through 9, and 10 through 12. However, the 2001 ESEA legislation does away with the grade clusters and phases-in an every-grade testing requirement at the elementary level. By the 2005–2006 school year, annual testing in math and reading or language arts must be implemented in Grades 3 through 8, and at least once in Grades 10 through 12. By the 2007–2008 academic year, science assessments must be added at least once in three Grade clusters, 3 through 5, 6 through 9. and 10 through 12, for all students. States must make the assessments available to all students including those with disabilities and students with limited English proficiency through reasonable accommodations and adaptations. The same tests and assessments must be administered to all children with no distinction between high and low achievers. In addition, starting with the 2002–2003 academic year, states must provide an annual assessment of English proficiency (speaking, reading, and writing) for all English-language learners.

Each state is required to adopt a set of challenging academic content standards, and provide evidence that the annual tests are aligned with the state's achievement (performance) standards. Such tests must be part of the state's *single* accountability system for *all students*, and must be administered to all or virtually all students in those grades. The law specifies that "… the same knowledge, skills, and levels of achievement [shall be] expected of all children" (P.L. 107-110, [2001] Sec. 1111, [b] [1] [C]).

The level of challenge for the state content standards is described as "coherent and rigorous" content that "encourages the teaching of advanced skills." For the achievement or performance standards, states are required to identify "two levels of high achievement (proficient and advanced)" and a third but lower level of performance (basic) in order to provide a complete picture of the state's performance, including the progress of those students that have not yet reached the two higher levels. States are also given the option of revising both their content and performance standards over time as needed.

As states implement NCLB they are not required to adopt the language of the law such as *Basic, Proficient,* or *Advanced* that are terms used by NAEP to define the performance standards on that assessment. The states are also not required to define whatever terms they do use in the same way as NAEP or each other, or at the same level as NAEP or each other. In other words, each state can use its own discretion to define what *it* means by the three levels it must set in meeting the performance levels required by the law.

However, a system of checks and balances was built into the law. Specifically, if a local education agency (LEA) receives Title 1 funding, it must, if selected into the sample, participate in the NAEP assessments (in Grades 4 and 8 math and reading). This means that the results of a statistically sound sample drawn from each state can be used to compare the state's NAEP results to the state's annual testing results in the same subjects. Consequently, if a state shows remarkable gains on its own annual tests, and demonstrates declines on the NAEP, the results on the state's tests would be called into question.

Accountability: Annual Yearly Progress (AYP)

The first part of the accountability component of the law is AYP. This is one area of the law that was unclear and ambiguous; it is also a complex and somewhat idiosyncratic part of the law that gives fairly broad latitude to the states. Each state must have a plan that demonstrates through a single, statewide accountability system how they will meet AYP in every district, across all schools (including charter schools), and for every public school elementary and secondary student. Although the Department of Education Regulations articulate some specifics, there is much that is still discretionary with the states.

Starting in the 2001–2002 academic year, states must gather baseline data as the "starting point" for calculating AYP. States are then given 12 years to reach a state-adopted "proficient" level, or until the end of the 2013–2014 academic year. States have some choices in how they plan on reaching the goal. They can strive for equally paced progress over the entire 12 years (called *12 equal goals*); or they can adopt an *adjustable mortgage* approach, with less progress expected initially and gradually increasing the expectations as the number of remaining years to reach "proficient" approaches (called the *accelerating curve*). In fact, about 20 states have selected this adjustable mortgage approach (Olson, 2003). In either case the regulations require equal increments over the period covered by the time line. However, the first incremental increase need not take effect until 2004–2005, and each subsequent progress benchmark can occur in increments of 3 years or less after the first (called *steady stair-step* approach). The regulations do not allow a *balloon mortgage* approach, that is, during the first few years little or no progress is made ("interest only"), whereas in the last few years much greater progress is made (*principal due*).

AYP must be tracked for students in several major subpopulations, including economically disadvantaged students, all major racial and ethnic groups, students with disabilities, and English-language learners. Such disaggregation is necessary to minimize the possibility that school populations might make progress toward the overall goals, but leave certain subpopulations of students behind.

The definition of AYP in the state plans must be based primarily on academic indicators such as test score results in mathematics and reading or language arts, and secondarily on other academic indicators such as other assessment results, retention rates, attendance rates, percentage of students completing gifted and talented, advanced placement, or college preparatory courses, and at the high school level, graduation rates. Such indicators must be reliable and valid, consistent with professional standards (if any), and consistent across the state within the grade spans.

There are a series of consequences for not meeting AYP at both the district and school levels. Schools/districts failing to meet AYP for 2 consecutive years are categorized as *needing improvement* and will be provided technical assistance. Those who fail to meet AYP for 3 consecutive years must offer the economically disadvantaged a variety of supplemental services. If they fail to meet AYP for 4 consecutive years, the school/districts must implement serious corrective action (e.g., replacing school staff, lengthening the school day or year, implementing a new curriculum, etc.). Finally, if a school/district fails to meet AYP after 5 years, the school or district must be totally restructured.

In addition, a series of incentives for successful schools/districts has been regulated including achievement awards for the successful, financial awards for teachers in successful schools, as well as school/district support systems for providing targeted assistance, and using outside consultants/consortia to provide technical assistance.

Accountability: State and District Report Cards

Beginning in the 2002–2003 academic year, states and districts must provide annual report cards on the achievement of students. State report cards must include among other specifics, disaggregated academic data using the state-defined performance levels, percentage of students not tested, statewide performance on secondary AYP indicators, information on schools not meeting AYP, and information on teacher qualifications and certification. District report cards must include information on schools classified as *needing improvement*, and comparative data on district and state performance levels. States not in full compliance with these requirements of the law will be subject to a penalty of withholding federal administrative funds from their Title 1 appropriation.

There are specific requirements for the minimum size of the groups to be included in the estimation of AYP, as well as the minimum size of reporting groups. In the first case, the regulations point only to group sizes that will yield statistically reliable information. In addition, at least 95% of the students enrolled in any one group must be included in the assessment. To meet such minimum requirements schools/districts are allowed to average data across school years or to combine data across grades (provided only students enrolled for the full academic year are included in the averages).

Teacher Competency

Another critical aspect of NCLB is the requirement of professional competency for both teachers and paraprofessionals in the classroom. The law stipulates that states have until the end of the 2005–2006 academic year to ensure that all teachers of core academic subjects (English, reading or language arts, mathematics, science, foreign languages, civics and government, economics, arts, history and geography) are *highly qualified*. Highly qualified is further defined as a teacher who has obtained full State certification (via a standard or alternative route); *or* has successfully completed a State certification examination; *and* who holds a license to teach (not including emergency, temporary, or provisional licenses).

Further, all new hires on or after the first day of the 2002–2003 academic year, must meet the *highly qualified* definition. All teachers at the elementary level must hold a bachelor's degree and successfully pass the state's rigorous test of subject knowledge and teaching skills in reading/language arts, writing, mathematics, and other areas of the elementary school curriculum. At the middle and secondary levels teachers may demonstrate their competency by passing a state licensing test or by successfully completing an undergraduate major in their teaching subject (or subjects); obtaining a graduate degree, completing coursework equivalent to an undergraduate degree, or obtaining advanced certification or credentialing.

The requirements for paraprofessionals are equally daunting. Currently, paraprofessionals in the classroom must have earned at least a secondary school diploma or a recognized equivalent. For all new hires after January 8, 2002, paraprofessionals must have successfully completed 2 years of postsecondary education; obtained an associate's or higher degree; and must have successfully completed a state assessment covering knowledge of reading and language arts, writing, mathematics, or in the case of early childhood education, reading readiness, writing readiness, and mathematics readiness. These new academic requirements will apply to all paraprofessionals in the classroom after January 8, 2006.

The Role of the National Assessment of Educational Progress (NAEP) in NCLB

The role of NAEP is remarkably different under NCLB than it was in the prior 40 years. NAEP began many years ago as a rather innocuous (i.e., low-stakes) measure of academic progress, reporting on student performance across the nation and in the four regions of the United States. It was only marginally helpful in informing educational policy at the national or regional levels. This changed in recent years as NAEP began in 1990 to report on academic progress in the states. Due to limited funding, however, NAEP's assessment schedule allowed testing only once every 4 years in some subjects (reading, mathematics, science, and writing), and every 6 to 10 years in other subjects (history, geography, civics, foreign language, economics, and the arts). NAEP has always been a voluntary test, with the assessment being administered at the national level by nonschool staff (and at the government's expense), and voluntarily administered in state sample schools by school staff (an in-kind contribution to the program).

With the advent of NCLB the reading and mathematics schedule in Grades 4 and 8 is now on a biennial basis in all states and the nation. All states must participate, and schools in districts that receive Title 1 funds must participate if selected into the sample. There is a single sample (samples are no longer divided as *national* and *state*), and the assessment in all schools is administered by nonschool staff (at the government's expense). Some 11,000 schools participated in the 2002 NAEP reading assessment.

In mid 2001, the National Assessment Governing Board, the independent board responsible for setting policy on NAEP, established an Ad Hoc Committee on Confirming Test Results (NAGB, 2002) to help structure NAEP's new role. The Committee received technical advice from a Planning Work Group. The overall results of this effort were distilled from an examination of extant NAEP results in three states and the advice of the Work Group. The work resulted in a set of principles for using NAEP to confirm state assessment results under NCLB. In general, the Committee concluded that:

- NAEP can be used as evidence to confirm the general trend of state results;
- Informed judgment and a "reasonable person" standard should be applied;
- Limitations in "confirming" process should be acknowledged explicitly;
- NAEP frameworks should continue to be developed using time-honored methods and should be stable;
- Statewide subgroup sampling procedures should be reliable. resulting in small standard errors;

- NAEP data releases should include methods for releasing understandable state results; and
- NAEP achievement level results should be augmented by full distribution data.

According to Reckase (2002) there are some issues that will need to be addressed as NAEP assumes responsibilities in its new role. First, there is the issue of content overlap between NAEP and the state assessments. In states where content standards and assessment frameworks reflect the NAEP, the joint interpretation of NAEP and state results will be more straightforward. Similarly, there is the issue of cut scores and definitions of performance levels. To the extent that there are not large variations between the NAEP definition of *proficient* and the state's definition, joint interpretation will be easier. Finally, there is the unmitigated issue of motivation. Although NAEP participation is mandatory it still does not take on the high-stakes nature that characterizes most state and local testing programs.

NAEP was first administered under the new law in 2002 in reading in fourth, eighth, and twelfth grades. The student sample sizes included 140,000 at Grade 4, 115,000 at Grade 8, and 15,000 at Grade 12 (where there is only a national sample). The results were reported in June, 2003. Forty-eight state results were reported for Grade 4 and 47 state results for Grade 8; the remaining two or three states did not have sufficient participation rates to meet the reporting requirements. The schedule calls for NAEP being administered on a biennial basis starting in 2003 up through 2013 in both reading and mathematics in Grades 4 and 8. The results of these assessments should be useful in helping the states and districts in developing their report cards.

EARLY IMPACT OF NCLB ON REFORM EFFORTS

The NCLB legislation is over 2 years old as of this writing. What is the early impact of the law at the school level? The intent and hope of the law is to have the requirements placed on the states and districts filter down to every school, and ultimately to every classroom in America. Because the primary goal of NCLB is to improve student learning, that means improving the inputs to the teaching–learning contract, including what and how curriculum is delivered, improving professional capacity in the schools through better qualified teachers and improved professional development, which in turn, should lead to better classroom–instructional decisions. Finally, improvements in student achievement should be more in evidence, so that no child is left behind. To what degree have the inputs to learning filtered down in the past 2 years, and how far down the road to success are we in turning around the lack-luster academic performance of students in the United States? This is the question that the next two sections of this chapter assesses.

School Reform and Curriculum

As indicated in the early part of this chapter, the locus of control for the NCLB law is the state. States have the responsibility of assuming their constitutional rights and providing leadership in the implementation of the law. State plans must be submitted for approval to the U.S. Department of Education; state time lines must meet the accountability requirements of the law, state assessments must measure progress each and every year, and state report cards must be published identifying schools that are poor performers. However, the human capital that really achieves the goals of the law interacts with students day in and day out, namely, the school staff and administrators who must deliver instruction to students. How much of the law has filtered down to that level? Are different instructional decisions being made today than were a few years ago?

Not many data exist to answer such questions, but some are intriguing. The NAEP reading assessments include a detailed questionnaire for teachers of the students in the NAEP samples. Several NAEP reading assessments posed background questions of teachers on similar, if not identical, topics. Where the wording of the question or the response options varied, both questions have been included in Table 12.1, with the older, alternate wording in italics. These questions were asked of teachers of fourth-grade students and focus on the language arts program as a whole, including both the reading and writing components.

Although it may be difficult to interpret the data unequivocally, there appears to be some evidence of trends. First, over the past decade, there has been a move to use both basal readers and trade books for instructional materials in the classroom. For example, in 1992 about one half of the teachers responding said they used a combination of materials, contrasting with about two thirds in 2002. Second, integration of the reading and writing components into a holistic language-arts approach seems to be less prevalent in 2002 than in 1998 and 2000. Third, time devoted to reading instruction increased on both a daily and weekly basis, and the amount of time devoted to teaching reading strategies also increased from 40%, reported in 1992, to about 62% in 2002. These data would suggest that different instructional decisions are being made in the classrooms of America in 2003 than a decade ago. Probably none of these changes can be directly ascribed to NCLB, but certainly state accountability programs and state standards and assessments have played a role. What gets tested gets taught. State programs have refocused on reading and mathematics especially. As a consequence, reading performance seems to be moving in the right direction. The

TABLE 12.1
Percentages of Fourth Grade Teachers Whose Students Were in the NAEP Sample Responding to Selected Reading Questionnaire Topics Across Several NAEP Cycles

Topic/Response Options	1992	1994	1998	2000	2002	2003
Materials that form core of reading program						
Primarily basal	33%	18%	20%	16%	13%	
Primarily trade book	13	20	17	20	16	
Both basal and trade	51	59	58	59	67	
Other	3	3	4	5	5	
Integrated reading and writing instruction						
Yes, central part		65	71			
Yes, supplemental part		34	28			
No			1	1		
How language arts is organized						
Primarily integrated					18	17
Some is integrated					77	77
Discrete subject				5	5	5
Time devoted to reading strategies						
Almost all the time	40					
Some of the time	58					
Never or hardly ever	2					
Time spent on reading skills and strategies						
More than 90%					6	
61–90%					18	
41–60%					38	
11–40%					35	
1–10%					3	
None					0	
Time per day on reading instruction						
30 minutes	5	5				
45 minutes	24	42				
60 minutes	52	44				
90 minutes or more	19	19				

(continued)

239

TABLE 12.1   (*continued*)

Topic/Response Options	1992	1994	1998	2000	2002	2003
Time per day on reading instruction						
Less than 30 minutes			1	1		
30–44 minutes			17	14		
45–59 minutes			42	31		
60–90 minutes			35	42		
Time spent on reading at grade 4						
Less than 1 hour			1			
At least 1 hour			13			
At least 2 hours			10			
3 hours or more			76			
Time spent on language arts						
Less than 7 hours				7	8	8
7–9.9 hours					28	26
10–12.9 hours					43	43
13 hours or more				21	20	23

Source. U.S. Department of Education, Institute of Education Sciences, National Center for Education Statistics, National Assessment of Educational Progress (NAEP), 2002, 2000, 1998, 1994 and 1992 Reading Assessments.

percentage of students in Grade 4 at the national level who are at or above the NAEP *Proficient* achievement level is significantly greater in 2002 than in either 1998 or 1992, according to the National Center for Education Statistics (2003). Similarly, the percentage of students below the *Basic* level in 2002 is significantly less than it was in 1994, 1998, and 2000. Results are not different for Grade 8 students. Unfortunately, the 2002 results described here are somewhat mitigated by the recently reported 2003 results, which show little change over the entire decade.

Reform Efforts in Professional Development

Any reform effort to improve student achievement must deal with one of the essential inputs of the leaning process, namely the quality of teaching to which students are exposed. NCLB articulates some very stringent requirements for teachers and paraprofessional in the classrooms of the future. The law insists on a quality teacher in every classroom. This means, of course, that noncertified teachers as well as those holding emergency and temporary or provisional certificates will not be good enough. Just as no one wants to receive health care from an unlicensed doctor, neither should we want our students to receive their education from unlicensed professionals.

Seastrom, Gruber, Henke, McGrath, and Cohen (2002) recently reported on the qualifications of the public school workforce using data from the School and Staffing Survey (SASS) conducted by NCES. The Seastrom et al. report focuses on the percentage of students in classes with a teacher teaching outside their field. Table 12.2 provides a summary of this percentage in two content areas, English and mathematics for the 1999–2000 school year compared to the 1987–1988 school year.

At the middle school level (Grades 5–9) approximately 6 out of every 10 students were taught English by teachers who held neither certification nor a major in English. Similarly, about 17% of students were in English classes with teachers who had neither a major nor minor nor held certification in English. These percentages declined measurably from those in the survey completed in the 1987–1988 school year when about 65% of students had teachers at the middle school level who held no major or certification in English, and nearly 20% held no major, minor, or certification.

In mathematics the picture is similar. Seven out of every 10 students sat in the classes of teachers without the appropriate major or certification, and 22% of the students had teachers without appropriate major, minor, or certification. Countering the overall trend, the percentage of students in this last category increased slightly from 1987–1988 to 1999–2000.

TABLE 12.2

Percentage of Public School Students by Grade Level Taught and Teacher's Qualification Status in English and Mathematics: 1987–1988 and 1999–2000

	Grades 5–9				Grades 10–12			
	No Major & Certification		No Major, Minor, or Certification		No Major & Certification		No Major, Minor, or Certification	
Subject Field	87–88	99–00	87–88	99–00	87–88	99–00	87–88	99–00
English	64.6	58.3	19.5	17.4	38.2	29.8	13.0	5.6
Mathematics	69.9	68.5	17.2	21.9	37.4	31.4	11.1	8.6

Note. The data in Rows 1 and 2 are from Seastrom et al. (2002), op.cit, p. 10. *Source.* U.S. Department of Education, National Center for Education Statistics, Schools and Staffing Survey, 1987–1988 "Public Teacher Survey," 1999–2000 "Public Teacher Survey," and 1999–2000 "Public Charter School Teacher Survey."

At the high school level, the percentage of students exposed to less than fully qualified teachers is lower than at the middle school level. This is what might be expected because courses at the high school level tend to be more specialized and more unambiguously require specialists to teach them. However, the percentage of students exposed is still higher than acceptable under the NCLB legislation. In the year 1999–2000, 3 out of every 10 students sat in classes taught by underqualified teachers with no major or certification in English and mathematics. This does not differ from the 1987–1988 school year.

An examination of the data from the state NAEP assessment background questions over the last decade in reading and mathematics show similar evidence for underqualified teachers in the classrooms. Table 12.3 presents some data from the teacher-reported questionnaires (completed by teachers whose students were selected into the NAEP sample between 1990 and 2000) in Grade-8 mathematics. Table 12.4 presents data from the Grade-8 reading questionnaires.

In mathematics, only about 4 in 10 teachers reported having an undergraduate major in mathematics, and from 1990 to 2000 the number of teachers holding a graduate degree in mathematics actually has decreased from 21% to 15%. However, as recently as 2000, 82% reported holding a state certification in middle or junior high or secondary mathematics. About one third had been in the mathematics classroom for more than 10 years. Teachers reported being more knowledgeable of local standards (66% reported "very knowledgeable") than they are of state standards (56% reported "very knowledgeable").

In reading, fewer than 6 of 10 teachers reported having an undergraduate major or minor in English or in a language-arts related subject, and even fewer, only 2 in 10, reported a graduate major or minor in English. Yet, many of those same teachers held a state certification to teach English in Grade 8, and had been in the classroom for more than two decades.

Improvement of Student Achievement

At this writing, few Annual Yearly Progress (AYP) data are available on a state-by-state basis to make any judgment about individual state results and student progress in those states. However, some states reported in 2003 their rather disquieting first year results. Among the 14 states, Florida led the pack with 87% of its schools not meeting the AYP target. Alaska, Delaware, and Pennsylvania, with 58%, 57%, and 51%, respectively, followed. West Virginia and California were tied at 45%, and Georgia followed at 42% not making AYP. The remaining seven states ranged from a low of 8% in Minnesota to a high of 32% in Oregon (Adequate Yearly Progress, 2003).

TABLE 12.3
Percentages of Eighth Grade Teachers Whose Students Were in the NAEP Sample Responding to Selected Mathematics Questionnaire Topics Across Several NAEP Cycles

Topic/Response Options	1990	1992	1996	2000
Undergrad major in mathematics				
Yes	42%	45%	47%	44%
No	58	55	53	56
Undergrad minor in mathematics				
Yes			23	22
No			77	78
Undergrad major in math education				
Yes		27	23	27
No		73	77	73
Graduate major in mathematics				
Yes	21%	16	18	15
No	79	84	82	85
Certification in middle/junior high/secondary math				
Yes		86%	89%	82%
No		13	10	15
Years taught mathematics				
2 years or less			11	17
3–5 years			14	16
6–10 years			21	19
11–24 years			37	32
Knowledgeable about local math standards				
Very				66
Somewhat				27
Little or no				4
No local standards				3
Knowledgeable about state math standards				
Very				56
Somewhat				39
Little or no				4
No state standards				1

Source. U.S. Department of Education, Institute of Education Sciences, National Center for Education Statistics, National Assessment of Educational Progress (NAEP), 2000, 1996, 1992 and 1990 Mathematics Assessments.

TABLE 12.4
**Percentages of Eighth-Grade Teachers Whose Students Were
in the NAEP Sample Responding to Selected Reading Questionnaire
Topics Across Several NAEP Cycles**

Topic/Response Options	1994	1998	2002	2003
Undergraduate major in English				
Yes	59%			
No	41			
Undergraduate major reading or language arts				
Yes	24			
No	76			
Undergraduate major/minor English				
Major		57%	51%	47%
Minor/special emphasis		19	20	21
No, not in this subject		24	27	32
Undergraduate major/minor in other language-arts related subject				
Major			11	11
Minor/special emphasis			18	19
No			71	71
Undergraduate major/minor in reading, language arts or literacy education				
Major		14	18	18
Minor/special emphasis		19	26	28
No, not in this subject		67	56	53
Graduate major English				
Yes	23			
No	77			
Graduate major reading or language Arts				
Yes	24			
No	76			
Graduate major/minor English				
Major		19	17	15
Minor/special emphasis		10	12	13
No, not in this subject		71	71	71

Topic/Response Options	1994	1998	2002	2003
Graduate major/minor in other language-arts related subject				
Major			7	6
Minor/special emphasis			10	11
No			84	83
Graduate major/minor in reading, language arts, or literacy education				
Major		15	21	19
Minor/special emphasis		10	18	18
No, not in this subject		75	61	63
Certification in English				
Yes	75			
No	23			
Not offered in state	1			
Certification in middle/junior high English				
Yes	81			
No	16			
Not offered in state	3			
Years taught English				
Not taught		2		
2 years or less		16		
3–5 years		15		
6–10 years		17		
Years taught reading				
2 years or less	18	21		
3–5 years	16	14		
6–10 years	17	18		
11–24 years	37	N/A		

Source. U.S. Department of Education, Institute of Education Sciences, National Center for Education Statistics, National Assessment of Educational Progress (NAEP), 2003, 2002, 1998, and 1994 Reading Assessments.

EARLY ASSESSMENT OF STATE PROGRESS

Shortly after the NCLB legislation went into effect, according to the Education Commission of the States Clearinghouse (a grantee of the Department of Education that tracks and reports on state compliance with NCLB), only

18 jurisdictions had annual reading tests in Grades 3 to 8, 15 jurisdictions had annual tests in mathematics, whereas 24 jurisdictions had annual science tests in each of the grade clusters required by NCLB, only seven jurisdictions than currently met the reading, mathematics, and science assessment requirements of NCLB (Cracium, 2002).

Since then, states have supplemented already existing testing programs, or designed new programs that meet the requirements of the new law. Initially, about one half of the states were not even in compliance with the 1994 ESEA law and were operating under a time-line waiver. However, most waivers were scheduled for termination during the summer and fall of 2003, with one extending no later than January 2004 (Ohio), as states scrambled to meet the requirements.

Some states initiated their NCLB-related reform efforts at different points in time, some earlier, some later. Those with an early start could outpace the late starters, at least initially. The size of the state also could impact progress. For example, small states with more limited resources could very well be disadvantaged by comparison to larger states with many resources; or larger states could be bogged down by the bureaucracy in the state, whereas smaller states are able to change state policies more easily. The following section looks at some comparative data from contrasting groups of states: large–small, lower SES–higher SES, and early reform–late reform. Much of the information provided in this next section comes primarily from two sources: the state comparative database developed by ECS (2003) and data compiled by Education Week (Olson, 2003).

Large Versus Small States

Selecting states to examine in this case is somewhat arbitrary. However, for purposes of this discussion the author has elected to look at two large states, New York and Oregon, and two small states, Rhode Island and Delaware. Only one state, Oregon, had an accountability plan fully approved by the Department of Education.

In terms of the NCLB standards and assessments, there are perhaps more commonalities than differences. Of the four states, Oregon appears to have some of the largest departures from the requirements. For example, Oregon still allows exclusions for LEP students and for students with disabilities, and currently they have no assessment for English-language learners. Despite Oregon's departures from the legislative requirements, they were one of the first five states to be fully approved by the Department of Education on July 1, 2003, along with Connecticut, Hawaii, Illinois, and Texas (Olson, 2003).

In terms of measuring AYP, Oregon has a district-level accountability system, and it is unclear whether it applies to all schools. Both Delaware and Oregon seem to provide no evidence that their students will reach 100% proficiency by 2013–2014, and Oregon currently has no clear definition of AYP in their plan. Two states, Oregon and Delaware, provide no evidence that 95% of the students in the various subpopulations required under the law will be included in the tested population. Oregon's liberal policy of exclusions militates against a 95% inclusion rate; the reasons are not clear in Delaware.

The quality of state/district reports cards vary substantially in these four states. New York State, for example, provides raw numbers for students not tested but not the percentage of the population that those numbers represent. Oregon provides a more complete disaggregation of the data (except for LEP students) but does not report on percentage of emergency teacher certifications, or on actual versus target student performance. Delaware reports dropout rates not graduation rates, and although Rhode Island disaggregates the data for gender, race and ethnicity, disability, and limited-English proficiency (LEP), it does not do so for migrant status or SES, and it does not compare actual to target student performance.

None of the four states currently provides any evidence that they will achieve the goal of a highly qualified teacher in every classroom by 2005–2006, and they do not seem to be working on providing professional development for teachers to reach such a goal by that date.

Low-SES Versus High-SES States

Again the choice of states is quite arbitrary, however, using the government free or reduced-price lunch program as a proxy for socioeconomic status (SES), Alabama and New Mexico, are two states with some of the highest percentages of students in Grades 4 and 8 eligible for the lunch program and New Hampshire and Minnesota, are two states with fairly low percentages of eligible students in Grades 4 and 8. None of these states has a fully approved accountability plan.

Annual assessments in reading and mathematics vary from state to state. New Mexico has the most clearly defined testing program currently in place, with either a norm-referenced or state standards-based test for all students in Grades 3 to 9. The Alabama testing plan is being developed and will include standard-based tests in reading and mathematics by 2004. New Hampshire has a testing program in grade clusters, and the state legislation only "encourages" districts to implement plans that will augment the state testing in place. Minnesota also has grade-cluster testing and is currently piloting at least one new test in Grade 7.

Alabama has no test for LEP students in place and only encourages those students to take advantage of the state-testing opportunities without the support of state policies to require the inclusion of these students. Minnesota and New Mexico require participation in testing by LEP students, as does New Hampshire, with only a few exceptions (allowable under state statutes). Only one state, New Mexico, has firm inclusion rules for all migrant students. The remaining three states do not.

All four states appear to be in compliance with the disaggregation requirements for the state/district report cards, providing data for required subpopulations of students, with the exception that New Hampshire does not require disaggregation by gender or migrant status. Similarly, there is a single accountability system for all students in the state, except for New Hampshire, where it is unclear whether the system applies to all schools in the state. Surprisingly, none of the four states has an AYP plan that targets 100% proficiency by 2013–2014 or that even spells out incremental targets over time, except in the most general of terms.

In terms of teacher quality, Alabama continues to allow emergency certification, and a new subject-matter portfolio assessment currently under development will be voluntary for both those currently employed teachers and new teachers in the system. The state also allows National Board accreditation to substitute for a major in the subject or demonstrated competency in the subject. New Mexico's plan for teacher quality includes the elimination of the substandard teaching license by 2006. New Hampshire has a subject-matter examination required for all new teachers, and they are currently collecting baseline data to ensure a highly qualified teacher in every classroom by 2005–2006. In addition, the state also has a comprehensive statewide professional development plan.

Early-Reform Versus Late-Reform States

The criteria for selecting the states in these contrasting groups were: (1) whether the state met the requirements of the 1994 ESEA legislation, and (2) whether the state would be able to test in Grades 3 through 8 and high school in reading and mathematics by 2003–2004. Two states, Colorado and Indiana, both met the 1994 legislation testing requirements, and are testing all students in reading and mathematics in the 2003–2004 school year. Two contrasting states, Ohio and Iowa, are under time line waivers until late 2003 or early 2004 and will not test students in reading and mathematics in Grades 3 through 8 and high school in the 2003–2004 school year. None of these states currently has a fully approved accountability plan.

All four states are doing very well with respect to NCLB standards and assessments. All states have reading and mathematics standards, as well as annual assessments in reading, mathematics, science, or are well on the way to such assessments. Ohio, however, does not require the inclusion of LEP students in the testing.

All four states report as required on AYP. The first big difference occurs in the disaggregation of results. Colorado neither disaggregates by subpopulations nor does it have a single accountability system because some schools are exempted, for example, alternative education schools. Graduation rates are included in their respective annual report cards.

Iowa seems to have the most stringent requirements for highly qualified teachers in the classroom, with a triennial evaluation based on the Iowa Teaching Standards for all teachers. Ohio follows as a close second in terms of high standards for teachers in the classroom. Surprisingly, Colorado accepts the equivalent of a minor in the subject matter (or 24-semester hours) as its *highly qualified* definition. None of the four has annual measurable objectives for teachers to ensure they reach the goal by 2005–2006, and they do not have high-quality professional development goals in place.

CONCLUSION

Where will NCLB be 1 year from now? Or 2 years from now? With the proverbial crystal ball to gaze into the author could accurately predict what will happen to the legislation, and to the lives of the children and school staff it affects. However, if a lesson can be learned from the history of national educational policy in the United States, there are some indications already in the wind. The Center on Education Policy (2004) recently completed a comprehensive report on the second year of implementation for NCLB. The CEP report, together with some understanding of history, plays a pivotal role in describing what the future of NCLB might be like.

In the past several months, the Federal Regulations for NCLB published by the USDOE are gradually being relaxed. The Department has made a series of moves described by the U.S. Secretary of Education as "common sense solutions" in order to be responsive to the mounting complaints about the requirements of the law (Dobbs, 2004). The complaints started when states began to realize the real burden of the accountability component under NCLB (Archer, 2003).

Burden is like beauty, found mostly in the eye of the burdened. What is burdensome for one state may not be for another, for a number of reasons. Take for example the notion of annual testing. Some states have already in place an annual testing system instituted as part of their response to the 1994 ESEA legislation. These same states may have plans for expanding their statewide system to include other subjects and grades in the next several years. They have planned sufficient resources to reach their long-term goals. For them, the annual testing requirement may not be burdensome, and may even provide some leverage in the public arena (e.g., State Board of Education, local school boards, or parent and teacher groups) to stay the course. For other states that started from behind and are still playing catch-up, the annual testing requirement may truly be burdensome, with lack of time, resources, and public support all playing a role. The burden is usually described by states as lack of sufficient funding, or even unfunded mandates by the federal government. At a recent meeting of the National Governor's Association, the NGA called for changes to NCLB, and is crafting its position on the federal law based on their discussions (Richard & Robelen, 2004).

As early as the summer of 2003 the state of Vermont considered refusing federal Title 1 funds in order to be free of the NCLB requirements. In the last analysis, the state did not refuse the funding. However, some regional school districts in the state have redirected Title 1 funds away from those schools that are most at risk of being classified as *in need of improvement*. In addition, according to the CEP report, three districts in Connecticut (Cheshire, Somers, and Marlborough) have refused Title 1 funding. Similarly, several states have introduced pieces of legislation that would allow the state to formally opt out of NCLB funding altogether, including Utah, Virginia, New Jersey, New Hampshire, and others. Currently, though, no state legislatures have passed such legislation. A closely watched case is the one in Utah, where a final vote in the state Senate is expected soon (Huff, 2004), as of this writing. Other community groups are also thinking about the difficulties of implementing the law. At a meeting of the Business Roundtable in late 2003, participants addressed some of the challenges that NCLB is facing in the coming months and years, with a few ideas on how to fix it (*Education Law*, 2003).

There have also been some dozen or more attempts at the federal level to amend the law, dealing with such issues as eliminating annual testing, deferring sanctions, or modifying teacher requirements. None of these amendments has made it through the legislative process but could get through in the future, perhaps attached to some omnibus appropriations bill. In the meantime, the regulatory process for interpreting the intent of the law plays a crucial role in crafting these common-sense solutions (as described by Secretary Rod Paige).

There is no doubt in the author's mind that the intent of the law is a laudable goal for American public education. In this, the most developed and richest nation in the world, we should not leave any child behind. We should want our future citizens to be well-educated, no matter what their gender, race, linguistic origins, disability, or economic disadvantage. We should offer all children equal opportunities to reach their highest potential as human beings. That does not mean that all children will achieve equally. It does mean, however, that we need to strive to eliminate achievement gaps between various subgroups in the school-age population. Our children deserve the best teaching and learning experiences in the classroom that we can possibly provide. Whatever needs to be done to structure the environment to achieve that goal is our responsibility as citizens. In this author's view, this means rethinking issues such as accountability, teacher preparation and certification, sanctions for school failures, and a host of other uncomfortable and controversial topics.

It also means rethinking the title of this chapter, "Leave no standardized test behind." This is a clear and unabashed defense of testing as a mechanism for achieving accountability from those who are responsible for guiding the learning process and measurable achievement from those who are learners.

Will NCLB help us achieve these laudable goals? And if we agree that NCLB is the right tool for the job, the next question is, will the future leaders and those who set national education policy have enough political strength to pursue the goals, although tough to reach, without watering down the means to the end? The author's hunch is that NCLB will not make it through the political fire unscathed, if at all.

The course that the regulatory process is on right now points in the direction of softening the law. Call it what you will, but "common-sense solutions" translates into chipping away at the essence of the legislation until it is weakened and has lost its backbone for exacting real and measurable change in American public education. During late 2003 and into early 2004, several new rules were announced by the USDOE, including final rules on alternate assessments for students with disabilities (Fact Sheet, 2003), and the assessment of English language learners (Fact Sheet, 2004a), on the requirements for highly qualified teachers in rural schools, and for teachers of science and multisubjects (Fact Sheet, 2004b). The political periscope is up and searching for other issues that might be targets for the "common-sense solutions" to ease the burdens of NCLB. In 2004 or 2005, the focus could be on AYP, or subgroup definitions, or minimum participation rates. None of this bodes well for a strong piece of legislation with enough clout to ensure full implementation in the most intractable venues.

Lessons learned from how the political winds can shift and change the "directions of the fire" are also playing out during the 2004 presidential campaign. Had the results of the election been different it was not clear what the outcome for NCLB would have been. As of this writing however, the longevity of NCLB seems to be assured. If confirmed by the Senate, the new Secretary of Education will undoubtedly be a strong and passionate supporter of the law. Spellings is closely tied to the Texas dress-rehearsal and a crafter of the details of the law that seems to be making a difference in American public education. We can only hope that the spirit, if not the letter, of the law will remain intact and American education will enjoy, at some future moment, the success we need to meet the needs of all our children well into the twenty-first century.

REFERENCES

Adequate Yearly Progress. (2003, September 30). *Education Week*. Retrieved March 1, 2004, from http://www.edweek.org

Archer, J. (2003, November 19). Survey: Administrators vexed by mandates. *Education Week*. Retrieved March 1, 2004, from http://www.edweek.org

Center for Education Policy. (2004, January). *From the capital to the classroom: Year 2 of the No Child Left Behind Act*. Washington, DC: Author.

Cracium, K. (2002, March). *State assessment programs in grades and subjects required under ESEA*. Retrieved February 1, 2003, from http://www.ecs.org

Dobbs, M. (2004, March 16). Federal rules for teachers relaxed. *Washington Post*. Retrieved March 16, 2004, from http://www.washingtonpost.com

Education Commission of the States. (2003). *State database*. Retrieved October 1, 2003, from http://www.ecs.org

Education law faces 2004 challenges, speakers say. (2003, December 10). *Education Week*. Retrieved February 1, 2004, from http://www.edweek.org

Education Week. (1991, April 24). Excerpt from Bush administration's plan to revamp schools. Retrieved February 1, 2003, from http://www.edweek.org

Education Week. (2001, November 28). Seven years and counting. Retrieved September 1, 2003, from http://www.edweek.org

Fact Sheet. (2003, December 9). *No Child Left Behind provision gives schools new flexibility and ensures accountability for students with disabilities*. Retrieved March 1, 2004, from http://www.ed.gov

Fact Sheet. (2004a, February 19). NCLB provisions ensure flexibility and accountability for limited English proficient students. Retrieved March 1, 2004, from http://www.edu.gov

Fact Sheet. (2004b, March 15). No Child Left Behind flexibility: Highly qualified teachers. Retrieved March 1, 2004, from http://www.ed.gov

Grissmer, D., Flannagan, A., Kawata, J., & Williamson, S. (2000). *Improving student achievement: What state NAEP test scores tell us*. Santa Monica, CA: RAND.

Haney, W. (2000). The myth of the Texas miracle in education. *Educational Policy Analysis Archives, 8*(41). Retrieved March 1, 2003, from http://epaa.asu.edu/epaa/v8n41

Hoff, D. (2004, February 28). Utah House softens stand on federal education law. *Education Week*. Retrieved February 1, 2004, from http://www.edweek.org

Klein, S. P., Hamilton, L. S., McCaffrey, D. F., & Stecher, B. M. (2000). *What do test scores in Texas tell us?* Issues Paper 202. Washington, DC: RAND. Retrieved March 1, 2003, from http://www.rand.org/publications/IP

Miller, J. A. (1991, April 24). Bush strategy launches 'crusade' on education. *Education Week*. Retrieved February 1, 2004, from http://www.edweek.org

National Assessment Governing Board. (2002). *Using the National Assessment of Educational Progress to confirm state test results: A report of the ad hoc committee on confirming test results*. Washington, DC: Author.

National Center for Education Statistics. (2003). Retrieved October 1, 2003, from http://www.nces.ed.gov/nationsreportcard/naepdata/

National Commission on Excellence in Education. (1983). *A nation at risk: The imperative for educational reform.* Washington, DC: U.S. Department of Education.

National Goals Panel. (1993). *Promises to keep: Creating high standards for American students.* Washington, DC: National Goals Panel.

National Governors Association. (1991). *Educating America: State strategies for achieving the national education goals.* Washington, DC: Author.

Olson, L. (2003a, June 18). Education Department accepts variety of strategies. *Education Week.* Retrieved March 1, 2004, from http://www.edweek.org

Olson, L. (2003b, August 6). 'Approved' is relative term for Ed. Dept. *Education Week.* Retrieved March 1, 2004, from http://www.edweek.org

P.L. 107-110. *No Child Left Behind Act of 2001.* Section 602. Retrieved February 1, 2003, from http://www.nagb.org/about/plaw.html

P.L. 103-227. (1994). *Goals 2000: Educate American act.* Washington, DC.

Reckase, M. (2002, February). *Using NAEP to confirm state test results: An analysis of issues.* Paper presented at a conference of the Thomas B. Fordham Foundation, Washington, DC.

Richard, A., & Robelen, E. W. (2004, March 3). Federal law is questioned by governors. *Education Week.* Retrieved March 3, 2004, from http://www.edweek.org

Robelen, E. W. (2001, December 18). Congress passes education reform bill. *Education Week.* Retrieved March 1, 2003, from http://www.edweek.org

Seastrom, M. M., Gruber, K. J., Henke, R., McGrath, D. J., & Cohen, B. A. (2002). *Qualifications of the public school workforce: Prevalence of out-of-field teaching 1987–88 to 1999–2000.* Washington, DC: National Center for Education Statistics. Retrieved March 1, 2003, from http://www.nces.ed.gov

Title 1 – Improving the Academic Achievement of the Disadvantaged; Final Rule, Fed. Reg. 71710 (2002) (to be codified at 34 CFR § 200).

Wong, K. K. (1998). Political institutions and educational policy. In G. J. Cizek (Ed.), *Handbook of educational policy* (pp. 297–324). San Diego: Academic Press.

APPENDIX A

Polls and Surveys That Have Included Items About Standardized Testing, in Reverse Chronological Order: 1954 to Present

Sponsoring Organization	Poll/Survey Organization/ Individuals	Title/Subject of Poll/Survey (If Any)	Survey/ Polling Dates	Respondent Groups (Sample is National Unless Otherwise Indicated)	Number of Respondents (Margin of Error p > .95)*	Resp. Rate %	# Items
Broad, Fordham, Hewlett, & Weinberg Foundations	Public Agenda	Stand by me	Spring 2003	teachers	1345 (3%)		4
Educational Testing Service	Hart & Teeter	Quality, affordability, and access …	May 2003	adults, college faculty & students, biz	1003 A (3.1%)		1
Business Roundtable	Business Roundtable	What parents, studs, teachers think …	Mar 2003	summary of data from other polls			
National Education Association	Greenberg Quinlan Research, Tarrance Group		Feb 2003	registered voters, parent voters os	1000 (^4%), 200 parent-voter		5
Atlantic Philanthropies Foundation	NBETPP, Lych School of Ed, Boston College	Perceived effects of testing …	Jan-Mar 2003	teachers in U.S.; & in MA, MI, & KS	4195 US (^1%), 360 M,M,K(^7%)	35	3
Public Education Network, *Education Week*	Lake, Snell, Perry & Associates	Demanding quality education in …	Jan 2003	voters, with Black & Latino os	1050 V (3.5%) 125 B, 125 L		2
	Jones, Egley	The carrot and the stick …	2003	FL teachers (grades 3–5)	708 (1.3%)	45 of cntys	3

(continued)

Sponsoring Organization	Poll/Survey Organization/ Individuals	Title/Subject of Poll/Survey (If Any)	Survey/ Polling Dates	Respondent Groups (Sample is National Unless Otherwise Indicated)	Number of Respondents (Margin of Error p > .95)*	Resp. Rate %	# Items[1]
Phi Delta Kappa	Gallup	Attitudes toward public schools	2003	adults		>50	
	Jones, Johnson	The effects of high-stakes testing …	2002	NC tchrs (grds 1–5) in 5 schls in 1 county	23 (^3%)	>50	2
	McDonald	Perceived role of diploma examinations	2002	Alberta tchrs, admins in 71 high schls	364 tchrs (^6%) 40 admins	85	3
Public Ed Network/ EdWeek		Accountability for all: What voters want …	2002	adults			1
Americans for Better Education	Winston Group	Support for ed reforms stronger …	Dec 2002	adults	1100 (^4%)		2
Blair Center of Southern Politics and Society	U. Arkansas Survey Research Center	Arkansas Poll	Oct 2002	AR adults	768 (^4%)		1
Chicago Tribune	Market Shares Corporation		August 2002	IN teachers (public schools)	600 (^5%)		4
CA Business for Ed. Excellence	Fairbanks, Maslin Maullin & Assoc.	Benchmark CA voter survey	August 2002	CA registered, active voters	800 (3.5%)		11
Quinnipiac University	Quinnipiac University Polling Institute	Quinnipiac University Poll	July 2002	NYC adults	932 (^4%)		

					>50	5
Phi Delta Kappa	Gallup	Attitudes toward public schools	June 2002	adults	1,020 (^4%)	5
Horatio Alger Association	Horatio Alger Association	State of our nation's youth	May 2002	students (high school)	1003 (3.1%)	2
Virginia Tech U.	Center for Survey Research		Apr-Jun 2002	VA adults	769 (^4%)	1
Educational Testing Service	Hart & Teeter	A national priority: Americans speak on teacher quality	Apr-May 2002	adults, parents, teachers, policy makers	1003A (3.2%) 407P (5) 409T (5%) 203PM (7)	7
Public Policy Institute (CA)	Public Policy Institute (CA)	Californians and their government	Dec-Jan 2002	CA adults, voters	2056A (2%), 1503V (2.5%)	4
Mass Insight	Opinion Dynamics	Taking charge	Jan-Feb 2002	at-risk students	140 (interviews) (8.3%)	3
	Ryan, McGinn Samples Research	West Virginia Poll	Jan 2002	WV adults	400 (^6%)	1
Minority Student Achievement Network			2002	students		1
Horatio Alger Association	Horatio Alger Association	State of our nation's youth	May 2001	students (high school)	1014 (3.1%)	2
	Lumley, Yen	Impact of writing assessment …	Apr 2001	PA teachers	168 (^8%)	1
	Roderick, Engel	Grasshopper and ant	2001	Chicago at-risk 6th- and 8th-graders	102 (^10%)	1

(continued)

Sponsoring Organization	Poll/Survey Organization/ Individuals	Title/Subject of Poll/Survey (If Any)	Survey/ Polling Dates	Respondent Groups (Sample is National Unless Otherwise Indicated)	Number of Respondents (Margin of Error $p > .95$)*	Resp. Rate %	# Items[1]
Public Policy Institute (CA)	Public Policy Institute (CA)		Dec 2001	CA adults	2000 (^2%)		2
Public Agenda, Ed Week, Pew Trust, GE Fund	Public Agenda	Reality check 2002: Where is backlash?	Nov-Dec 2001	studs empls profs parents tchrs	600S,T,Pa(4%) 250E,Pr(6%)	> 50	14
U. North Carolina, Chapel Hill	Odum Institute for Research	Carolina poll	Fall 2001	NC adults	648 (^4%)		1
National Post	COMPAS	Global poll on ed performance	Sept 2001	Canadian adults			2
Wisconsin Policy Research Institute	Wisconsin Policy Research Institute		Sept 2001	WI adults	1002 (^4%)		1
Education Week	Beldon Russonello & Stewart	Quality counts	Sept 2001	teachers			17
	Market Shares Corporation		August 2001	IL(Cook, DuPage, McHenry) adults	1196 (^3.5%)		1
U. New Hampshire	U. New Hampshire Survey Center		August 2001	NH adults	400 (^6%)		2
Associated Press	International Communications Research		July-Aug 2001	adults	1006 (^4%)		4
Fox News	Opinion Dynamics	Fox News, Opinion Dynamics poll	July 2001	registered voters	900 (4%)		1

Sponsor	Organization	Title	Date	Population	Sample (margin)	Result	N
Wallace, *Reader's Digest* Funds	Public Agenda	Trying to stay ahead of the game	Jul-Aug 2001	principals, superintendents	909 principals, 853 sups (3%)	34%S 23%P	3
Kaiser Family Foundation		Public perspectives survey	June 2001	adults, politicians, media	1807:1206A (^3.5%), 300P,M		1
NBC News, Wall Street Journal	Hart & Teeter		June 2001	adults			1
CBS News, New York Times	*New York Times, CBS News*		June 2001	adults	1050 (^4%)		2
Virginia Tech University	Center for Survey Research		June 2001	VA adults	686 (^4.5%)		1
Phi Delta Kappa	Gallup	Attitudes toward the public schools	May-Jun 2001	adults	1108 (3.5%)	> 50%	5
Business Roundtable	Business Roundtable	Assessing testing backlash	Spring 2001	summary of data from other polls			
Educational Testing Service	Hart & Teeter, Coldwater Corporation	A measured response: Americans speak on ed reform	Apr-May 2001	adults, parents os, ed policy makers, teachers, admins	1054A (3.1%), 431P,200T,A,Ep		13
CBS News, New York Times	*CBS News, New York Times*	*CBS News, New York Times* poll	March 2001	adults	1105 (^4%)		3
Los Angeles Times	*Los Angeles Times*		March 2001	adults	1449 (^3%)		1
Harris	Institute for Social Research	The Harris Poll	Mar 2001	adults	1008 (^4%)		5

(continued)

Sponsoring Organization	Poll/Survey Organization/ Individuals	Title/Subject of Poll/Survey (If Any)	Survey/ Polling Dates	Respondent Groups (Sample is National Unless Otherwise Indicated)	Number of Respondents (Margin of Error $p > .95$)*	Resp. Rate %	# Items[1]
Quinnipiac University	Quinnipiac University Polling Institute		Mar 2001	NYC adults	1087 (^4%)		2
Harris	Harris Interactive		Feb–Mar 2001	adults	1008 (^4%)		7
National Endowment for the Arts	The Tarrance Group, Inc.		Feb 2001	registered voters, parent-voters os	1200 (^3.5%)		4
National Education Association	Greenberg, Quinlan & Tarrance Group	Education top priority	Feb 2001	voters, parent os	1200 (3.1%)		5
Newsweek	Princeton Survey Research		Feb 2001	adults	1000 (^4%)		1
	Ryan, McGinn Samples Research	West Virginia Poll	Feb 2001	WV adults	401 (^6%)		1
Public Policy Institute (CA)	Public Policy Institute (CA)		Jan 2001	CA adults	2011 (^2%)		1
CNN, USA Today	Gallup		Jan 2001	adults	1018 (^4%)		2
CBS News, New York Times	CBS News, New York Times		Jan 2001	adults	1086 (^4%)		3
Ohio state legislature	Legislative Office of Education Oversight	Proficiency testing, achieve- ment, and …	2000	teachers (8th grade)	~570 (^5%)		2

Source	Title	Date	Population	Sample	Confidence	No.
Education Week, Pew Charitable Trust, GE Fund	Reality check 2001	Nov–Dec 2000	adults, professors, employers, parents	602 Pa (^5%), 251 E, 254 Pr	> 60%	14
Gallup	Gallup poll	Oct 2000	adults	1004 (^4%)	> 50%	2
Beldon Russonello & Stewart	*Education Week* Making the grade; A better balance	Sept 2000	teachers (public schools)	1019 (3.1%)		15
Public Agenda	Parents of public school students …	Sept 2000	parents (K-12 public schools)	803 (^4%)	> 60%	5
Public Agenda	… Little sign of backlash …	Sept 2000	adults, parents, teachers	590 tchrs, 527 parents (^5%)	> 60%	16
Ohio Commission for Student Success		August 2000	OH adults	1002 (^4%)		8
Beldon Russonello & Stewart		August 2000	MS adults, parent os	306 adults (^7%)		5
Beldon Russonello & Stewart		August 2000	VA adults, parent os	315 adults (^7%) 111prnts (^10%)		4
Beldon Russonello & Stewart		August 2000	WV adults, parent os	295 adults (^7%)		4
Beldon Russonello & Stewart		July 2000	NY adults, parent os	356 adults (^6%)		4
Beldon Russonello & Stewart		July 2000	IN adults, parent os	331 adlts (^6.5%)		5
Beldon Russonello & Stewart		July 2000	IL adults, parent os	331 adlts (^6.5%)		3

(continued)

Sponsoring Organization	Poll/Survey Organization/ Individuals	Title/Subject of Poll/Survey (If Any)	Survey/ Polling Dates	Respondent Groups (Sample is National Unless Otherwise Indicated)	Number of Respondents (Margin of Error $p > .95$)*	Resp. Rate %	# Items[1]
The Business Roundtable	Beldon Russonello & Stewart		Jul-Aug 2000	adults			1
American Assn of School Administrators	Lake, Snell, Perry	Voters give testing an "F" (parents poll)	Spring 2000	parents (public schools)			2
American Assn of School Administrators	Luntz, Lazlo	Voters give testing an "F" (high-stakes poll)	May 2000	registered voters	800 (3.5%)	< 20%	4
U. Maryland	Program on Int'l Policy Attitudes	Education survey	Jun-Jul 2000	adults	650 (^4.5%)		2
Phi Delta Kappa	Gallup	Attitudes toward public schools	June 2000	adults, parents	1093 (3.5%)	> 50%	7
U. North Carolina, Chapel Hill	Odum Institute for Research	Carolina Poll	Spring 2000	NC adults	652 (^4.5%)		1
	Angus Reid Group		May 2000	(Ontario) adults	525 (^5.5%)		2
U. Connecticut, Rutgers University	Center for Survey Research, Heldrick Center	Attitudes about work, employers & gov't	May 2000	employed adults	1014 (3.5%)		1
Assn. of American Publishers	J.D. Franz Research	Parents survey	Apr-June 2000	parents	1023 (3.1%)	67%	20
American Viewpoint	American Viewpoint	National monitor survey	April 2000	"likely" voters	800 (^4%)		24

Arizona Republic, Phoenix Gazette	*Arizona Republic, Phoenix Gazette* research dept		April 2000	AZ registered voters	801 (^4%)		3
Sylvan Learning Centers	Harris Interactive	State-mandated ed assessments	April 2000	parents (public schools, ex. NE, IA)	606 (4%)	n/a	17
SmarterKids.com	Opinion Research Corporation Int'l	... Parental confusion over ... tests	April 2000	parents (public schools)	1011 (^4%)	19	3
Assn for Supervision and Curriculum Development	Harris Interactive, Sylvan Learning Center	Nat'l survey gauges parent perceptions...	April 2000	parents	600 (^5%)	41	5
ABC News, Washington Post	*ABC News, Washington Post*		Mar-Apr 2000	adults, parents os	1011 (^4%), 192 parent		3
MI Assn Early Childhood Teacher Educators	Adams, Karabenick	Impact of ... testing Much pain, no gain?	early 2000	MI teachers	1656 (^3%)		1
Democratic Leadership Council	Penn, Schoen & Berland		Jan 2000	registered voters	1000 (^4%)		1
The Advocate (Baton Rouge)	*The Advocate* (Baton Rouge)		Jan 2000	LA (Ascension Parish) adults	350 (^6.5%)		1
American Federation of Teachers	Albert Shanker Institute		1999-2000	teachers (AFT members)			2
Media General	Media General	Virginia's SOL exams	Dec 1999	VA adults	541 (^5.5%)		2
Public Agenda	Public Agenda	Reality check 2000	Oct-Nov 1999	teachers, employers parents, professors	600 T, Pa (^5%), 250E, Pr (^7.5%)	> 60%	1

(continued)

Sponsoring Organization	Poll/Survey Organization/ Individuals	Title/Subject of Poll/Survey (If Any)	Survey/ Polling Dates	Respondent Groups (Sample is National Unless Otherwise Indicated)	Number of Respondents (Margin of Error $p > .95$)*	Resp. Rate %	# Items[1]
American Assn of School Administrators	Lake, Snell, Perry		Oct 1999	parents (public school)	750 (^4%)		2
National Education Summit	Public Agenda	Standards: Where the public stands	Sept 1999	summary of data from other polls			
NPR, Kennedy School, Kaiser Foundation	International Communications Research	NPR, Kaiser, Kennedy School ed survey	Jun-Jul 1999	adults, parents	1,422 (^3%)		6
Democratic Leadership Council	Penn, Schoen & Berland	A hunger for reform	June 1999	registered voters	502 (^5.5%)		4
Phi Delta Kappa	Gallup	Attitudes toward the public schools	May-Jun 1999	adults	1,103 (3.5%)	> 50%	3
	Lane, Parke, Stone		Apr 1999	MD tchrs, studs, principals	161 T (^9%) 103 elem, 58 middle		2
Metro Education Research Consortium	McMillan, Myran, Workman	Impact of mandated testing on …	April 1999	VA teachers	802 T (^4%) 722 yr 1, 80 yr 2		1
Marist Institute			1998				4
National Education Goals Panel	Public Agenda	Summing it up	1998	summary of data from other polls			
Zogby International	Zogby International	Zogby's real America	Dec 1998	adults	1003 (^4%)	<20%	1

Public Agenda	Public Agenda	Reality check parent survey	Oct-Nov 1998	parents, tchrs, studs, employers, profs	700 Pa, T, & S (^4%), 250 E, Pr	> 60%	2
NAACP Defense Fund	Louis Harris	Unfinished agenda on race	Jun-Sept 1998	adults			1
Democratic Leadership Council	Penn, Schoen & Berland	Active center holds survey	Jul-Aug 1998	registered voters	1400 (^3%)		2
Phi Delta Kappa	Gallup	Attitudes toward public schools	June 1998	adults	1151 (3.5%)	> 50%	1
W. K. Kellogg, Surdna, & Rockefeller Foundations	Public Agenda	Time to move on	Mar-Apr 1998	parents	1600 (3%)	>60	3
Public Education Network	Public Agenda	An agenda for public schools	Mar-Apr 1998	adults	1220 (^3.5%)	>60	1
Newsweek, Kaplan Education Center	Princeton Survey Research		March 1998	adults, parents	750 A (^4%), 407 P (^6%)		3
CT Dept of Ed, Council Chief State Schl Officers	Behuniak, Chudowsky, Dirir	Consequences of Assessment …	1997	CT teachers	731 (^4%)	58	2
Montana State U., Billings	Montana State U., Billings		Nov 1997	MT adults	420 (^6%)		1
CNN, USA Today	Gallup	Gallup, CNN, USA Today poll	Oct 1997	adults	872 (^4%)		4
Time, CNN	Yankelovich Partners	Time, CNN, Yankelovich poll	Sept 1997	adults, "active" adults os	1282 (^3.5%) 251AA (^8)		1
NBC News, Wall Street Journal	Hart and Teeter	NBC News, Wall Street Journal poll	Sept 1997	adults	2004 (^2%)		2

(continued)

Sponsoring Organization	Poll/Survey Organization/ Individuals	Title/Subject of Poll/Survey (If Any)	Survey/ Polling Dates	Respondent Groups (Sample is National Unless Otherwise Indicated)	Number of Respondents (Margin of Error $p > .95$)*	Resp. Rate %	# Items[1]
Public Agenda, Education Week, Pew Trusts	Public Agenda	Reality Check	Sep-Oct 1997	parents, studs, profs tchrs, employers	700Pa,S,T (4%), 250Pr,E (7%)	> 60%	1
Public Agenda	Public Agenda	Getting by	1997	students	1000 (^4%)	60%	6
Fordham Foundation	Public Agenda	Different drummers	Jul-Sep 1997	education professors	900 (3%)	17%	6
Democratic Leadership Council	Penn, Schoen & Berland	New democratic electorate survey	July 1997	registered voters	1009 (^4%)		2
Phi Delta Kappa	Gallup	Attitudes toward public schools	June 1997	adults, parents (public school)	1,517 A (3%), 1,017 P (4%)	> 50%	3
South Carolina Department of Education	Public Agenda	South Carolinians look at …	May 1997	SC adults, educators, leaders	800A (3%), 225E, 182L	38%E 23%L	2
Nat'l Assn. Elem. School Principals	NAESP	Tough discipline policies a must …	April 1997	principals (NAESP members)	1,350 (^3.5%)	45%	3
NBC News, Wall Street Journal	Hart and Teeter	NBC News, Wall Street Journal poll	March 1997	adults	2010 (^2%)		7
Wirthlin	Wirthlin Quorum Survey		Feb 1997	adults	1002 (^4%)		2
American Viewpoint	American Viewpoint	National monitor poll	Feb 1997	registered voters	1000 (^4%)		2

Sponsor	Pollster	Title	Date	Population	Sample (%)	Response	
Horatio Alger Assn, Nat'l Assn Sec Schl Principals	NFO Research	The mood of American youth	1996	high school students	1000 (3%)		3
	Public Agenda	Committed to change	1996	MO adults			5
Carnegie, USWest, PTA, NEA, AFT, Gund, Morris, Rockefeller, Hewlett, Mills	Public Agenda	Given the circumstances	1996	teachers (Black, Hispanic os)	1164, 800 in-depth (3.4%)	> 60%	
Public Agenda	Public Agenda	America's views on standards	1996	summary of data from other polls			
	Marist Institute		1996	adults			1
American Federation of Teachers	Peter Hart	Teachers favor standards …	1996	teachers (AFT members)			2
NBC News	Blum & Weprin Associates	NBC News Poll	Apr 1996	adults	504 (^5.5%)		1
US News & World Report	Tarrance; Mellman, Lazurus & Lake	U.S. News & World Report poll	March 1996	adults	1000 (^4%)		2
	Din	Impact of testing on practices …	Feb 1996	KY teachers, principals	180 (^8%)		1
Nat'l Assn. Elem. School Principals	NAESP	Standardized tests useful, but …	1995	principals (NAESP members)	1139 (^4%)	~38%	1

(continued)

Sponsoring Organization	Poll/Survey Organization/ Individuals	Title/Subject of Poll/Survey (If Any)	Survey/ Polling Dates	Respondent Groups (Sample is National Unless Otherwise Indicated)	Number of Respondents (Margin of Error $p > .95$)*	Resp. Rate %	# Items[1]
Public Agenda; Inst for Ed Leadership; 5 Foundations	Public Agenda	Assignment incomplete	1995	parents, politicians, adults, tchrs, civic leaders	1200A (3.4%) 439Pa, 237T, 1151CL (^4%)	> 60% 32%CL	3
American Federation of Teachers	Peter D. Hart	Academic standards & discipline ...	Oct 1995	teachers (AFT members)			2
Phi Delta Kappa	Gallup	Attitudes toward public schools	May-Jun 1995	adults, parents	1311 Adults (^3.5%)	> 50%	3
National Alliance of Business	Scholastic, Inc.	Education in the U.S	April 1995	business leaders, teachers, admins.	1050T, 910A (^4%), 620 B	12B 21T 18A	1
Time, CNN	Yankelovich Partners		Mar 1995	adults, with Blacks os	1060 (^4%)		1
Metropolitan Life	Louis Harris	Survey of the American Teacher	1995	teachers (public schools)	1011 (^4%)	~30%	3
American Assn of School Administrators	Public Agenda	The broken contract	1994	CT adults			1
Amer. Federation of Teachers	Peter D. Hart	Valuable views	Apr 1994	teachers (AFT members)	800 (^4%)		3
8 different foundations, Business Roundtable	Public Agenda, CRC	First things first	August 1994	adults, parents (Black, Christian os)	1198 adults, 724 parents (3%)	> 60%	4

Organization	Pollster	Title	Date	Population	Sample (design effect)	Response rate	#
Phi Delta Kappa	Gallup	Attitudes toward public schools	1994	adults, parents	1,326 adults (^3.5%)	>55%	3
Amer. Federation of Teachers	Peter D. Hart	Valuable views	April 1994	teachers (AFT members)	800 (^4%)		9
National Assn of Music Merchants	Gallup	Amer. attitudes toward music	Mar-Apr 1994			>55%	1
	Jett, Schafer	Teachers attitudes toward …	Apr 1993	MD teachers	538 (^5%)	~44%	1
	Market Strategies		Sept 1993	MI registered voters	800 (^4%)		1
Phi Delta Kappa	Gallup	Attitudes toward public schools	May-Jun 1993	adults, parents	1306 (4%)	>55	7
Newsweek, National PTA	NU Stats, Inc.	Third PTA nat'l education survey	Feb 1993	adults, with minority (Black, Hisp) os	1148 (^3.5%): 562W, 280B,H		1
Metropolitan Life		Survey of the American teacher	1993	teachers (public schools)	1000 (^4%)		1
Phi Delta Kappa	Gallup	Attitudes toward public schools	Apr-May 1992	adults, parents	1306 (4%)	>55	7
Life Magazine	Gallup	If women ran America	Mar-Apr 1992	adults	1222 (^3.5%)		1
	Ryan McGinn Samples Research	West Virginia Poll	Mar 1992	WV adults	412 (^6%)		1
National Assn. of Elem. School Principals	NAESP		Mar 1992	principals	800 (^4%)	~30	2

(continued)

269

Sponsoring Organization	Poll/Survey Organization/ Individuals	Title/Subject of Poll/Survey (If Any)	Survey/ Polling Dates	Respondent Groups (Sample is National Unless Otherwise Indicated)	Number of Respondents (Margin of Error $p > .95$)*	Resp. Rate %	# Items[1]
Charles F Kettering Foundation, Public Agenda	Public Agenda	Ed reform: Players and politics	Jan-Mar 1992	tchrs, admins, board members, biz execs	803:T(6%) A(8%) Bo(12%) Bi(8%)	35	2
U.S. General Accounting Office	U.S. GAO	Survey on systemwide testing	1991-2	state, district administrators	48 states (0%) 370 districts (3%)	100 74	4
	Stake, Theobald	Teachers' views of testing's impact …	1991	teachers in 7 states	285 (^6%)	?	1
	Bond, Cohen		1991	IN administrators	211 (^8%)	21	2
Kansas state Department of Education	Glassnapp, Poggio, Miller		1991	KS studs, parents, board, tchrs, admins	12802S, 3938P (^1%) 1250 T, A (^3%) 441B	~55A	1
Agenda Magazine	Louis Harris	School reform: Public perceptions	Oct-Nov 1991	adults	1252 (^3.5%)		2
	Louis Harris	An assessment of American ed …	Sept 1991	adults, parents, biz, higher ed, grads			
Newsweek, National PTA, Chrysler	ICR Survey Research Group	Chrysler national parent survey	May-Jun 1991	parents	792 (^4%)		1
Agenda Magazine	Louis Harris	Does school budgeting add up?	May-Jun 1991	adults, board prezs, admins, union reps	1254 Al (^3.5%) 200B,An,U (^8%)		2

Organization	Investigator	Title	Date	Population	Sample (response rate)		No.
Times Mirror News	Princeton Survey Research	*Times Mirror* Interest Index	May 1991	adults	1206 (^3.5%)		1
Phi Delta Kappa	Gallup	Attitudes toward public schools	May-Jun 1991	adults	1500 (3%)	> 55	8
Gallup	Gallup	Gallup Poll	Apr-Jun 1991	adults, Black os	1005 (3.5%) 303 B (^6%)		1
NBC News, Wall Street Journal	Hart and Teeter		May 1991	adults	1508 (^3%)		1
Indiana Youth Poll	Indiana Youth Institute		1991	IN students	1560 (3%)		2
Metropolitan Life		Survey of the American teacher	1991	teachers	1007 (^4%)		1
	Delong	Perceptions of quality indicators …	1990	CA principals and admins.	80 school districts		1
Alberta Teachers' Association	Calder	Impact of diploma examinations on …	1990	AL teachers, students	135 T (^9%), 238 S (^7%)	50% schls	8
British Columbia Ministry of Education	Anderson, Muir, Bateson, Blackmore, Rogers	Impact of provincial examinations on …	1990	BC teachers, studs, parents, principals	1833S (^2.5) 947T,608P (^4%) 160 Prin (^8%)	~50	13
Fayetteville Graduate Center	Flynn	Community attitudes toward the state MCT	1990	NC adults (in 4 counties)	150 (^8%)	> 80	3

(continued)

Sponsoring Organization	Poll/Survey Organization/Individuals	Title/Subject of Poll/Survey (If Any)	Survey/Polling Dates	Respondent Groups (Sample is National Unless Otherwise Indicated)	Number of Respondents (Margin of Error $p > .95$)*	Resp. Rate %	# Items
Carnegie Foundation		The condition of teaching	1990	teachers	21,389 (^0.2%)	54%	3
National Science Foundation	Boston College Center for Study of Testing, Education, and Policy	Influence of testing on teaching math and science, grades 4–12	1990	teachers, principals	4,950 teachers (^0.5%)	45%	>5
CBS News	CBS News		May-Jun 1990	adults	1107 (^4%)		2
ABC News	ABC News		Feb 1990	adults	766 (^4%)		1
	Ryan McGinn Samples Research	West Virginia Poll	Jan 1990	WV teachers (public schools)	200 (^8%)		1
South Carolina state Department of Education	Division of Public Accountability	The Exit Exam	1989	students (grades 8 and 11)			2
William T Grant & Nat'l Science Foundations	Stevenson, Chen, Uttal	Beliefs & achievement	1989	Chicago parents, students (20 schls)	968P 1161S (^4%)	40%	1
Texas A&M University	Public Policy Resources Lab	Texas Poll	July 1989	TX adults	1007 (^4%)		1
Phi Delta Kappa	Gallup	Attitudes toward public schools	May-Jun 1989	adults	1584 (3%)	>60%	1
Assoc. Press, Media General	Assoc. Press, Media General		May 1989	adults	1084 (^4%)		1

Sponsor	Researcher	Title	Date	Population	Sample	%	
University of Louisville	Urban Research Institute		May 1989	KY (Oldham County) adults	589 (^5%)		1
	Green, Williams	Student test use by classroom teachers	May 1989	WY, LA teachers	555 WY (2.5%), 253 LA (2.6%)	81%W 54%L	2
Assoc. Press, Media General	Assoc. Press, Media General		March 1989	adults	1108 (^4%)		1
	O'Sullivan	Teacher perceptions of effects of testing …	Feb 1989	NC teachers (in 19 districts)	139 (^7%)		3
Metropolitan Life		Survey of the American teacher	1988	teachers			1
NAACP Legal Defense Fund	Louis Harris	Unfinished agenda on race	Jun-Sept 1988	adults (White, Black, Asian-Amer)	3123(^1%) 110A 2008W, 1005B		1
Phi Delta Kappa	Gallup	Attitudes toward public schools	April 1988	adults, parents	2118 (2%)	> 60%	2
	Yoong	Teachers' perceptions … toward MCT …	1987	Bloomington IN teachers	27 (^15%)	100%	1
East Texas State U.	Lutz, Maddirala; Center for Rsrch and Policy Studies	State mandated testing in TX …	1987	TX teachers	797 (^4%)	23%	3
Eagleton Institute of Politics	Eagleton Institute of Politics		May 1987	NJ teachers	800 (^4%)		1

(continued)

Sponsoring Organization	Poll/Survey Organization/ Individuals	Title/Subject of Poll/Survey (If Any)	Survey/ Polling Dates	Respondent Groups (Sample is National Unless Otherwise Indicated)	Number of Respondents (Margin of Error $p > .95$)*	Resp. Rate %	# Items'
Phi Delta Kappa	Gallup	Attitudes toward public schools	April 1987	adults, parents	1571 adults (3%)	> 60%	3
Research for Better Schools	Corbett, Wilson	Raising the stakes	winter 1987	MD, PA teachers, admins.	277 PA & 23 MD districts		4
University of Nevada, Las Vegas	Center for Survey Research		1986	NV (Las Vegas, Carson City, Washoe) adults			1
Council ... Advance/Support Education	Opinion Research Corporation		Dec 1986	adults	1010 (^4%)		1
Arizona Republic, Phoenix Gazette	Arizona Republic, Phoenix Gazette		Oct 1986	AZ adults	1007 (^4%)		1
University of Maryland	Survey Research Center		July 1986	MD (Prince Georges County) adults	525 (^5%)		1
	Talmey-Drake Research & Strategy		April 1986	CO adults	510 (^5.5%)		1
Phi Delta Kappa	Gallup	Attitudes toward public schools	April 1986	adults, parents	1552 (3%)	> 60%	6
	Ryan McGinn Samples Research	West Virginia Poll	Jan 1986	WV adults	500 (^5.5%)		1
Texas A&M University	Public Policy Resources Lab	Texas Poll	1986	TX adults	1000 (^4%)		1

National Institute of Education	Market Opinion Research	Academic standards	Nov-Jan 1985-6	adults	1200 ($\hat{}$3.5%)		6
Phi Delta Kappa	Gallup	Public attitudes toward schools	May 1985	adults, parents	1528 (3%)	> 60%	2
National Institute of Education	Market Opinion Research	Academic standards	Nov-Jan 1984-5	adults	1200 ($\hat{}$3.5%)		6
	Higginbotham	Perceptions of the Arkansas …	1984	AR legislators, admins, tchrs	all L, 100A, 100T	50L 70A,T	1
Metropolitan Life		Survey of the American teacher	1984	teachers	1000 ($\hat{}$4%)	35%	1
University of South Dakota	Gullickson	Teacher perspectives … use of tests	1984	SD teachers	391 (1.5%)	87%	4
Associated Press, Media General	Associated Press, Media General		June 1984	adults	1243 ($\hat{}$3.5%)		3
Phi Delta Kappa	Gallup	Public attitudes toward schools	May 1984	adults, parents	1515 ($\hat{}$3%)	> 60%	2
	Aiken, Romen	Attitudes, experiences concerning testing	Apr 1984	summary of data from other polls			
WY Dept of Education, U. of Wyoming	Stager, Green	Wyoming teachers' use of tests	Feb 1984	WY teachers	555 (3%)	81%	1

(continued)

Sponsoring Organization	Poll/Survey Organization/ Individuals	Title/Subject of Poll/Survey (If Any)	Survey/ Polling Dates	Respondent Groups (Sample is National Unless Otherwise Indicated)	Number of Respondents (Margin of Error p > .95)*	Resp. Rate %	# Items[1]
National Assn Secondary School Principals			1983	high school students			2
National Education Association	NEA Research	Nationwide teacher opinion poll	Sept 1983	teachers (NEA members)	1596 (^3%)	80%	2
Newsweek	Gallup		June 1983	adults, parents	760 (^4%)		1
Phi Delta Kappa	Gallup	Attitudes toward public schools	May 1983	adults, parents	1540 (^3%)	> 65%	2
National Institute of Education	Estes, Demaline	MCT clarification process	1982	adults	385	77%	2
UCLA	Center for the Study of Evaluation	Test use project	1982	teachers, administrators	851T (^4%) 486 elem, 365 secon	60%E 48%S	8
	Wood	Role of standardized … tests in …	Jan 1982	MD teachers, admins (1 county)	215 T, 120 A (^8%)	50% T	1
	Peterson		1981	districts admins.	29	97	1
Nat'l Institute of Education, UCLA	Yeh, Herman, Rudner	Teachers and testing: Survey of test use …	1981	CA teachers	256 (^7%)		2
UCLA	Center for the Study of Evaluation	Test use project	1981	CA teachers, students (9 schools)	60 S (^13%), 91 T (^10%)		4

Organization	Researcher	Title	Date	Population	Sample (^%)	>65%	
Phi Delta Kappa	Gallup	Public attitudes toward education	1981	adults	(^4%)	>65%	4
ABC News, Washington Post	ABC News, Washington Post		Sept 1981	adults, principals (high school)	1501 A (^3%) 303 P		4
Newsweek	Gallup		March 1981	adults	1103 (^4%)		1
	G. B. Johnson	Perceptions ... toward minimum competency testing program	Jan 1981	DODS—Europe studs, admins, parents, teachers	100 S, P, T (^10%), 57 A	100S, 96A,63P, 80T	5
	Edelman	Impact of the mandated testing program ...	1980	CA teachers (3rd grade, 39 schls)	104 (^10%)	66%	1
	Horn	Competency-based testing in NV	Aug 1980	NV tchrs, legltrs, admins, board prez	311 (^7%)	55%	4
Charles F. Kettering Foundation	Gallup	Public attitudes toward education	May 1980	adults		>65%	1
	Karmos & Karmos	Attitudes toward standardized ...	April 1980	IL students (3 school in south IL)	356 (^6%)		
Educational Testing Service	Yankelovich, Skelly & White	Parents attitudes toward tests	Jan-Feb 1980	parents, high school graduates	1008 (^4%)		8

(continued)

277

Sponsoring Organization	Poll/Survey Organization/ Individuals	Title/Subject of Poll/Survey (If Any)	Survey/ Polling Dates	Respondent Groups (Sample is National Unless Otherwise Indicated)	Number of Respondents (Margin of Error $p > .95$)*	Resp. Rate %	# Items[1]
Psychological Corporation	Beck, Stetz	Teacher and student attitudes	1978-80	teachers, students (in norming sample) NCME members	71763 S (.2%) 3306 T (1%) 284M	95 T 88 S 57 M	3
U. Pittsburgh, Learning R&D Center	Salmon-Cox		1979	teachers (elementary school)			1
Amer. Federation of Teachers	UCLA Center for the Study of Evaluation	Teachers and testing	Fall 1979	teachers (AFT members)	209 (8%)	26%	2
Charles F. Kettering Foundation	Gallup	Public attitudes toward education	May 1979	adults	1511 (3%)	> 65	3
	Olejnik	Standardized ... testing ... viewed from the ...	April 1979	FL teachers, counselors, admins	137 (9%)	69†a 86c	1
	Down	Implications of MCT for minority students	1979	adults, Blacks			
UCLA	Center for the Study of Evaluation		1978	CA teachers (19 elementary schools)	256 (6.5%)	60	1
CBS News	CBS News		June 1978	adults	1622 (3%)		3

NY State Board of Regents	NY State Education Department	Report: Competency Testing Program ...	May 1978	NY principals and admins			1
Charles F. Kettering Foundation	Gallup	Public attitudes toward education	Apr-May 1978	adults	1539 (^3%)	> 65%	4
	Shab	Who wants minimal competencies?	Jan 1978	GA studs, tchrs, admins, parents			
Washington Post	George Fine Research		Jan 1978	adults	1519 (^3%)		1
Charles F. Kettering Foundation	Gallup	Public attitudes toward education	1977	adults	1506 (^3%)	> 70%	1
Charles F. Kettering Foundation	Gallup	Public attitudes toward education	April 1976	adults	1549 (^3%)	> 70%	2
National Assn Secondary School Principals			1974	high school students			2
Charles F. Kettering Foundation	Gallup	Attitudes toward public schools	April 1971	adults	1625 (^3%)	> 70%	1
Charles F. Kettering Foundation	Gallup	Public attitudes toward schools	April 1970	adults	1592 (^3%)	> 70%	2
C.F.K. Ltd.	Gallup	Attitudes toward public schools	Feb 1969	adults	1505 (^3%)	> 70%	2

(continued)

Sponsoring Organization	Poll/Survey Organization/Individuals	Title/Subject of Poll/Survey (If Any)	Survey/Polling Dates	Respondent Groups (Sample is National Unless Otherwise Indicated)	Number of Respondents (Margin of Error p > .95)*	Resp. Rate %	# Items[!]
Washington Post	Louis Harris		Feb 1967	adults			1
	Gallup-American Institute of Public Opinion		Sept 1962	adults	1701 (^3%)	>70%	1
	Gallup-American Institute of Public Opinion		Mar 1961	adults	1608 (^3%)	>70%	1
	Gallup-American Institute of Public Opinion		1958	adults			1
	Gallup-American Institute of Public Opinion		July 1954	adults	1500 (^3%)	>70%	4
2 other pre-1967 items	both Gallup		<1967	adults			

*Margin of error indicated is for percentages of responses near 30 or 70 percent. Very low or very high percentages of responses (e.g., below 20% or above 80%) would have a lower margin of error. Mid-range percentages of responses (e.g., about 50%) would have a higher margin of error. See, for reference, the "Sampling Tolerances" table used by Gallup in the *Phi Delta Kappan*, v.81, n.1, p.29 of 34, at www.pdkintl.org/kappan/kpol0090.htm

[!] That is, the approximate number of items reviewed for the purpose of this study. Poll or survey might have contained additional items on the general topic of testing.

^Upper bound estimate based on size of response sample, used if source does not indicate the margin of error. See, for reference, the "Sampling Tolerances" table used by Gallup in the *Phi Delta Kappan*, v.81, n.1, p.29 of 34, at www.pdkintl.org/kappan/kpol0090.htm

"os" = oversample

Appendix B

Some Studies Revealing Testing Achievement Benefits, by Methodology Type

Note. Listings representing multiple studies (e.g., meta-analyses, research syntheses) in bold.

Author, Year	Topic or Location	Method
Theoretical Models & Literature Reviews		**Type**
Adams, Chapman, 2002	**education quality studies**	**literature review**
Behuniak, 2002	**consumer-reference testing**	**conceptual model**
Roueche, Roueche, 1999	**mastery learning in developmental education**	**review of studies**
Marion, Sheinker, 1999*	**minimum competency testing**	**literature review**
Lane, Parke, Stone, 1998	statewide performance assessment	conceptual framework for examining consequences
McCabe, McCabe, & Day, 1998, 2000	**U.S. postsecondary developmental education**	**review of mastery learning**
O'Neill, 1998	**writing assessment**	**literature review, historical analysis**
Black, Wiliam, 1998	**classroom assessment**	**literature review**
Somanathan, 1996	education standards & earnings	mathematical model
Bailey,1996	**washback in language testing**	**literature review**
Cross, Cross, & Steadman, 1996, 1997	**assessment in U.S. higher education**	**literature review**
Betts, 1996	education standards & earnings	mathematical model
Wiliam, Black, 1996	**relationship between formative and summative assessment**	**conceptual model**
Costrell, 1995	national education standards	mathematical model

Author, Year	Topic or Location	Method
Cameron, Pierce, 1994, 1996	meta analysis	studies on effect of extrinsic rewards
Costrell, 1994	college admission standards	mathematical model
Schanker, 1994	need for high standards and tests	conceptual model
Covington, 1993	college students	review of research on motivation in college study
Southern Regional Education Board, 1993	U.S. Southern states	review of SREB studies
Costrell, 1993	education standards	mathematical model
Thomas, 1992	relationship between effort, expectations, & achievement	literature review
Kulik, Kulik, 1991	multiple (frequent testing = more achievement gains)	meta-analysis of developmental instruction
Northwest Regional Lab, 1990	effective schools	literature review
Cotton, 1990	effective schools	literature review
Becker, Rosen, 1990	learning effect of assessment	mathematical model
Levine, Lezotte, 1990	many U.S. studies	research synthesis of school effectiveness studies
Duran, 1989	dynamic assessment with at-risk Hispanic children	literature review and conceptual model
Hughes, 1989, 1993	how washback effect works and how to measure it	conceptual model
Crooks, 1988	multiple	literature review on relationship between testing and outcomes
Hillocks, 1987	multiple	research synthesis of studies on teaching writing
Popham, Kirby, 1987	teacher re-certification tests	conceptual model
Kulik, Kulik, 1987	multiple (frequent testing = more achievement gains)	meta-analysis of 49 experiments and quasi-experiments
U.S. ED, 1987	teaching & learning	literature review
Kang, 1985	incentives provided by testing	mathematical model
Taylor, Valentine, Jones, 1985	effective schools studies	literature review
Corcoran, 1985	competency testing & at-risk youth	conceptual model
Dawson, Dawson, 1985	minimum competency testing	conceptual model
Kiemig, 1983	U.S. higher education	review of effectiveness studies
Hoegl, 1983	legal & administrative rationales for standards	conceptual model

Author, Year	Topic or Location	Method
Purkey, Smith, 1983	U.S.	review of effective schools studies
Milton, 1981	U.S.	review of testing studies
Popham, 1981	minimum competency testing	conceptual model
Mallory, 1980	minimum competency testing	annotated bibliography
Hawisher, Harper, 1979	minimum competency testing	annotated bibliography
ERIC, 1978	minimum competency testing	annotated bibliography
Jackson, Battiste, 1978	minimum competency testing	annotated bibliography
Fincher, 1978	minimum competency testing	conceptual model
Riley, 1977	n/a	historical analysis
Stanley, 1976	accelerated learning for advanced students	conceptual model
Bloom, 1976	mastery learning	conceptual model
Anderson, 1976	multiple	effect of frequency of testing in mastery learning
Block, Tierney, 1974	multiple	methodological study of mastery learning experimental design
Staats, 1973	experiments on classroom reinforcement systems	literature review
Anderson, 1973	multiple	review of mastery testing experiments
Kazdin, Bootzin, 1972	experiments on classroom reinforcement systems	literature review
Bloom, 1971	mastery learning	conceptual model
O'Leary, Drabman, 1971	experiments on classroom reinforcement systems	literature review
Kirkland, 1971	controlled experiments	literature review of 200 studies on effect of tests on students, schools
Homme, Csanyi, Gonzales, Rechs, 1969	experiments on classroom reinforcement systems	literature review
Keller, 1968	developed mastery learning system with frequent testing	process model
Bloom, 1968	mastery learning	conceptual model
Carroll, 1963	mastery learning	conceptual model
Tyler, 1959	influence of tests on teaching & student effort	review of studies and conceptual models
Tyler, 1949	influence of tests on teaching & student effort	conceptual model
Brereton, 1944	Great Britain	literature review

Author, Year	Topic or Location	Method
Consultative Committee on Examinations, 1910	Great Britain	literature review

Controlled Experiments		Type
Ogden, Thompson, Russell, Simons, 2003***	university screening test for supplemental instruction	test group received mastery learning SI, higher performance, lower retention
Locke, Latham, 2002	multiple	meta-analysis of over 3 decades of experiments
Fuchs, Fuchs, Karns, Hamlett, Katzaroff, 1999	16 teachers and their classes	group using performance assessments improved on several measures
Ross, Rolheiser, Hoaboam-Gray, 1998	300 grade 5 and 6 students in Ontario schools	controlled experiment between continuously evaluated group and controls
Tuckman, Trimble, 1997	41 8th grade science students	controlled experiment comparing effect of homework and quizzes
Ramirez, 1997***	university screening test for supplemental instruction	test group received mastery learning SI, higher performance, lower retention
Cross, Cross, & Steadman, 1996, 1997	assessment in U.S. higher education	literature review
Egeland, 1995	fifth-graders in a suburban school district	controlled experiment (3 groups: control, Hawthorne, and tested group)
Wolf, Smith, 1995	158 undergraduates	controlled experiment comparing graded testing to nongraded testing
Tuckman, 1994	226 undergraduates	controlled experiment comparing homework to weekly quizzes
Chao-Qun, Hui, 1993	Fuxin City, China	comparison of student score gains of teacher tested group against control
Ritchie, Thorkildsen, 1994	96 fifth-graders in 4 classrooms	comparison of mastery learning group to a traditional learning group
Cameron, Pierce, 1994, 1996	meta analysis	studies on effect of extrinsic rewards
Brown, Walberg, 1993	406 Chicago elementary students	controlled experiment on test motivation (stakes vs. no stakes)
Toppino, Luipersbeck, 1993	160 college students	students learn incorrect test items in retests, (i.e., they learn while taking tests)
Jones, 1993	18 upper-level high school math classes, 546 students	experiment on second-chance option of final test score replacing earlier scores
Brooks-Cooper, 1993	high school students	group offered money for correct answers did better on test than controls

Author, Year	Topic or Location	Method
Kika, McLaughlin, Dixon, 1992	two classes of grade 11 algebra students	weekly tested students learned more than bi-weekly tested students
Khalaf, Hanna, 1992	2,000 Saudi 10th grade biology students	controlled experiment comparing students tested monthly and semimonthly
Bangert-Drowns, Kulik, Kulik, 1991	multiple	**meta-analysis of 35 studies on testing frequency effects on achievement**
Kulik, Kulik, 1991	multiple (frequent testing = more achievement gains)	**meta-analysis of developmental instruction**
Thompson, 1990	multiple	**calculation of comparative costs of mastery testing to control**
Csikszentmihalyi, 1990	multiple	**review of psychology studies on human productivity**
Duran, 1989	at-risk Hispanic children	experiment with "dynamic" assessment used with treatment group
Kulik, Kulik, 1989	multiple	**meta-analysis of mastery testing experiments and quasi-experiments**
Stark, Shaw, Lowther, 1989	multiple	**review of research between length of goal horizon and motivation**
Crooks, 1988	multiple	**meta-analysis on classroom evaluation experiments from 14 research fields**
Friedman, 1987	college mathematics courses	contrasting groups given multiple tests throughout course to one given one at end
Hillocks, 1987	multiple	**research synthesis of studies on teaching writing**
Kulik, Kulik, 1987	multiple	**meta-analysis of 49 experiments and quasi-experiments**
Guskey, Gates, 1986	multiple	**research synthesis of 25 studies on mastery learning**
Marsh, 1984	ten classes from five universities	contrasting of achievement gains with take-home and in-class exams
Natriello, Dornbusch, 1984	multiple	**review of controlled experiments and quasi-experiments**
Kulik, Kulik, Schwalb, 1983	multiple	**meta-analysis of**
Locke, Shaw, Saari, Latham, 1981	multiple	**review of research on relationship between motivation and goals**
Good, Grouws, 1979	**Missouri 4th-grade mathematics classrooms**	**effectiveness study**
Kulik, Kulik, Cohen, 1979	multiple (frequent testing = increased achievement)	**meta-analysis of studies of Keller's mastery learning process**

Author, Year	Topic or Location	Method
Chamberlin, et al., 1978	**AP students at Indiana U. and their matched pairs**	**AP students took more courses and achieved better grades**
Goodson, Okey, 1978	**college science students**	**controlled experiment on using test results diagnostically throughout course**
McMillan, 1977	undergraduates classes	controlled experiment comparing effects of high- and low-effort assignments & praise
Abbott, Falstrom, 1977	**multiple**	**controlled experiments**
Engel, 1977	alternative schools	controlled experiments
Rosswork, 1977	**multiple**	**review of controlled experiments, sensitivity analysis**
Block, Burns, 1976	**multiple**	**mastery learning experiments**
McWilliams, Thomas, 1976	elementary students	controlled experiment
Poggio, 1976	Kansas mathematics students	long-term controlled experiments of mastery learning methods
Swanson, Denton, 1976	high school chemistry students	controlled experiment on use (or non-use) of test results in remediation
Cross, 1976	**multiple**	**review of mastery learning research**
Gaynor, Millham, 1976	students in college psychology courses	controlled experiment, one group with weekly tests during term, other just two
Anderson, 1976	**multiple**	**effect of frequency of testing in mastery learning**
Burrows, Okey, 1975	4th and 5th graders	controlled experiment on mastery learning and testing versus controls
Okey, 1974, 1975		mastery learning study
Davis, 1975	U.S. university	mastery testing requirement improves test performance
Glasnapp, Poggio, Ory, 1975	Kansas classrooms	effect of mastery learning methods
Fiel, Okey, 1974	U.S.	effect of evaluation component in mastery learning
Roueche, Kirk, 1974	**community college remediation programs**	**frequent testing improved student mastery and program success**
Kim, Cho, Park, Park, 1974	20 Korean classrooms	mastery learning study in moral education
Jones, 1974	20 classrooms	mastery learning study in algebra
Hymel, 1974	**Louisiana**	**study of mastery learning methods**
Resnick, Robinson, 1974	**review of literacy research**	**motivational effect of requirements**

Author, Year	Topic or Location	Method
Staats, 1973	multiple	controlled experiments on classroom reinforcement programs
Roueche, Wheeler, 1973	community college remediation programs	frequent testing improved student mastery and program success
Block, 1973b	multiple	mastery learning experiments
Anderson, 1973	multiple	review of mastery testing experiments
Roueche, 1973	community college remediation programs	frequent testing improved student mastery and program success
Wentling, 1973	U.S. classrooms	experiment comparing mastery to nonmastery methods
Block 1973a	multiple	mastery learning experiments
Kazdin, Bootzin, 1972	multiple	controlled experiments on classroom reinforcement programs
Block, 1972	multiple	mastery learning experiments
Lee, Kim, Kim, Park, Yoo, Chang, Kim, 1971	179 classrooms	mastery learning study in math and science
O'Leary, Drabman, 1971	multiple	controlled experiments on classroom reinforcement programs
Kirkland, 1971	multiple	review of 200 studies on effects of tests on students and schools
Block, 1971	multiple	mastery learning experiments
Homme, Csanyi, Gonzales, Rechs, 1969	multiple	controlled experiments on classroom reinforcement programs
Somerset, 1968	Ugandan primary and secondary schools	national exams improved school management, learning
Roueche, 1968	community college remediation programs	frequent testing improved student mastery and program success
Westbrook, 1967	U.S. classrooms	effect of test reporting (versus no information about test performance)
Wrightstone, 1963	multiple	contrasting gains between controls and students frequently tested w/ feedback
Carroll, 1955	University and military language programs	review of many controlled experiments
Skinner, 1954	multiple	frequent testing increased learning in controlled experiments
Pollaczek, 1952	multiple	contrasting gains between controls and students getting feedback from tests

Author, Year	Topic or Location	Method
Ross, Henry, 1939	multiple	contrasting gains between controls and students frequently tested
Kirkpatrick, 1934	multiple	contrasting gains between controls and students frequently tested
Keys, 1934	multiple	contrasting gains between controls and students frequently tested
Turney, 1931	multiple	contrasting gains between controls and students frequently tested
Panlasigui, Knight, 1930	2 matched groups, 358 studs in 56 4th grade math classes	contrasting gains, controls with students comparing their test results to standards
Hurlock, 1925	effect of incentives on IQ scores	controlled experiments

Quasi Experimental Designs		Type
Ellet, Teddlie, 2003	U.S. teacher evaluation and school effectiveness	review of studies of relations between the two
Reynolds, Mujis, Treharne, 2003	teacher evaluation and school effectiveness	review of studies of relations between the two
Langer, 2001	4 states, 25 schools, 44 teachers, 88 classes, 2 years	observations, interviews, documents, field notes
Phelps, 2001	TIMSS, 100+ other data sources	compared high-scoring to low-scoring TIMSS countries
Taylor, Pearson, Clark, Walpole, 1999	14 English schools, primary grades	compared school and classroom factors related to reading achievement
Designs for Change, 1997**	Chicago elementary schools, 1990–19977	compared improved schools to others, controlling for background factors
McCabe, McCabe, & Day, 2000	U.S. postsecondary developmental education	review of mastery learning
Morgan, Ramist, 1998	U.S.	differential success of AP students in college verifies "opt out" value of AP exam
Beardon, 1997	Dallas mathematics class	comparison of effective teachers' practices to other teachers'
Mullis, 1997	TIMSS	exploratory data analysis
Schonecker, 1996	Minnesota community colleges	students where testing (for remediation) mandatory do better than counterparts
Tanner, 1995	U.S. school district	effect of competency testing on instruction
Chen, Stevenson, 1995	East Asian & U.S. Caucasian, Asian-American students	motivation and mathematics achievement

Author, Year	Topic or Location	Method
Boylan, Bonham, Claxton, Bliss, 1992, 1994	**U.S. developmental education programs**	**mastery learning techniques produced higher grades and retention rates**
Morgan, Crone, 1993	U. California AP students compared to matched pairs	AP students took more courses, tougher courses, and received higher grades
Mattsson, 1993**	Sweden	comparison of variance in teacher marks in tested and non-tested subjects
Moore, 1991	79 classrooms in 13 schools in one district	MANCOVA used to compare four groups based on teacher attitudes to testing
Thompson, 1990	**multiple**	**calculation of comparative costs of mastery testing to control**
Levine, Lezotte, 1990	**many U.S. studies**	**research synthesis of school effectiveness studies**
LaRoque, Coleman, 1989	British Columbia	comparison groups (longitudinal and cross-sectional)
Mortimore, Sammons, Stoll, Lewis, Ecob, 1988	British junior schools	teacher effectiveness comparison at school and classroom levels
Willingham, Morris, 1986	U.S.	contrasts AP students' college progress to their matched counterparts'
Brooke, Oxenham, 1984	Ghana and Mexico	comparison of system with high standards and stakes (Ghana) to one without
Clark, Lotto, Astuto, 1984	**U.S.**	**review of effective schools studies**
Taylor, Valentine, Jones, 1985	**effective schools studies**	**literature review**
Rutter, 1983	**U.S.**	**review of effective schools studies**
Purkey, Smith, 1983	**U.S.**	**review of effective schools studies**
Brookover, Lezotte, 1979	8 elementary schools in Michigan	questionnaires, interviews, administrative records
Wellisch, MacQueen, Carriere, Duck, 1978	U.S.	paired comparison of 26 high- and low-achieving schools, pre-post testing
Foss, 1977	Great Britain	experimental design, comparison groups, pre-post, with interviews and surveys
Fillbrandt, Merz, 1977	one U.S. district	compares test performance of graduating seniors with "successful" job holders
Wildemuth, 1977	**U.S.**	**review of effective schools studies**
Jones, Gordon, Schechtman, 1975	U.S. community college	mastery testing study

Author, Year	*Topic or Location*	*Method*
Olmsted, 1957	**U.S. universities**	**review of testing studies**
Pressey, 1954	U.S. students from high school into adulthood	review of longitudinal studies of tested and accelerated cohort to matched pairs
Terman, 1954	U.S. students from high school into adulthood	longitudinal comparison of tested and accelerated cohort to matched pairs
Fund for the Advancement of Education, 1953	U.S. students from high school into adulthood	longitudinal comparison of tested and accelerated cohort to matched pairs
Wood, 1953	Ohio high school graduates through college	longitudinal comparison of tested to nontested students
Pressey, 1949	U.S. students from high school into adulthood	longitudinal comparison of tested and accelerated cohort to matched pairs
Terman, 1954	U.S. students from high school into adulthood	longitudinal comparison of tested and accelerated cohort to matched pairs
Tyler, 1941	3 locations: Columbus, OH; Rochester, NY; Chicago, IL	comparison groups/experimental studies

Case Studies & Structured Interviews		**Type**
Singh, McMillan, 2002	Virginia	case studies
Garcia, Rothman (Achieve) 2002	**Maryland, Massachusetts, Texas**	**case studies**
Denison University, 2002	freshman class	case study
Mass Insight, 2002	Massachusetts	surveys and interviews in urban areas
DeBard, Kubow, 2001	**Perrysburg Schools, OH**	**focus groups and surveys of teachers, administrators, students, support staff**
Cawelti, 2001	**6 U.S. school districts**	**case studies**
Henchey, et al., 2001	**Québec, British Columbia, Alberta**	**case studies of 12 secondary schools in low-income settings**
Hansen, 2001	Chicago	pre-post, case study
Anderson, 2001	Brazosport ISD, Texas	pre-post, case study
Milanowski, Heneman, 2001**	1 Midwestern school district	teacher interviews and survey
Chapman, Snyer, 2000	**country case studies**	**research synthesis**
Hogan, 2000	Texas	case study
Yussufu, Angaka, 2000	Kenya	case study of national test result-induced changes in local schools
Blum, 2000	Reynolds SD, Oregon	pre-post observations, review of admin. records, interviews, data analysis
van Dam, 2000	the Netherlands	case study of new national turnkey school-based assessment program

Author, Year	Topic or Location	Method
Beaudry, 2000**	Maine	case studies, teacher and administrator surveys, site visit observations
Chen, Chang, 1999	freshmen at CUNY	compared GPAs for 6 years of non-tested, to tested-remediated, to non-remediated
Schleisman, 1999	Minneapolis	structured interviews
Kelley, 1999	**Kentucky, Maryland, Charlotte, Douglas Cnty, CO**	**case studies with interviews, surveys, document analysis**
Greene, 1999	New York State	effects of new teacher certification tests
Goldberg, Roswell, 1999**	Maryland	case study, teacher survey
Southern Regional Education Board, 1998	**Hoke County, NC, and other Southern cities and districts**	**case studies of academic-vocational program**
Trelfa, 1998	Japan	case studies
Grissmer, Flanagan, 1998	NAEP, Texas & North Carolina	data analysis, review of administrative data
Powell, 1997	U.S.	history of original College Board system from 1900 to 1942
Miles, Bishop, Collins, Fink, Gardner, Grant, Hussain, et al., 1997	ten'All Regents' high schools in New York State	case studies
Aguilera, Hendricks, 1996	3 Texas school districts	case studies
Banta, Lund, Black, Oblander, 1996	**U.S. higher education programs**	**multiple case studies**
Oshiro, 1996	University of Hawaii–West Oahu	evaluation of senior project
Resnick, Nolan, Resnick, 1995	France and the Netherlands	case studies, content analysis
Stevenson, Lee, et al., 1995, 1997	**Japan, United Kingdom, France, Germany**	**literature reviews, interviews with students, parents, and teachers**
Prais, 1995	France, Germany, U.K.	comparative case studies
Bottoms, Mikos, SREB, 1995	7 high schools in the South	case studies of academic-vocational program
Bentz, 1994	Illinois	case study of the feedback effect of teacher testing on curriculum & instruction
Bishop, 1993	U.K., French, Dutch, U.S. documents	case studies
Bamberg, Medina, 1993**	**multiple**	**review of case studies**
Wolf, Rapiau, 1993	France and England	comparative case studies

Author, Year	Topic or Location	Method
U.S. General Accounting Office(a), 1993	Canadian Provinces	case studies, summary of program evaluations
Eckstein, Noah, 1993	8 countries	case studies
Nassif, 1992	Georgia, Illinois, Texas, West Virginia, New York State	case studies of teacher testing
Heyneman, Ransom, 1992	World Bank countries	case studies
Gibbs, 1992; Oxford Centre for Staff Development, 1992	redesigned courses over 2½ year period	ten case studies
Brown, 1992*, **	14 schools in states of IL, TN, and NY	structured interviews of 5th and 6th grade teachers and their principals
Whetton, National Foundation for Educational Research, 1992**	England & Wales	study of teachers' adaptations to national assessment
Steedman, 1992	France, Germany, U.K.	comparative case studies
Ferrara, Willhoft, Seburn, Slaughter, Stevenson, 1991	Maryland	survey, case studies, data analyses, with shadow test comparisons
Harnisch, Switzer, 1991	136 teachers in a Midwestern state	math and science teachers
Bude, 1989*	Kenya	case study of national testing program
O'Sullivan, 1989*	North Carolina	interviews with 139 K-12 teachers
Somerset, 1988	Kenya	case study
Corcoran, Wilson, 1986	U.S.	case studies of secondary schools in recognition program
Resnick, Resnick, 1985	England & Wales	observations, interviews, and literature review
Natriello, Dornbusch, 1984	U.S.	observations of 38 classrooms
Brooke, Oxenham, 1984	Ghana and Mexico	comparison of system with high standards and stakes (Ghana) to one without
Oxenham, 1984	several Asian countries	comparative case studies
Ogle, Fritz, 1981**	Skokie, IL	case study
Popham, Rankin, 1981	Detroit, MI	case study
Rentz, 1979	Georgia	case study, surveys, interviews
Findley, 1978	Westside H.S., Omaha, NE	case study
Schab, 1978	one U.S. school district's minimal competency testing	case study
Neal, 1978	Denver	case study

Author, Year	Topic or Location	Method
Foss, 1977	Great Britain	experimental design, comparison groups, pre-post, with interviews and surveys
Engel, 1977	alternative schools	case study
Solberg, 1977	Netherlands	case study
Estes, Colvin, Goodwin, 1976	Phoenix SD	case study of district designed testing program
Lortie, 1975	**multiple**	**case studies of school teachers, including study of how some succeed**
Rist, 1970	U.S.	administrative records and case studies on tests as "second chance" option
Feldhusen, 1964	U.S.	student survey and interviews

Program evaluations		type of evaluation
Ferman, 2004	Israel	surveys, interviews, document analysis
Jones, Jones, Hargrove, 2003*	North Carolina, Florida	teacher surveys and interviews
Jones, Egley, 2003*	North Carolina	teacher survey
Standards Work, 2003	Virginia	mixed-mode, with shadow test comparison
Jones, Johnston, 2002*	North Carolina	teacher surveys and interviews
McDonald, 2002	Alberta	teachers, administrators, survey, pre-post
Dougherty, Collins, 2002	Texas	school administrators survey
Achieve, 2001**	Massachusetts	program evaluation, content analysis
Guth, Holtzman, Schneider, et al. (WestEd), 2001	California	teacher and administrator surveys
Gipps, 2000	32 English schools	classroom observations, interviews, surveys, data analysis of admin records
Legislative Office of Education Oversight, 2000	Ohio	shadow measures comparison, case studies, surveys, interviews, ...
Beaudry, 2000	Maine	case studies, teacher and administrator surveys, site visit observations
Bergeson, Fitton, Bylsma, Neitzel, 2000**	Washington State	interviews, surveys, data analysis, review of administrative records
Goldberg, Roswell, 1999**	Maryland	case study, teacher survey
Boylan, Saxon, 1998	**Texas developmental education programs**	**document summary, interviews, surveys, etc.**

Author, Year	Topic or Location	Method
Neville, 1998**	Chicago (2 elementary schools)	observations, interviews, surveys, data and content analysis of admin. records
Florida Office of Program Policy Analysis, 1997	Florida	analysis of administrative records, surveys, 27 school site visits
Anderson, Artman, 1972	one university	mastery learning program in physics
Clarke, Stephens, 1996	Victoria State, Australia	document content analysis, surveys & interviews with teachers, admin. survey
Abar, 1996	Massachusetts	interviews, survey
Boylan, 1996	**Texas Academic Skills Program**	**document summary, interviews, surveys, etc.**
U.S. General Accounting Office(a), 1993	**Canadian Provinces**	**interviews, literature review, summary of program evaluations**
Wilson, Corbett, 1991*	Maryland & Pennsylvania	teacher, administrator surveys
Ferrara, Willhoft, Seburn, Slaughter, Stevenson, 1991	Maryland	survey, case studies, data analyses, with shadow test comparisons
Anderson, Muir, Bateson, Blackmore, Rogers, 1990	British Columbia	mixed-mode evaluation, surveys of teachers, students, parents, employers, principals
Pine, 1989**	New Jersey schools	change in instruction after addition of testing requirement
Stevenson, Chen, Uttal, 1989	Cook County, IL	parents, students, analysis of student records
Heyneman, 1987, 1988	**World Bank countries**	**summary of program evaluations**
Somerset, 1987	Kenya case study	evaluation of change in national testing program
Kellaghan, Madaus, Airasian, 1982*	Ireland	teacher survey and more
Peterson, 1981	several U.S. large city school districts	effect of minimum competency testing
Venezky, Winfield, 1979	several low SES Delaware elementary schools	site visits, observations, interviews, administrative records, work logs
Abramowitz, 1978	U.S.	survey of public and private high schools regarding early graduation policies
Fisher, 1978	Florida	program evaluation, data analysis
Foss, 1977	Great Britain	experimental design, comparison groups, pre-post, with interviews and surveys

Author, Year	Topic or Location	Method
Polls and Surveys **(only items pertaining to link between tests and improved achievement, motivation, alignment)**		**Population Surveyed**
Bradshaw, 2002	21 north-eastern North Carolina districts	teachers
Mass Insight, 2002	Massachusetts	students in urban areas, survey and interviews
Public Agenda, 2002	U.S.	students, employers, parents, teachers, college professors
Educational Testing Service, Hart & Teeter, 2002	U.S.	adults, parents, teachers, policy makers
Public Education Network, *EdWeek*, 2002	U.S.	teachers
Educational Testing Service, Hart & Teeter, 2001	U.S.	public and parents
Business Roundtable, 2001	U.S.	parents
Quinnipiac University, 2001	New York City	adults
Lumley, Yan, 2001	Pennsylvania	teachers
Public Agenda, 2000	U.S	public, parents
EdWeek, Beldon, Russonello, & Stewart, 2000*	U.S.	teachers
Banerji, 2000**	Florida	survey of districts regarding alignment of district activities with state initiatives
Earl, Torrance, 2000**	Ontario	survey of 2,400 elementary schools
Amer Assn School Admins., Lake, Snell, & Perry, 2000	U.S.	parents
McMillan, Myran, Workman, 1999**	Virginia	teachers (722 in year 1; 80 in year 2) regarding changes in instruction
Lane, Parke, Stone, 1999	Maryland	teachers, students, principals
Heneman, 1998	Charlotte-Mecklenburg SD, North Carolina	teachers
CNN, USA Today, Gallup, 1997	U.S.	adults
Boylan, Bliss, Bonham, 1997, 1999	**U.S. developmental education programs**	**students (N = 6,000)**
NBC, Wall Street Journal, Hart & Teeter, 1997	U.S.	adults

Author, Year	Topic or Location	Method
Phi Delta Kappa, Gallup, 1997	U.S.	public, parents (public schools)
Behuniak, Chudowsky, Dirir, 1997	Connecticut	teachers
Din,1996**	Kentucky	teachers, principals
Phi Delta Kappa, Gallup, 1995	U.S.	public, parents (public schools)
Public Agenda, 1994	U.S.	public, parents
American Federation of Teachers, 1994	U.S.	teachers (AFT members)
Loerke, 1993	Alberta	teachers, administrators
Jett, Schafer, 1993	Maryland	teachers
Newsweek, PTA, NU Stats, 1993	U.S.	adults
U.S. General Accounting Office(b), 1993	U.S. states and districts	district and state administrators
Bond, Cohen, 1991	Indiana	school and district administrators
Stake, Theobold, 1991*	7 U.S. states	teachers and administrators
Perrin, 1991	Geneva Canton (Switzerland)	students
Calder, 1991*	Alberta	teachers, students
Glasnapp, Poggio, Miller, 1991	Kansas	students, parents, teachers, board members, administrators
Phi Delta Kappa, Gallup, 1991	U.S.	public, parents
NBC News, Wall Street Journal, Hart & Teeter, 1991	U.S.	adults
Flynn, 1990	4 North Carolina counties	public, parents
Delong, 1990	California	school and district administrators
South Carolina DOE, 1990	South Carolina	students, teachers, public, parents
CBS News, 1990	U.S.	adults
Green, Williams, 1989*	Wyoming, Louisiana	teachers
Lutz, Maddirala, 1987	**Texas**	**teachers**
Phi Delta Kappa, Gallup, 1987	U.S.	public, parents
Stager, Green, 1984*	Wyoming	teachers
Gullickson, 1984	a rural Midwestern state	elementary and secondary teachers
Herman, Dorr-Bremme, 1983*	U.S.	teachers
Clark, Guskey, Benninga, 1983***	a rural Midwestern state	teacher survey, ratings, and weekly logs

Author, Year	Topic or Location	Method
Estes, Demaline, 1982	NIE Hearing on minimum competency testing	adults in audience
Johnson, 1981	U.S. DOD schools	students, parents, teachers, administrators
Ward, Gould, AFT, 1980	U.S. AFT members	teachers (AFT members)
Horn, 1980	Nevada	teachers, administrators, board presidents, legislators
Karmos, Karmos, 1980	U.S.	students, teachers
Down, 1979	U.S. minorities	adults
Center for Research & Evaluation, UCLA, 1979*	U.S.	teachers
Shab, 1978	Georgia	students, teachers, parents, administrators
Feldhusen, 1964	U.S.	students

Benefit-Cost Analyses/Data Analyses of Administrative Records		Type
Johnson, Treisman, Fuller, 2000	Texas	literature review and data analyses
Toenjes, Dworkin, Lorence, Hill, 2000	Texas	data analysis, critique of literature, with shadow test comparison
Phelps, 2000	Texas	data analysis, critique of literature, with shadow test comparison
Lane, Parke, Stone, 1999	Maryland	data analysis (longitudinal)
Magruder, McManis, Young, 1997	Truman State University	twenty-year study, in several stages of implementation of campus-wide program
Bock, Wolfe, 1996	Tennessee	data analysis of administrative records
Phelps, 1996	Texas	benefit-cost analysis of teacher test
Phelps, 1994, 1998, 2002	U.S.	benefit-cost analysis of large-scale testing
Solmon, Fagnano, 1990	Texas	benefit-cost analysis of teacher test
Salmon-Cox, 1980*	U.S.	administrative records and case studies on tests as "second chance" option
Polgar, 1976	California	data analysis of budgetary records
Weinman, 1976	Massachusetts	data analysis of trends, content analysis of college catalogues, and interviews
Rist, 1970	U.S.	administrative records and case studies on tests as "second chance" option

Author, Year	Topic or Location	Method
New York State Regents, 1936**	New York State	pre-post testing, data analysis of administrative records

Multivariate Analysis		Type
Braun, 2003*	State NAEP	multiple regression (cross-sectional, pre-post)
Rosenshine, 2003	State NAEP	multiple regression (cross-sectional, pre-post)
Carnoy, Loeb, Smith, 2002	State NAEP	multiple regression (cross-sectional, pre-post)
Thompson, 2002	State NAEP	multiple anova and regression
Bishop, Mane, Bishop, Moriarty, 2001	**review of testing benefit studies**	**multiple regression**
Carnoy, Loeb, Smith, 2001	Texas	multiple regression
Wenglinsky, 2001	U.S. (1996 NAEP Mathematics)	multilevel structural equation model
Hannaway, McKay, 2001	Houston	regressions (longitudinal), with shadow test comparison
Betts, Costrell, 2001	Massachusetts	multiple regression
Woessman, 2000	TIMSS micro data	robust linear regression (cross sectional)
Massachusetts Finance Office, 2000	Massachusetts	multiple regression
Grissmer, Flanagan, Kawati, Williamson, 2000	State NAEP	multiple regression (longitudinal)
Bishop, 1999	TIMSS	multiple regression (cross sectional)
Ladd, 1999	Dallas	regressions (cross-sectional)
Mitchell, 1999	DeKalb SD, Georgia	multiple anova
Herrick, 1999	State NAEP	multiple regression (cross-sectional, pre-post)
J. Sanders, 1999	Tennessee	regression of teacher on later student scores
Bishop, 1998	New York & North Carolina	multiple regression (cross sectional)
Mendro, 1998	Dallas	multiple regression
Betts, 1998	U.S.	multiple regression (longitudinal)
Bishop, Moriarty, Mane, 1997	SAT-1 by state, 8th grade NAEP math	multiple regression
Webster, Mendro, Orsak, Weerasinghe, Bembry, 1997	Dallas	multiple regression (longitudinal)

Author, Year	Topic or Location	Method
Brookhart, 1997	U.S. (Longitudinal Study of American Youth)	path model analysis (fitted with stepwise regression)
Pomplun, 1997**	Kansas	path model analysis of teacher behavior
Schafer, Hultgren, Hawley, Abrams, Seubert, Mazzoni, 1997	Maryland	multiple regressions (cross-sectional)
Sanders, Rivers, 1996	Tennessee	regression of teacher on later student scores
Ferguson, Ladd, 1996	Alabama	multiple regressions of teacher factors on student achievement (cross-sectional)
Zigarelli, 1996	U.S. (NELS-88)	multiple regressions - tests of effective schools' constructs
Bishop, 1995	IEA-Reading	multiple regression (cross sectional)
Bishop, 1995	U.S.-NELS88 and High School & Beyond data sets	multiple regression (longitudinal)
Mullis, Jenkins, Johnson, 1994	U.S. Math NAEP	multiple regressions, multi-level
Frederiksen, 1994	U.S. states	pre-post & control group comparison
Bishop, 1994	IAEP (Canada)	multiple regression (cross sectional)
Bishop, 1993	IAEP	multiple regression (cross sectional)
Psacharopoulos, Velez, 1993	Bogota, Columbia	multiple regression (longitudinal) on records of individual students, graduates
Graham, Husted, 1993	SAT by state	multiple regression (cross sectional)
Richards, Shen, 1992	South Carolina	multiple regression (cross sectional)
Jacobson, 1992	U.S. states (NLS)	multiple regression (longitudinal) re: minimum comp.
Ferguson, 1991	Texas	multiple regression of teacher factors on student achievement (cross-sectional)
Winfield, 1990	National NAEP (Reading)	multiple regression with gain scores(cross-sectional)
Singh, Marimutha, Mukjerjee, 1990	Malaysia	factor analysis on sources of motivation
Fuller, 1987	**World Bank countries**	**meta-analysis of 60 multivariate studies**
Winfield, 1987	NAEP Reading and Writing	multiple regression with gain scores (cross sectional)
Fuchs, Fuchs, Tindal, 1986	two groups of first-grade students	mancova - mastery learning improves learning, especially for low-achievers

Author, Year	Topic or Location	Method
Strauss, Sawyer, 1986	North Carolina	multiple regression - effect of teacher test scores on student achievement
Mangino, Babcock, 1986	Austin, TX	multiple anova, pre-post testing
Rohm, Sparzo, Bennett, 1986	undergraduate students	multiple analysis of covariance with 5 different retesting methods
Walstad, 1984	Missouri	multiple regression (production function) and administrator survey
Parramore, 1980	North Carolina	multiple anova with administrative records
Moss, Kagan, 1961	U.S.	regressions (longitudinal)

Pre-Post Testing, With Controls for Background Trends		Type
S.R.E.B., Bradby, Dykman, 2002	Southern States	pre-post comparisons
Tobias, 2000	New York City	pre-post comparison
Strozeski, 2000	Texas	pre-post comparison
Heneman, 1998	Charlotte-Mecklenburg SD, North Carolina	pre-post survey on school performance reward program
Johnson, 1998	Texas	interrupted time series, with shadow test
Nolet, McLaughlin, 1997	2 classrooms of 5th grade students in urban school	pre-post on performance assessment intervention
Andrews, Fullilove, 1997	Hong Kong	after introduction of high stakes oral test, compared videotapes pre and post cohorts
Jones, 1996	developmental math courses at a university	introduction of motivational techniques with tests as the stimulator
Webb, 1996	1 hospital's nursing staff	students at end of training take job profiling test, contrast pre-post skills
Frederiksen, 1994	U.S. states	pre-post & control group comparison
Chao-Qun, Hui, 1993	Fuxin City, China	pre-post comparison of student scores with initiation of teacher test
Wall, Alderson, 1993**	Sri Lanka	site visits, classroom observations, interviews, data analysis of admin. records
Shohamy, 1993**	Israel	site visits, classroom observations, interviews, data analysis of admin. records
Alderson, Wall, 1993**	Sri Lanka	site visits, classroom observations, interviews, data analysis of admin. records

Author, Year	Topic or Location	Method
Rudger, 1991	Texas	pre-post comparisons, with controls
Johnstone, 1990**	Texas	pre-post comparisons of schools' response to availability of test results
Ligon, et al., 1990	Texas	pre-post comparisons with controls and shadow test comparisons
Hughes, 1988	Turkish higher education	pre-post comparisons with introduction of high-stakes test
Pennycuick, Murphy, 1988	England & Wales	pilot testing at school level, pre post comparisons
Losack, 1987	Florida	pre-post testing, with controls
Hess, Lockwood, 1986	Alabama	pre-post testing, with controls
Serow, 1982	North Carolina	pre-post testing, with controls
Parramore, 1980	North Carolina	multiple anova with administrative records, pre-post testing
Whiteley, 1980	Santa Cruz SD, CA	pre-post testing
Wellisch, MacQueen, Carriere, Duck, 1978	U.S.	paired comparison of twenty-six high- and low achieving schools, pre-post testing
Cronbach, 1960	**military training programs**	**data analysis, observations, interviews**
Stuit, 1947	**U. S. Navy training programs**	**data analysis, observations, interviews**

Interrupted Time Series With Shadow Measure		Type
Meisels, Atkins-Burnett, Xue, Nicholson, Bickel, Son, 2003	Pittsburgh	interrupted time series, with shadow test
Standards Work, 2003	Virginia	mixed-mode, with shadow test comparison
Toenjes, Dworkin, Lorence, Hill, 2000	Texas	data analysis, critique of literature, with shadow test comparison
Phelps, 2000, 2003	Texas	data analysis, critique of literature, with shadow test comparison
Kelleher, 2000	Massachusetts	interrupted time series with shadow tests
Fontana, 2000	New York State	pre-post comparison of schools "under review" with rise in standards
Johnson, 1998	Texas	interrupted time series, with shadow test
Manzo, 1997	Johnson County, North Carolina	improvement on state tests after introducing its own testing program

Author, Year	Topic or Location	Method
Schmoker, 1996	multiple	many case studies
Robertson, Simpson, 1996	Northern Virginia Community College	common final exams introduced, performance improved on other measures
Poje, 1996	University of Memphis	change in general education testing program, from no- to high-stakes
Waters, Burger, Burger, 1995	Weld County SD, Colorado	district introduced grade promotion exams and saw increases in NRT scores
Matthews, Matthews, & de la Garza, 1991, 1994	Texas	changes to retention & achievement levels after introduction of college entrance exams
Chao-Qun, Hui, 1993	Fuxin City, China	pre-post comparison of student scores with initiation of teacher test
Plazak, Mazur, 1992	Poland	change in sec. student achievement after introduction of university entrance exams
Grisay, 1991	Belgium (French Community)	interrupted time series, with shadow test
Ferrara, Willhoft, Seburn, Slaughter, Stevenson, 1991**	Maryland	survey, case studies, data analyses, with shadow test comparisons
Rodgers, et al., 1991	Austin, TX	mancova compares scores on shadow test before and after introduction of TEAMS
Corbett, Wilson, 1991**	Maryland & Pennsylvania	teacher and administrator surveys
Weston, 1991	England & Wales	change in student behavior after change in testing program
Ligon, Johnstone, Brightman, Davis, et al., 1990	Texas	pre-post comparisons with controls and shadow test comparisons
Lerner, N. J. ED, 1990	New Jersey	interrupted time series, with shadow test comparison
Hess, Lockwood, 1986	Alabama	pre-post testing, with controls
Stevens, 1984	Los Angeles, CA	interrupted time series, with shadow test comparison
Alexander, 1983	Dallas	one test used to provide information for another, whose scores then rose
Brunton, 1982	Parkrose SD, Oregon	interrupted time series, with shadow test comparison
Schlawin, 1981	New York	interrupted time series, review of records, interviews
Ogden, 1979	Austin, TX	interrupted time series with shadow test

Author, Year	Topic or Location	Method
Task Force on Educational Assessment Programs, 1979	Florida	administrative records on course selection changes after test introduction
Enochs, 1978	Modesto, CA	interrupted time series, with shadow test
Pronaratna, 1976	Sri Lanka	interrupted time series, with administrative records on course-taking, effort

* Study is one of two types: (1) overall results were mixed, but there was clear evidence or conviction that testing with stakes improved student learning or motivation; (2) argument in text implied negative results, but data show positive results for achievement and motivation effects.

** Study finds improvements in administrative, instructional, and curricular coordination, in quality control, and in organizational clarity and reliability of quality control measures. Such outcomes normally accompany improvements in academic achievement, but an independent conclusion regarding an improvement in achievement was not indicated.

*** Study finds better outcomes for group identified by screening test, the test being necessary to identify them. In all these cases, moreover, the test group participates in program modeled on mastery learning principles.

Appendix B References

Abar, S. H. (1996). *The perceived influences that prompt teachers to initiate changes in curriculum and instruction*. EdD , University of Massachusetts, Amherst.

Abbott, R. D., & Falstrom, P. (1977). Frequent testing and personalized systems of instruction, *Contemporary Educational Psychology, 2*, 251–257.

Abramowitz, S. (1978, March). *The selective applicability of education policy: The California High School Proficiency Exam*. Paper presented at the Annual Meeting of the American Educational Research Association, Toronto.

Achieve, Inc. (2001, October). *Measuring Up: A Report on Education Standards and Assessments for Massachusetts*. Washington, DC.

Adams, D., & Chapman, D. (2002). *The quality of education: Dimensions and strategies*. Manila: Asian Development Bank.

Alexander, C. R. (1983, September). A case study: Testing in the Dallas Independent School District. In W. E. Hathaway (Ed.), *Testing in the schools. New directions for testing and measurement* (No. 19). San Francisco: Jossey-Bass.

Alderson, J. C., & Wall, D. (1993). Does washback exist? *Applied Linguistics, 14*, 115–129.

American Association of School Administrators. (2000). *Parents Poll*. Washington, DC: Lake, Snell, Perry, & Associates, Inc.

American Federation of Teachers. (1994). *Valuable Views: A Public Opinion Research Report on the Views of AFT Teachers on Professional Issues*. Washington, DC: Author.

Anderson, G. E. (2001). Brazosport independent school district: Implementation of the Quality agenda to ensure excellence and equity for all students. In *Education Reform Success Stories*. Amherst, MA: National Evaluation Systems.

Anderson, J. O., Muir, W., Bateson, D. J., Blackmore, D., & Rogers, W. T. (1990, March 30). *The Impact of Provincial Examinations on Education in British Columbia: General Report*. British Columbia Ministry of Education.

Anderson, L. W. (1973). *Time and school learning*. PhD dissertation, University of Chicago.

Anderson, L. W. (1976, April). The effects of a mastery learning program on selected cognitive, affective and interpersonal variables in grades 1 through 6. Paper presented at the annual meeting of the American Educational Research Association, San Francisco.

Anderson, L. W. (1976). An empirical investigation of individual differences in time to learn. *Journal of Educational Psychology, 68*(2), 226–233.

Anderson, O. T., & Artman, R. A. (1972). A self-paced, independent study, introductory physics sequence-description and evaluation. *American Journal of Physics, 40*, 1737–1742.

Andrews, S., & Fullilove, J. (1997). The elusiveness of washback: Investigating the impact of a new oral exam on students' spoken language performance. Paper presented at the International Language in Education Conference, University of Hong Kong, Hong Kong.

Annotated bibliography on minimum competency testing. (1978). ERIC ED156186.

Aquilera, R.V., & Hendricks, J. M. (1996, September). Increasing standardized achievement scores in a high risk school district. *Curriculum Report, 26*(1). Reston, VA: National Association of Secondary School Principals.

Bailey, K. M. (1996, November). Working for washback: A review of the washback concept in language testing. *Language Testing, 13*(3).

Bamburg, J., & Medina, E. (1993). Analyzing student achievement: Using standardized tests as the first step. In J. Bamburg (Ed.), *Assessment: How do we know what they know?* Dubuque: Kendall-Hunt.

Banerji, M. (2000, April). Designing district-level classroom assessment systems. Paper presented at the annual meeting of the American Educational Research Association, New Orleans, LA.

Bangert-Drowns, R. L., Kulik, J. A., & Chen-Lin, C. (1991, November/December). Effects of frequent classroom testing. *Journal of Educational Research, 85*(2), 89–99.

Banta, T. W., Lund, J. P., Black, K. E., & Oblander, F. W. (1996). *Assessment in practice: Putting principles to work on college campuses.* San Francisco: Jossey-Bass.

Barrett, R. L. (1968). Changes in accuracy of self estimates. *Personnel and Guidance Journal, 47*, 353–357.

Beardon, D. (1997). *An overview of the elementary mathematics program 1996–97.* Research report REIS97-116-3. Dallas: Dallas Public Schools.

Becker, W., & Rosen, S. (1990, June). *The learning effect of assessment and evaluation in high school.* Paper #7, Economics Research Center, NORC Discussion. Chicago, IL.

Behuniak, P., Chudowsky, N., & Dirir, M. (1997, March). *Consequences of state assessment practices in Connecticut.* Paper presented at the annual meeting of the National Council on Measurement in Education, Chicago, IL.

Behuniak, P. (2002, November). Consumer-referenced testing. *Phi Delta Kappan, 84*(3), 199–207.

Bentz, S. K. (1994). The impact of certification testing on teacher education. *Continuing discussions in teacher certification testing.* Amherst, MA: National Evaluation Systems.

Betts, J. R. (1998). The Impact of educational standards on the level and distribution of earnings, mimeo. Department of Economics, University of California, San Diego.

Betts, J. R., & Costrell, R. M. (2001). Incentives and equity under standards-based reform, in D. Ravitch (Ed.), *Brookings Papers on Education Policy*. Washington, DC: Brookings Institute Press.

Beaudry, J. (2000, April). *The positive effects of administrators and teachers on classroom assessment practices and student achievement*. Paper presented at the annual meeting of the American Educational Research Association, New Orleans, LA.

Bergeson, T., Fitton, R., Bylsma, P., & Neitzel, B. (2000, July). *Organizing for success (updated): Improving mathematics performance in Washington State*. Olympia: Office of the Superintendent of Public Instruction.

Bishop, J. H. (1993, December). *Impact of curriculum-based examinations on learning in Canadian secondary schools*. Working Paper 94-30, Center for Advanced Human Resource Studies, New York State School of Industrial and Labor Relations, Cornell University, Ithaca, NY.

Bishop, J. H. (1994, December). *Impacts of school organization and signaling on incentives to learn in France, The Netherlands, England, Scotland, and the United States*. Working paper 94-30, Center for Advanced Human Resource Studies, New York State School of Industrial and Labor Relations, Cornell University, Ithaca, NY.

Bishop, J. H. (1995, Fall). The power of external standards. *American Educator, 19*(4), 10–14, 17–18, 42–43.

Bishop, J. H. (1999). Nerd harassment, incentives, school priorities, and learning. In S. Mayer & P. Peterson (Eds.), *Earning and Learning*. Washington, DC. Brookings Institute.

Bishop, J. H. (2000, Summer). Diplomas for learning: Not for seat time. *Economics of Education Review, 19*(4), 333–349.

Bishop, J. H., Mane, F., Bishop, M., & Moriarty, J. (2001). The role of end-of-course exams and minimum competency exams in standards-based reforms. In D. Ravitch (Ed.), *Brookings Papers on Education Policy*. Washington, DC: Brookings Institute.

Black, P., & Dylan, W. (1998, October). Inside the black box: Raising standards through classroom assessment. *Phi Delta Kappan, 80*(2), 139–144.

Block, J. H. (Ed.). (1971). *Mastery learning: Theory and practice*. New York: Henry Holt.

Block, J. (1972). Student learning and the setting of mastery performance standards. *Educational Horizons, 50*, 183–191.

Block, J. H. (1973a). Teachers, teaching and mastery learning. *Today's Education, 63*, 30–36.

Block, J. H. (1973b). *Mastery performance standards and student learning*. PhD dissertation, University of California, Santa Barbara.

Block, J. H. ,& Burns, R. B. (1975, March–April). *Time in school learning: An instructional psychologist's perspective*. Paper presented at the annual meeting of the American Educational Research Association. Washington, DC.

Block, J. H., & Burns, R. B. (1976). Mastery learning. In L. E. Shulman (Ed.), *Review of Research in Education* (pp. 3–49). Itasca, IL: F. E. Peacock.

Block, J.H. & Tierney, M. (1974). An exploration of two correction procedures used in mastery learning approaches to instruction. *Journal of Educational Psychology, 66*, 962–967.

Bloom, B. (1968). Learning for mastery. *Evaluation Comment, 1*(2), 2–13.

Bloom, B. (1971). Mastery learning. In J. H. Block (Ed.), *Mastery learning: Theory and practice.* New York: Henry Holt.

Bloom, B. (1976). *Human characteristics and school learning.* New York, NY: McGraw-Hill.

Blum, R. E. (2000). Standards-based reform: Can it make a difference for students? *Peabody Journal of Education, 75*(4), 90–113.

Bock, R. D., & Wolfe, R. (1996). Audit and review of the Tennessee Value-Added Assessment System (TVAAS): Final Report, Part 1. In R. D. Bock, F. Wolfe, & T. H. Fisher (Eds.), *A review and analysis of the Tennessee Value-Added Assessment System.* Nashville: Tennessee Comptroller of the Treasury, Office of Education Accountability.

Bond, L. A., & Cohen, D. A. (1991). The early impact of Indiana Statewide testing for educational progress on local education agencies. In R. G. O'Sullivan & R. E. Stake (Eds.), *Advances in Program Evaluation, 1*(B), 78–79, 86–87.

Bottoms, G., & Mikos, P. (1995). *Seven most-improved "High Schools that Work" sites raise achievement in reading, mathematics, and science: A report on improving student learning.* Atlanta, GA: Southern Regional Education Board.

Boudreau, J. W. (1988, December). *Utility analysis for decisions in human resource management.* Working Paper 88–21. Ithaca, NY: New York State School of Industrial and Labor Relations, Cornell University.

Boylan, H. (1999). Exploring alternatives to remediation. *Journal of Developmental Education.* 22(3), 2–11.

Boylan, H., Bliss, L., & Bonham, B. (1997). Program components and their relationship to student performance. *Journal of Developmental Education, 20*(3), 2–9.

Boylan, H., Bonham, B., Abraham, A., Anderson, J., Morante, E., Ramirez, G, & Bliss, L. (1996). *An evaluation of the Texas Academic Skills Program.* Austin, TX: Texas Higher Education Coordinating Board.

Boylan, H., Bonham, B., & Bliss, L. (1994, **month?**). *National study of developmental education: Characteristics of faculty and staff.* Paper presented at the National Association for Developmental Education Conference, Washington, DC.

Boylan, H., Bonham, B., Claxton, C., & Bliss, L. (1992, November). *The state of the art in developmental education: Report of a national study.* Paper presented at the First National Conference on Research in Developmental Education. Charlotte, NC.

Boylan, H., & Saxon, D. P. (1998). *An evaluation of developmental education in Texas colleges and universities.* Austin, TX: Texas Higher Education Coordinating Board.

Bradshaw, L. K. (2002). Local district implementation of state mandated teacher evaluation policies and procedures: The North Carolina case. *Journal of Personnel Evaluation in Education.* 16(2), 113–127.

Braun, H. (2004, January 5). Reconsidering the impact of high-stakes testing. *Education Policy Analysis Archives, 12*(1). Retrieved December 27, 2004 from http://epaa.asu.edu/epaa/v12n1/

Brereton, J. L. (1944). *The case for examinations.* London: Cambridge University Press.

Brickman, W. W. (1946). Preparation for the Regents' examination. *School and Society, 64,* 263.

Brooke, N., & Oxenham, J. (1984). The influence of certification and selection on teaching and learning. In J. Oxenham (Ed.), *Education versus qualifications? A study of relationships between education, selection for employment and the productivity of labor*. London: George Allen & Unwin.

Brookhart, S. M. (1997, July/August). Effects of the classroom assessment environment on mathematics and science achievement. *Journal of Educational Research, 90*(6), 323–330.

Brookover, W. B., & Lezotte, L. W. (1979, May). Changes in school characteristics coincident with changes in student achievement. *Occasional Paper No.17*. East Lansing: Institute for Research on Teaching, Michigan State University.

Brooks-Cooper, C. (1993, August). *The effect of financial incentives on the standardized test performance of high school students*. Unpublished master's thesis, Cornell University, Ithaca, NY.

Brown, D. F. (1992, April). *Altering curricula through state testing: Perceptions of teachers and principals*. Paper presented at the annual meeting of the American Educational Research Association, San Francisco, CA.

Brown, S. M., & Walberg, H. J. (1993, January/February). Motivational effects on test scores of elementary students. *Journal of Educational Research, 86*(3), 133–136.

Brunton, M. L. (1982, March). *Is competency testing accomplishing any breakthrough in achievement?* Paper presented at the Annual Meeting of the Association for Supervision and Curriculum Development, Anaheim, CA.

Bude, U. (1989). *The challenge of quality in primary education in Africa*. Bonn, Germany: German Foundation for International Development, Education, Science and Documentation Center.

Burrows, C. K., & Okey, J. R. (1975, April). *The effects of a mastery learning strategy*. Paper presented at the Annual Meeting of the American Educational Research Association. Washington, DC.

Business Roundtable. (2001, Spring). *Assessing and addressing the "Testing Backlash."*

Calder, P. (1990). *Impact of diploma examinations on the teaching-learning process*. A study commissioned by the Alberta Teachers Association. University of Alberta, Dept. of Educational Psychology and the Alberta Teachers' Association.

Cameron, J., & Pierce, W. D. (1994, Fall). Reinforcement, reward, and intrinsic and extrinsic motivation: A meta-analysis. *Review of Educational Research, 64*(3), 363–423.

Cameron, J., & Pierce, W. D. (1996, Spring). The debate about rewards and intrinsic, motivation: Protests and accusations do not alter the results. *Review of Educational Research; 66*(1), 39–51.

Carnoy, M., Loeb, S., & Smith, T. L. (2001, November). *Do higher state test scores in Texas make for better high school outcomes?* CPRE Research Report Series RR-047, Consortium for Policy Research in Education, University of Pennsylvania, Philadelphia.

Carroll, J. B. (1955). The Harvard foreign language aptitude tests in the *12th Yearbook of the National Council on Measurements Used in Education*, Part 2. Cleveland.

Carroll, J. (1963). A model of school learning. *Teachers College Record, 64*, 723–733.

Cawelti, G. (2001, Fall). *Six districts, one goal of excellence*. National Staff Development Council.

CBS News. (1990). CBS News Poll. New York: Author.

Center for the Study of Evaluation. *Testing in the nation's schools and districts: How much? What kinds? To what ends? At what costs?* Report No.194. Los Angeles: University of California.

Chao-Qun, W. & Hui, Z. (1993). Educational assessment in mathematics teaching: Applied research in China. In M. Niss (Ed.), *Cases of assessment in mathematics education: An ICMI study*. Boston: Kluwer Academic.

Chapman, D. W., & Snyder, C. W. (2000). Can high-stakes national testing improve instruction: Reexamining conventional wisdom. *International Journal of Educational Development, 20*, 457–474.

Chen, C., & Stevenson, H. W. (1995, August). Motivation and mathematics achievement: A comparative study of Asian-American, Caucasian-American, and East Asian high school students. *Child Development, 66*(4), 1215–1234.

Chen, S., & Chang, D. (1999, June). *Remedial education and grading: A case study approach to two critical issues in American higher education*. New York, NY: The Research Foundation of the City University of New York.

Chicago elementary schools with a seven-year trend of improved reading achievement: What makes these schools stand out? (1997, October). *Designs for Change*. Chicago: Author.

Clark, C. R., Guskey, T. R., & Benninga, J. S. (1983, March/April). The effectiveness of mastery learning strategies in undergraduate education. *Journal of Educational Research, 76*(4), 210–214.

Clark, D. L., Lotto, L. S., & Astuto, T. A. (1984, Summer). Effective schools and school improvement: A comparative analysis of two lines of inquiry. *Educational Administration Quarterly, 20*(3), .41–68.

Clarke, D., & Stephens, M. (1996). The ripple effect: The instructional impact of the systemic introduction of performance assessment in mathematics. In M. Birenbaum & F. Dochy (Eds.), *Alternatives in assessment of achievements, learning processes and prior knowledge*. Evaluation in Education and Human Services. Boston: Kluwer Academic.

CNN, *USA Today*, & Gallup Corporation. (1997). Gallup, CNN, *USA Today* Poll. New York: Author.

Consultative Committee on Examinations. (1910). *Report*. Great Britain.

Corbett, H. D., & Wilson, B. (1989). *Raising the stakes in statewide mandatory minimum competency testing*. Research for Better Schools, Philadelphia.

Corbett, H. D., & Wilson, B. L. (1991). *Two state minimum competency testing programs and their effects on curriculum and instruction*. (ERIC ED377251)

Corcoran, T. B. (1985). *Competency Testing and At-Risk Youth*. Philadelphia: Research for Better Schools.

Corcoran, T. B., & Wilson, B. L. (1986). *The search for successful secondary schools: The first three years of the secondary school recognition program*. Philadelphia: Research for Better Schools.

Costrell, R. M. (1993, November). *Can national educational standards raise welfare?* Mimeo.

Costrell, R. M. (1994, September). A simple model of educational standards. *American Economic Review. 84*(4), 956–971.

Costrell, R. M. (1995). An Economic Analysis of College Admission Standards. *Education Economics, 1*(3), 227, 241.

Cotton, K. (1995). *Effective schooling practices: A research synthesis 1995 update.* Northwest Regional Education Laboratory.

Covington, M. V. (1993). A motivational analysis of academic life in college. In J. C. Smart (Ed.), *Higher education: Handbook of theory and research, 9,* 50–93. New York: Agathon Press.

Cronbach, L. J. (1960). *Essentials of psychological testing.* New York: Harper & Row.

Crooks, T. J. (1988, Winter). The impact of classroom evaluation practices on students. *Review of Educational Research. 58*(4), .438–481.

Cross, K. P. (1976). *Accent on learning.* San Francisco, CA: Jossey-Bass.

Cross, K. P., & Steadman, M. H. (1996). *Classroom research: Implementing the scholarship of teaching.* San Francisco: Jossey-Bass.

Cross, K. P. (1997). *Developing professional fitness through classroom assessment and classroom research. The Cross Papers, Number 1.* Mission Viejo, CA: The League for Innovation in the Community College.

Czikszentmihalyi, M. (1990). *Flow: The psychology of optimal experience.* New York: Harper Perennial.

Davis, M. L. (1975). Mastery test proficiency requirement affects mastery test performance. In J. M. Johnston (Ed.), *Behavior research and technology in higher education.* Springfield, IL: Charles C. Thomas.

Dawson, K. S., & Dawson, R. E. (1985). *Minimum competency testing and local schools* [mimeograph].

DeBard, R., & Kubow, P. K. (2001). Impact of proficiency testing: A collaborative evaluation. In R. Nata (Ed.), *Progress in Education, 2,* 1–55. Huntington, NY: Nova Scientific Publisher.

Delong, J. W. (1990). Perceptions of relationships of quality indicators to improvement of California high schools. Unpublished EdD dissertation, University Park: University of Southern California.

Denison University. (2002, April). Freshmen improve grades through assessment. *First-Year Experience Newsletter. 7*(2), 3.

Din, F. S. (1996, February). *The impact of Kentucky state testing on educational practices in Kentucky public schools.* Paper presented at the Annual Meeting of the Eastern Educational Research Association, Cambridge, MA. (ERIC: ED405352)

Down, A. G. (1979, April). *Implications of minimum-competency testing for minority students.* Paper presented at the annual meeting of the National Council on Measurement in Education, San Francisco, CA.

Dougherty, C., & Collins, S. (2002, January). *Use of the 'Just for the Kids' data by Texas elementary schools,* Technical Report No.1. National Center for Educational Accountability.

Duran, R. P. (1989). Assessment and instruction of at-risk Hispanic students. *Exceptional Children, 56*(2), 154–158.

Earl, L., & Torrance, N. (2000). Embedding accountability and improvement into large-scale assessment: What difference does it make? *Peabody Journal of Education, 75*(4), 114–141.

Eckstein, M. A., & Noah, H. J. (1993). *Secondary school examinations: International perspectives on policies and practice.* New Haven: Yale University Press.

Edmonds, R. R., & Frederiksen, J. R. (1979). *Search for effective schools: The identification and analysis of city schools that are instructionally effective for poor children.* Washington, DC: Educational Resources Information Center.

Egeland, P. C. (1995). *The effect of authentic assessments on fifth-grade student science achievement and attitudes.* PhD dissertation, Northern Illinois University, DeKalb.

Ellet, C. D., & Teddlie, C. (2003). Teacher evaluation, teacher effectiveness and school effectiveness: Perspectives from the USA. *Journal of Personnel Evaluation in Education, 17*(1), 101–128.

Engel, G. S. (1977, March/April). One way it can be. *Today's Education, 66*, 50–52.

Enochs, J. C. (1978, May). Modesto, California: A return to the four Rs. *Phi Delta Kappan,* 609–610.

Estes, G. D., Colvin, L. W., & Goodwin, C. (1976, April). *A criterion-referenced basic skills assessment* . Paper presented at the annual meeting of the American Educational Research Association, San Francisco.

Estes, G. D., & Demaline, R. (1982, January). *Phase II: Final evaluation report of minimum competency testing clarification process.* Northwest Regional Education Laboratory.

Feldhusen, J. F. (1964, February). *Student perceptions of frequent quizzes and post-mortem discussion of tests.* Paper presented at the Annual Meeting of the National Council on Measurement in Education, Chicago.

Ferguson, R. F. (1991). Paying for public education: New evidence on how and why money matters. *Harvard Journal on Legislation, 28*(2), 465–498.

Ferguson, R. F., & Ladd, H. F. (1996). How and why money matters: An analysis of Alabama schools. In H. F. Ladd (Ed.), *Holding schools accountable: Performance-based reform in education* (pp. 265–298). Washington: Brookings.

Ferman, I. (2004). The washback of an EFL national oral matriculation test to teaching and learning. In L. Cheng, Y. Watanabe, & A. Curtis (Eds), *Washback in language testing: Research Contexts and Methods* (pp. 191–210). Mahwah, NJ: Lawrence Erlbaum Associates.

Ferrara, S., Willhoft, J., Seburn, C., Slaughter, F., & Stevenson, J. (1991). Local Assessments designed to parallel statewide minimum competency tests: Benefits and drawbacks. In R. G. O'Sullivan & R. E. Stake (Eds.), *Advances in program evaluation: Effects of mandated assessment on teaching* (pp. 41–74). JAI Press.

Fiel, R. L., & Okey, J. R. (1974). The effects of formative evaluation and remediation on mastery of intellectual skills. *The Journal of Educational Research, 68*, 253–255.

Fillbrandt, J. R., & Merz, W. R. (1977, Spring). The assessment of competency in reading and mathematics using community based standards, *Educational Research Quarterly, 2*, 3–11.

Fincher, C. (1978, October). *Beyond Bakke: The positive benefits of testing.* Paper presented at a Seminar for State Leaders in Postsecondary Education, New Orleans, LA.

Findley, J. (1978, May). Westside's minimum competency graduation requirements: A program that works. *Phi Delta Kappan,* 614–618.

Fisher, T. H. (1978, May). Florida's approach to competency testing. *Phi Delta Kappan, 59*, 599–602.

Flynn, T. M. (1990). *Community attitudes toward the high school minimum competency test*. Fayetteville State University Graduate Center, Fayetteville, NC.

Fontana, J. (2000, June). New York's test-driven standards. In A. Glatthorn & J. Fontana (Eds.), *Coping with standards, tests, and accountability: Voices from the classroom*. Washington, DC: NEA Teaching and Learning Division.

Foss, O. (1977, May 23–28). A new approach: Vocational foundation courses and examinations . In F. M. Ottobre (Ed.), *Criteria for awarding school leaving certificates: An international discussion* (pp. 191–209). Based on the Proceedings of the 1977 Conference of the International Association for Educational Assessment held at the Kenyatta Conference Center, Nairobi.

Frederiksen, N. (1994). *The influence of minimum competency tests on teaching and learning*. Princeton, NJ: Educational Testing Service.

Friedman, H. (1987). Repeat examinations in introductory statistics. *Teaching of Psychology, 14*, 20–23.

Fuchs, L. S., Fuchs, D., & Tindal, G. (1986, May/June). Effects of mastery learning procedures on student achievement. *Journal of Educational Research, 79*(5), 286–291.

Fuchs, L., Fuchs, D., Karns, K., Hamlett, C. L., & Katzaroff, M. (1999). Mathematics performance assessment in the classroom: Effects on teacher planning and student problem solving. *American Educational Research Journal, 35*(3), 609–645.

Fuller, B. (1987). What school factors raise achievement in the Third World? *Review of Educational Research, 57*(3), 255–292.

Fund for the Advancement of Education. (1953). *Bridging the gap between school and college*. New York.

Garcia, J., & Rothman, R. (2001). *Three paths, one destination: Standards-based reform in Maryland, Massachusetts, and Texas*. Washington, DC: Achieve.

Gaynor, J., & Millham, J. (1976). Student performance and evaluation under variant teaching and testing methods in a large college course. *Journal of Education Psychology, 68*, 312–317.

Gibbs, G. (1992). *Improving the quality of student learning*. Bristol, England: Technical and Educational Services.

Gipps, C. (2000). Findings from large scale assessment in England. *The effects and related problems of large scale testing in educational assessment*. Foreign Language Teaching and Research. Vienna, Austria: IAEA.

Glasnapp, D. R., Poggio, J. P., & Ory, J. C. (1975, March/April). *Cognitive and affective consequences of mastery and non-mastery instructional strategies*. Paper presented at the annual meeting of the American Educational Research Association, Washington, DC.

Glasnapp, D., John, R., Poggio, P., & Miller, M. D. (1991). Impact of a "Low Stakes" state minimum competency testing program on policy, attitudes, and achievement. In R. G. O'Sullivan & R. E. Stake (Eds.), *Advances in program evaluation: Effects of mandated assessment on teaching* (pp. 41–74). Greenwich, CT: JAI Press.

Goldberg, G., & Roswell, B. S. (2000). From perception to practice: The impact of teachers' scoring experience on performance-based instruction and classroom assessment. *Educational Assessment, 6*(4), 257–290.

Good, T. L., & Grouws, D. A. (1979). The Missouri Mathematics Effectiveness Project: An experimental study in fourth grade classrooms. *Journal of Educational Psychology, 71*(3), 355–362.

Goodson, M. L., & Okey, J. R. (1978, November). The effects of diagnostic tests and help sessions on college science achievement. *Journal of College Science Teaching, 8,* 89–90.

Gould, J., & Ward, J. (1980, July). *Teachers and tests: The teacher union response.* Paper presented at the annual Summer Instructional Leadership Conference of the American Association of School Administrators, Chicago, IL.

Graham, A., & Husted, T. (1993). Understanding state variation in SAT scores. *Economics of Education Review, 12*(3), 197–202.

Green, K. E., & Williams, J. E. (1989, March). *Standardized test use by classroom teachers: Effects of training and grade level taught.* Paper presented at the annual meeting of the National Council on Measurement in Education, San Francisco.

Greene, H. (1999). Seeking common ground: One New York experience. *Teacher preparation assessment: The hows and whys of new standards* (pp. 116–118). Amherst, MA: National Evaluation Systems.

Grisay, A. (1991, September 12–15). Improving assessment in primary schools: "APER" research reduces educational failure rates. In P. Weston (Ed.), *Assessment of pupil achievement: Motivation and school success: Report of the Educational Research Workshop held in Liège, Belgium.* Council of Europe. Swets & Zeitlinger, Amsterdam.

Grissmer, D., & Flanagan, A. (1998, November). *Exploring rapid score gains in Texas and North Carolina.* Santa Monica, CA: RAND National Education Goals Panel.

Grissmer, D. W., Flanagan, A., Kawata, J., & Williamson, S. (2000, July). *Improving student achievement: What NAEP state test scores tell us.* Santa Monica, CA: RAND.

Gullickson, A. R. (1984, March/April). Teacher perspectives of their instructional use of tests. *Journal of Educational Research, 77*(4).

Guskey, T. R., & Gates, S. L. (1986). Synthesis of research on the effects of mastery learning in elementary and secondary classrooms. *Educational Leadership, 43*(8), 73–80.

Guth, G., Holtzman, D., Schneider, S., Carlos, L., Smith, J., Hayward, G., & Calvo, N. (2001, August). *Evaluation of California's standards based accountability system.* Final report, November 1999. San Francisco: WestEd.

Hannaway, J., & McKay, S. (2001, October 23–24). School accountability and student achievement: The case of Houston. Paper presented at "Making the grade: Assessing the reform of Houston's public schools" conference, sponsored by the University of Houston, the Houston Independent School District, and the Houston Annenberg Challenge.

Hansen, P. (2001). Chicago public schools: Improvement through accountability. *Education Reform Success Stories.* Northampton, MA: National Evaluation Systems.

Harnisch, D., & Switzer, D. (1991). Teachers' perceptions of the instructional uses of tests. In R. G. O'Sullivan & R. E. Stake (Eds.), *Advances in program evaluation: Effects of mandated assessment on teaching* (pp. 163–188). Greenwich, CT: JAI Press.

Hawisher, M., & Harper, M. J. (1979). *Competency testing: Bibliography.* Competency Testing Project, Winthrop College, Rock Hill, SC.

Henchey, N., Dunnigan, M., Gardner, A., Lessard, C., Muhtadi, N., Raham, H., & Violato, C. (2001, November). *Schools that make a difference: Final report: Twelve Ca-*

nadian secondary schools in low-income settings. Society for the Advancement of Excellence in Education, Kelowna, British Columbia.

Heneman, H. G., III. (1998). Assessment of the motivational reactions of teachers to a school-based performance award program. *Journal of personnel evaluation in education, 12,* 143–159.

Herman, J. L., & Dorr-Bremme, D. W. (1983). Uses of testing in the schools: A national profile. In W. E. Hathaway (Ed.), *Testing in the schools.* San-Francisco: Jossey-Bass.

Herrick, M. L. (1999). *State-level performance assessments and consequential validity.* PhD dissertation, University of Maryland, College Park.

Hess, A.C., & Lockwood, R. E. (1986, April). *The relationship of a basic competency education program to overall student achievement: A state perspective.* Paper presented at the annual meeting of the National Council on Measurement in Education (NCME), San Francisco.

Heyneman, S. (1987). *Uses of examinations in developing countries: Selection, research, and education sector management.* Seminar Paper No.36, Economic Development Institute, The World Bank, Washington, DC.

Heyneman, S. P., & Ransom, A. (1992). Using examinations and testing to improve educational quality. In M. A. Eckstein & H. J. Noah (Eds.), *Examinations: Comparative and international studies.* Oxford: Pergamon Press.

Hilloks, G., Jr. (1987). Synthesis of research on teaching writing. *Educational Leadership, 44*(8), pp. 71–82.

Hoegl, J. (1983, August). *Educational standards, accountability, and student achievement: Legal and administrative considerations for competency testing.* Unpublished manuscript. (ERIC ED 265648)

Hogan, K. (2000, June). Educational reform in Texas. In A. Glatthorn & Fontana, J. (Eds.), *Coping with standards, tests, and accountability: Voices from the classroom.* Washington, DC: NEA Teaching and Learning Division.

Homme, L., Csanyi, A. P., Gonzales, M. A., & Rechs, J. R. (1969). *How to use contingency contracting in the classroom.* Champaign, IL.: Research Press.

Horn, N. (1980, August). *Competency-based testing in Nevada: Perceptions of legislators, school district superintendents, local school board presidents, and third grade teachers.* EdD dissertation, University of Nevada, Las Vegas.

Hughes, A. (1988). Introducing a needs-based test of English language proficiency into an English-medium university in Turkey. In A. Hughes (Ed.), *Testing English for university study* (pp. 134–153). London: Modern English Publications.

Hughes, A. (1989). *Testing for language learners.* Cambridge: Cambridge University Press.

Hughes, A. (1993). *Backwash and TOEFL 2000.* Unpublished manuscript, University of Reading, Berkshire, UK.

Hurlock, E. B. (1925, September). The effects of incentives on the constancy of the I.Q. *Pedagogical Seminary, 32,* 422–434.

Hymel, G. M. (1974). *An investigation of John B. Carroll's model of school learning as a theoretical basis for the organizational structuring of schools.* Final Report. NIE Project No. 3-1359. New Orleans, LA: University of New Orleans.

Jackson, M., & Battiste, B. (1978). *Competency testing: An annotated bibliography.* Unpublished manuscript. (ERIC ED167503)

Jacobson, J. (1992, October 29). *Mandatory testing requirements and pupil achievement.* PhD dissertation. Cambridge, MA: Massachusetts Institute of Technology.

Jett, D. L., & Schafer, W. D. (1993, April). *High school teachers' attitudes toward a statewide high stakes student performance assessment.* Paper presented at the Annual Meeting of the American Educational Research Association, Atlanta.

Johnson, G. B. (1981). *Perceptions of students, parents, teachers, and administrators in District I, Department of Defense Dependents' Schools Europe, toward a minimum competency testing program.* EdD dissertation, University of Southern California, Los Angeles.

Johnson, J. F, Jr. (1998). The influence of a state accountability system on student achievement in Texas. *Virginia Journal of Social Policy & the Law, 6*(1).

Johnson, J., Treisman, U., & Fuller, E. (2000, December). Testing in Texas. *School Administrator, 57*(11), 20–24, 26.

Johnstone, W. (1990, January 25–27). Local school district perspectives. In G. Ligon et al. (Eds.), *Statewide testing in Texas.* A symposium presented at the annual meeting of the Southwest Educational Research Association, Austin, Texas.

Jones, B., & Johnston, A. (2002). *The effects of high-stakes testing on instructional practices.* Paper presented at the Annual Meeting of the American Educational Research Association, New Orleans.

Jones, B., & Egley, R. (2003). *The carrot and the stick: How testing affects teachers' job satisfaction and motivation.* Paper presented at the annual meeting of the Eastern Educational Research Association, New Orleans.

Jones, E. L., Gordon, H. A., & Schechtman, G. 1975. *A strategy for academic success in a community college.* Unpublished manuscript. Chicago: Olive-Harvey College.

Jones, F. G. (1974). *The effects of mastery and aptitude on learning, retention, and time.* PhD dissertation, University of Georgia, Athens.

Jones, J. B. (1993). *Effects of the use of an altered testing/grading method on the retention and success of students enrolled in college mathematics.* EdD dissertation, East Texas State University, Texas A&M, Commerce.

Jones, J., et al. (1996, Fall). Offer them a carrot: Linking assessment and motivation in developmental Mathematics. *Research and Teaching in Developmental Education, 13*(1), 85–91.

Jones, M, Jones, B., & Hargrove, T. (2003). *The unintended consequences of high-stakes testing.* Lanham, MD: Rowman & Littlefield.

Kang, S. (1985). A formal model of school reward systems. In J. Bishop (Ed.), *Incentives, learning, and employability.* Ohio State University, National Center for Research in Vocational Education.

Karmos, J. S., & Karmos, A. H. (1980). *Attitudes toward standardized achievement tests and relationships to achievement test performance.* Paper presented at the 64th Annual Meeting of the American Educational Research Association, Boston, MA.

Kazdin, A., & Bootzin, R. (1972). The token economy: An evaluative review. *Journal of Applied Behavior Analysis, 5*, 343–372.

Kellaghan, T., Madaus, G., & Airasian, P. (1982). *The effects of standardized testing.* Boston: Kluwer-Nijhoff Publishing.

Kelleher, J. (2000, June). Developing rigorous standards in Massachusetts. In A. Glatthorn & J. Fontana (Eds.), *Coping with standards, tests, and accountability: Voices from the classroom.* Washington, DC: NEA Teaching and Learning Division.

Keller, F. (1968). Goodbye teacher. *Journal of Applied Behavioral Analysis, 1*(2), 79–89.

Kelley, C. (1999). The motivational impact of school-based performance awards. *Journal of Personnel Evaluation in Education, 12*(4), 309–326.

Keys, N. (1934). The influence on learning and retention of weekly tests as opposed to monthly tests. *Journal of Educational Psychology, 25*, 427–436.

Khalaf Abdulkhalig, S. S., & Hanna, G. (1992, January). The impact of classroom testing frequency on high school students' achievement. *Contemporary Educational Psychology, 17*(1), 71–77.

Kiemig, R. (1983). *Raising academic standards: A guide to learning improvement.* Washington, DC: Association for the Study of Higher Education/Educational Resource Information Center.

Kika, F., McLaughlin, T., & Dixon, J. (1992, January/February). Effects of frequent testing of secondary algebra students. *Journal of Educational Research, 85*(3), 159–162.

Kim, Y., Cho, G., Park, J., & Park, M. (1974). *An application of a new instructional model.* Research report No. 8. Seoul, Korea: Korean Educational Development Institute.

Kirkland, M. C. (1971). The effects of tests on students and schools. *Review of Educational Research, 41*, 303–350.

Kirkpatrick, J. E. (1934). The motivating effect of a specific type of testing program. *University of Iowa Studies in Education, 9*, 41–68.

Kulik, C.-L., & Kulik, J. (1987). Mastery testing and student learning: A meta-analysis. *Journal of Educational Technology Systems, 15*, 325–345.

Kulik, J., & Kulik, C.-L. (1989). Meta-analysis in education. *International Journal of Education Research, 13*(3), 221–340.

Kulik, J., & Kulik, C.-L, (1991). *Developmental instruction: An analysis of the research.* Boone, NC: National Center for Developmental Education.

Kulik, J., Kulik, C.-.L, & Cohen, P. A. (1979). A meta-analysis of outcomes studies of Keller's Personalized System of Instruction. *American Psychologist, 34*, 307–318.

Kulik, J., Kulik, C.-L., & Schwalb, B. (1983). College programs for high risk and disadvantaged students: A meta-analysis of findings. *Review of Educational Research, 53*(3), 297–414.

Ladd, H. F. (1999). The Dallas school accountability and incentive program: An evaluation of its impacts on student outcomes. *Economics of Education Review, 18*, 1–16.

Lane, S., Parke, C., & Stone, C. (1999). *MSPAP Impact Study, Volume 1: Mathematics.* U.S. Department of Education and Maryland Assessment System Project.

Langer, J. (2001). Beating the odds: Teaching middle and high school students to read and write well. *American Educational Research Journal, 38*(4), 837–880.

LaRoque, L., & Coleman, P. (1989). Quality control: School accountability and district ethos. In M. Holmes, K. Leithwood, & D. Musella, (Eds.), *Educational Policy for Effective Schools.* Toronto: Ontario Institute for Studies in Education.

Lee, Y. D., Kim, C. S., Kim, H., Park, B. Y., Yoo, H. K., Chang, S. M., & Kim, S. C. (1971, April–November). *Interaction improvement studies on the mastery learning project. Final report on Mastery Learning Program.* Seoul, Korea: Educational Research Center, Seoul National University.

Legislative Office of Education Oversight. (2000, October). *Proficiency testing, student achievement, and local educational practices.* State of Ohio, Columbus.

Lerner, B. (1990, March). Good news about American education. *Commentary*, *91*(3).

Levine, D. U., & Lezotte, L. W. (1990). *Unusually effective schools: A review and analysis of research and practice*. The National Center for Effective Schools Research and Development. Madison, WI.

Ligon, G., et al. (1990, January 25–27). *Statewide testing in Texas*. A symposium presented at the annual meeting of the Southwest Educational Research Association, Austin, Texas.

Locke, E., & Latham, G. (2002, September). Building a practically useful theory of goal setting and task motivation: A 35-year odyssey. *American Psychologist, 57*, 705–717.

Locke, E. A., Shaw, K. N., Saari, L. M., & Latham, G. P. (1981). Goal setting and task performance: 1969-1980. *Psychological Bulletin, 90*(1), 125–152.

Loerke, D. (1993). Perceptions of the use of diploma examination results in teacher evaluation. Master's Thesis, University of Alberta, Edmonton, Alberta, Canada.

Lortie, D. C. (1975). *Schoolteacher: A sociological study*. Chicago: University of Chicago Press.

Losack, J. (1987, January). *Mandated entry- and exit-level testing in the state of Florida: A brief history, review of current impact, and a look to the future*. Miami-Dade Community College and Florida Office of Institutional Research.

Lumley, D., & Wenfan Y. (2001, April). *The Impact of state mandated, large-scale writing assessment policies in Pennsylvania*. Paper presented at the Annual Meeting of the American Educational Research Association Seattle.

Lutz, F., & Maddirala, J. (1987, July). *State mandated testing in Texas: The teacher response*. (Monograph No. 4). Center for Policy Studies and Research in Elementary and Secondary Education, East Texas State University, Commerce, TX.

Magruder, J., McManis, M., &Young, C. (1997, Winter). The right idea at the right time: Development of a transformational assessment culture. In P. Gray & T. Banta (Eds.), *The campus-level impact of assessment: Progress, problems, and possibilities. New directions for higher education, 1000*. San Francisco: Jossey-Bass.

Making the grade: A better balance. (2000, September). *Education Week; Beldon, Russonello, & Stewart*, Washington, DC: Author.

Mallory, A. (1980). *Competency Testing*. CEMREL, Paper 2.

Mangino, E., & Babcock, M. (1986, April). *Minimum Competency Testing: Helpful or Harmful for High Level Skills*. Paper presented at the annual meeting of the American Educational Research Association, San Francisco.

Manuel, H. T. (1952). Results of a half-century experiment in teaching a second language. *Modern Language Journal, 36*, 74–76.

Manzo, K. (1997, October 22). High stakes: Test truths or consequences. *Education Week on the Web* (pp. 1–2). Retrieved January 6, 2005 [on-line] from www.edweek.com

Marion, S., & Sheinker, A. (1999). *Issues and consequences for state-level minimum competency testing programs*. State Assessment Series, Wyoming Report 1. National Center of Educational Outcomes, Minneapolis.

Marsh, R. (1984, November/December). A comparison of take-home versus in-class exams. *Journal of Educational Research, 78*(2), 111–113.

Mass Insight Education. (2002). Taking charge: Urban high school students speak out about MCAS, academics and extra-help programs. *Mass Insight*. Retrieved January 6, 2005 [on-line] from www.massinsight.org

Matthews, J. (1994). The effectiveness of TASP-induced remediation among Texas's tri-ethnic population. *Continuing discussions in teacher certification testing*. Amherst, MA: National Evaluation Systems.

Matthews, J., & de la Garza, E. (1991). After implementation: The role of the state. In J. Matthews, R. Swanson, & R. Kerker (Eds.), *From politics to policy: A case study in educational reform*. New York: Praeger.

Mattsson, H. (1993). *Impact of assessment on educational practice and student behavior in the Swedish schools system* (pp. 175–182). In school-based and external assessments: Uses and issues. Papers presented at the 19th annual Conference of the International Association for Educational Assessment, Mauritius.

McCabe, R. (2000). *No one to waste: A report to public decision makers and community college leaders*. Washington, DC: Community College Press.

McCabe, R., & Day, P. (1998). *Developmental education: A twenty-first century social and economic imperative*. Mission Viejo, CA: League for Innovation in the Community College.

McDonald, M. (2002, September/October). The perceived role of diploma examinations in Alberta, Canada. *Journal of Education Research, 96*(1), 21–36.

McKenzie, D. E. (1983, April). Research for school improvement: An appraisal of some recent trends. *Educational Researcher, 12*(4), 5–17.

McMillan, J. (1977, Summer). The effect of effort and feedback on the formation of student attitudes. *American Educational Research Journal, 14*(3), 317–330.

McMillan, J., Myran, S., & Workman, D. (1999, April). *The impact of mandated state-wide testing on teachers' classroom assessment and instructional practices*. Paper presented at the annual meeting of the American Educational Research Association, Montréal, Québec.

McWilliams, J., & Andrew, T. (1976, September/October). The measurement of students' learning: An approach to accountability. *Journal of Educational Research, 70*, 50–52.

Measured response, A: American speak on education reform. (2001, April/May). Educational Testing Service; Hart & Teeter. Princeton, NJ: Author.

Meisels, S., Atkins-Burnett, S., Xue, Y., Nicholson, J., DiPrima Bickel, D., & Son, S.-H. (2003, February 28). Creating a system of accountability. *Education Policy Analysis Archives, 11*(9). Retrieved June 1, 2004 from http://epaa.asu.edu/epaa/v11n9

Mendro, R. (1998). Student achievement and school and teacher accountability. *Journal of Personnel Evaluation in Education, 12*(3), 257–267.

Milanowski, A., & Heneman, H. G., III. (2001). Assessment of teacher reactions to a standards-based teacher evaluation system: A pilot study. *Journal of Personnel Evaluation in Education, 15*(3), 193–212.

Milton, O. (1981). *Will that be on the final?* Springfield, IL: Charles C. Thomas.

Mitchell, F. M. (1999, April). *All students can learn: Effects of curriculum alignment on the mathematics achievement of third-grade students*. Paper presented at the Annual Meeting of the American Educational Research Association, Montréal, Québec, Canada.

Moore, W. P. (1991). *Relationships among teacher test performance pressures, perceived testing benefits, test preparation strategies, and student test performance.* PhD dissertation, University of Kansas, Lawrence.

Morgan, R., & Crone, C. (1993). *Advanced placement examinees at the University of California: An examination of the freshman year courses and grades of examinees in biology, calculus, and chemistry.* Statistical Report 93-210. Princeton, NJ: Educational Testing Service.

Morgan, R. & Ramist, L. (1998, February). *Advanced placement students in college: An investigation of course grades at 21 colleges.* Educational Testing Service, Report No. SR-98-13. Princeton: ETS.

Mortimore, P., Sammons, P., Stoll, L., Lewis, D., & Ecob, R. (1988). *School matters: The junior years.* Salisbury: Open Books.

Moss, H. A., & Kagan, J. (1961). Stability of achievement in recognition setting behaviors from early childhood through adulthood. *Journal of Abnormal and Social Psychology, 62,* 504–513.

Mullis, I. V. S., Jenkins, F., & Johnson, E. G. (1994, October). *Effective schools in mathematics: Perspectives from the NAEP 1992 Assessment.* U.S. Education Department, National Center for Education Statistics.

Mullis, I. V. S. (1997, April). *Benchmarking toward world-class standards: Some characteristics of the highest performing school systems in the TIMSS.* Paper presented at panel "International Benchmarking: New Findings," at the Annual Meeting of the American Educational Research Association, Chicago, IL.

Murnane, R. J. (1981, Fall). Interpreting the evidence on school effectiveness. *Teachers College Record, 83*(1), 19–35.

Nassif, P. (1992). Aligning assessment and instruction: Can teacher testing result in better teaching? *Current topics: Teacher certification testing.* Amherst, MA: National Evaluation Systems.

National priority, A: Americans speak on teacher quality. (2002, April/May). Educational Testing Service; Hart & Teeter. Princeton, NJ: Author

Natriello, G., & Dornbusch, S.M. (1984). *Teacher evaluative standards and student effort.* Longman: New York.

NBC News, *Wall Street Journal,* Hart & Teeter. (1991). NBC News - *Wall Street Journal* Poll. New York: Author.

NBC News, *Wall Street Journal,* Hart & Teeter. (1997). NBC News - *Wall Street Journal* Poll. New York: Author.

Neal, B. (1978). Denver, Colorado: A 17-year old minimum competency testing program. *Phi Delta Kappan, 59,* 610–611.

Neville, L. B. (1998). *Quality assurance and improvement planning in two elementary schools: Case studies in Illinois school reform.* PhD dissertation, Illinois State University, Normal.

Newsweek, PTA, NU Stats. (1993). *Third PTA national education survey.* Washington, DC: Author.

Nolet, V., & McLaughlin, M. (1997). Using CBM to explore a consequential basis for the validity of a statewide performance assessment. *Diagnostique, 22*(3), 147–163.

Northwest Regional Educational Laboratory. (1990, April). *Effective schooling practices: A research synthesis,* 1990 update. Portland: Author.

Office of Program Policy Analysis and Government Accountability, The Florida Legislature. (1997, June). *Improving student performance in high-poverty schools.*

Ogden, J. (1979, April). *High school competency graduation requirements: Do they result in better graduates?* Paper presented at the Annual Meeting of the American Educational Research Association, San Francisco.

Ogden, P., Thompson, D., Russell, A., & Simons, C. (2003, Spring). Supplemental instruction: Short/long-term impact on academic performance. *Journal of Developmental Education, 26*(3), 2–9.

Ogle, D., & Fritts, J., (1981). Criterion-referenced reading assessment valuable for process as well as for data. *Phi Delta Kappan, 62*(9), 640–641.

Okey, J. R. (1974). Altering teacher and pupil behavior with mastery teaching. *School Science and Mathematics, 74,* 530–535.

Okey, J. R. (1975, August). *Development of mastery teaching materials. Final evaluation report,* USOE G-74-2990. Bloomington: Indiana University.

Olmsted, J. W. (1957). Tests, examinations, and the superior college student. *The effective use of measurement in guidance* (pp. 17–20). The Sixth Annual Western Regional Conference on Testing Problems, Educational Testing Service, Los Angeles, CA.

O'Leary, K. D., & Drabman, R. (1971). Token reinforcement programs in the classroom: A review. *Psychological Bulletin, 75,* 379–398.

O'Neill, P. (1998, July). *Writing assessment and the disciplinarity of composition.* PhD dissertation, University of Louisville.

Oshiro, E. (1996). Evaluation of the senior project. In T. W. Banta, J. P. Lund, K. E. Black, & F. W. Oblander (Eds.), *Assessment in practice: Putting principles to work on college campuses* (pp. 177–179). San Francisco: Jossey-Bass.

O'Sullivan, R. G. (1989, February). *Teacher perceptions of the effects of testing on students.* Paper presented at the Annual Meeting of the National Council on Measurement in Education, San Francisco, CA.

Oxenham, J. (1984). *Education versus qualifications?* London: Unwin Education.

Oxford Centre for Staff Development. (1992, March). *Improving student learning.* Oxford, England: Oxford Centre for Staff Development, Oxford Brookes University.

Panlasigui, I., & Knight, F. B. (1930). The effect of awareness of success or failure. In F. B. Knight (Ed.), *Twenty-ninth yearbook of the National Society for the Study of Education: Report of the society's committee on arithmetic.* Chicago: University of Chicago Press.

Parramore, B. M. (1980, November). *Effects of mandated competency testing in North Carolina: The Class of 1980.* Paper presented at the Annual Meeting of the Evaluation Research Society, Washington.

Pennycuick, D., & Murphy, R. (1988). *The impact of graded tests.* London: Falmer Press.

Perrin, M. (1991). Summative evaluation and pupil motivation. In P. Weston (Ed.), *Assessment of pupil achievement: Motivation and school success: Report of the Educational Research Workshop held in Liège [Belgium] 12–15 September.* Council of Europe. Amsterdam: Swets & Zeitlinger.

Peterson, S. J. (1981). *The uses of minimum competency testing in large city school districts of the nation,* EdD dissertation, North Texas State University.

Phelps, R. P. (1994a). *Benefit-cost analyses of testing programs*. Paper presented at the annual meeting of the American Education Finance Association, Nashville, TN.

Phelps, R. P. (1994b). *The economics of standardized testing*. Paper presented at the annual meeting of the American Education Finance Association, Nashville, TN.

Phelps, R. P. (1996, March). Test basher benefit-cost analysis. *Network News & Views, Educational Excellence Network* (pp. 1–16).

Phelps, R. P. (1998). *Benefit-cost analysis of systemwide student testing*. Paper presented at the annual meeting of the American Education Finance Association, Mobile, AL.

Phelps, R. P. (2000, September–October). Walt Haney's Texas mirage, Parts 1–4. *EducationNews.org; Commentaries and Reports*.

Phelps, R. P. (2001, August). Benchmarking to the world's best in mathematics: Quality control in curriculum and instruction among the top performers in the TIMSS. *Evaluation Review, 25*(4), 391–439.

Phelps, R. P. (2002, February). Estimating the costs and benefits of educational testing programs. *Education Consumers Clearing House*.

Phelps, R. P. (2003). *Kill the messenger: The war on standardized testing*. New Brunswick, NJ: Transaction Publishers.

Phi Delta Kappa. (1987). The 19th annual Phi Delta Kappa/Gallup poll of the public's attitudes toward the public schools. *Phi Delta Kappan, 69*, 21–34.

Phi Delta Kappa. (1991). The 23rd annual Phi Delta Kappa/Gallup poll of the public's attitudes toward the public schools. *Phi Delta Kappan, 73*(1), 20–29.

Phi Delta Kappa. (1995). The 27th annual Phi Delta Kappa/Gallup poll of the public's attitudes toward the public schools. *Phi Delta Kappan, 77*(1), 41–56.

Phi Delta Kappa. (1997). The 29th annual Phi Delta Kappa/Gallup poll of the public's attitudes toward the public schools. *Phi Delta Kappan, 79*(1), 46–59.

Pine, C. (1989). Using assessment to improve instruction: The New Jersey algebra project. In R. T. Alpert, W. P. Gorth, & R. G. Allan (Eds.), *Assessing basic academic skills in higher education: The Texas approach*. Hillsdale, NJ: Lawrence Erlbaum Associates.

Plazak, T., & Mazur, Z. (1992). University entrance in Poland. In P. Black (Ed.), *Physics examinations for university entrance: An international study. Science and technology education*. Document series, No. 45. Paris: UNESCO.

Poggio, J. (1976, April). *Long-term cognitive retention resulting from the mastery learning paradigm*. Paper presented at the annual meeting of the American Educational Research Association, San Francisco.

Poje, D. J. (1996). Student Motivation and Standardized Testing for Institutional Assessment. In T. W. Banta, J. P. Lund, K. E. Black, & F. W. Oblander (Eds.), *Assessment in practice: Putting principles to work on college campuses* (pp. 179–182). San Francisco: Jossey-Bass.

Polgar, E. (1976). *The California high school proficiency exam.*

Pollaczek, P. P. (1952). A study of malingering on the CVS abbreviated individual intelligence scale. *Journal of Clinical Psychology, 8*, 75–81.

Pomplun, M. (1997). State assessment and instructional change: A path model analysis. *Applied Measurement in Education, 10*(3), 217–34.

Popham, W. J., & Rankin, S. C. (1981, May). Minimum competency tests spur instructional improvement. *Phi Delta Kappan, 62*(9), 637–39.

Popham, W. J. (1981, October). The case for minimum competency testing. *Phi Delta Kappan, 63*(2), 89–91.

Popham, W. J., & Kirby, W. N. (1987, September). Recertification tests for teachers: A defensible safeguard for society. *Phi Delta Kappan*, pp. 45–49.

Powell, A. G. (1997, Fall). Student incentives and the college board system. *American Educator*. American Federation of Teachers.

Prais, S. (1995). *Productivity, education and training. Vol. II.* London: National Institute for Economic and Social Research.

Pressey, S. L. (1949). *Educational acceleration: Appraisals and basic problems.* Columbus, OH: Ohio State University.

Pressey, S. L. (1954). Acceleration: Basic principles and recent research. In A. Anastasi (Ed.), *Testing problems in perspective: Twenty-fifth anniversary volume of topical readings from the Invitational Conference on Testing Problems.* American Council on Education.

Pronaratna, B. (1976). *Examination reforms in Sri Lanka. Experiments and innovations in education,* No. 24. International Bureau of Migration Series. Asian Centre of Educational Innovation for Development (Bangkok), Paris: UNESCO.

Psacharopoulos, G., Velez, E., & World Bank. (1993, April). Educational quality and labor market outcomes: Evidence from Bogota, Columbia. *Sociology of Education, 66*(2).

Public Agenda. (1994). *First things first: What Americans expect from the public schools.* New York: Author.

Public Agenda Online. (2000, September). Survey finds little sign of backlash against academic standards or standardized tests. New York: Author.

Public Agenda. (2002). *Stand by me.* New York: Author.

Public Education Network, Education Week. (2002). *Accountability for all: What voters want from education candidates.* Washington, DC: Author.

Purkey, S. C., & Smith, M. S. (1983). Effective schools: A review. *The Elementary School Journal, 83*(4), 427–452.

Quinnipiac University Polling Institute. (2001, March). *Poll of New York City Adults.* Hamden, CT: Quinnipiac University.

Ramirez, G. M. (1997, Fall). Supplemental instruction: The long-term impact. *Journal of Developmental Education, 21*(1), 2–11.

Rentz, R. R. (1979). Testing and the college degree. In W. B. Schrader (Ed.), *Measurement and educational policy: New directions for testing and measurement,* (1).

Resnick, L. B., & Robinson, B. H. (1974). *Motivational aspects of the literacy problem.* University of Pittsburgh, Learning Research and Development Center.

Resnick, D. P., & Resnick, L. B. (1985). Standards, curriculum, and performance: A historical and comparative perspective. *Educational Researcher, 14*(4), 5–20.

Resnick, L. B., Nolan, K. J., & Resnick, D. P. (1995). Benchmarking education standards. *Educational Evaluation and Policy Analysis, 17*(4), 438–461.

Reynolds, D., Mujis, D., & Treharne, D. (2003). Teacher evaluation and teacher effectiveness in the United Kingdom. *Journal of Personnel Evaluation in Education, 17*(1), 83–100.

Richards, C. E., & Shen, T. M. (1992, March). The South Carolina school incentive reward program: A policy analysis. *Economics of Education Review, 11*(1), 71–86.

Riley, B. E. (1977). *Accountability in Education: A Recurring Concept.*

Rist, R. C. (1970). Student social class and teacher expectations: The self-fulfilling prophecy in ghetto education. *Harvard Educational Review, 40,* 411–451.

Ritchie, D., & Thorkildsen, R. (1994). Effects of accountability on students' achievement in mastery learning. *Journal of Educational Research, 88*(2), 86–90.

Robertson, S. N., & Simpson, C. A. (1996). In T. W. Banta, J. P. Lund, K. E. Black, & F. W. Oblander (Eds.), *General education discipline evaluation process for the community college. Assessment in practice: Putting principles to work on college campuses,* (pp. 190–194). San Francisco: Jossey-Bass.

Rodgers, N. et al. (1991, April 3–7). *High stakes minimum skills tests: Is their use increasing achievement?* Paper presented at the Annual Meeting of the American Educational Research Association, Chicago, IL.

Rohm, R. A., Sparzo, F. J., & Bennett, C. M. (1986 , November/December). College student performance under repeated testing and cumulative testing conditions: Report on five studies. *Journal of Educational Research, 80*(2), 99–104.

Rosenshine, B. (2003, August 4). High-stakes testing: Another analysis. *Educational Policy Analysis Archives, 11*(24). Retrieved August 7, 2003 from http://epaa.asu.edu/epaa/v11n24/

Ross, C. C., & Henry, L. K. (1939). The relation between frequency of testing and learning in psychology. *Journal of Educational Psychology, 69,* 710–715.

Ross, J. A., Rolheiser, C., & Hoaboam-Gray, A. (1998). *Impact of self-evaluation training on mathematics achievement in a cooperative learning environment.* Social Science and Humanities Research Council of Canada, Ottawa.

Rosswork, S. G. (1977). Goal setting: The effects of an academic task with varying magnitudes of incentive. *Journal of Educational Psychology, 69,* 710–715.

Roueche, J. (1968). *Salvage, redirection, or custody?* Washington, DC: American Association of Junior Colleges.

Roueche, J. (1973). *A modest proposal: Students can learn.* San Francisco, CA: Jossey-Bass.

Roueche, J., & Kirk, R. (1974). *Catching up: Remedial education.* San Francisco, CA: Jossey-Bass.

Roueche, J., & Roueche, S. (1999). *High stakes, high performance: Making remedial education work.* Washington, DC: American Association of Community Colleges.

Roueche, J., & Wheeler, C. (1973, Summer). Instructional procedures for the disadvantaged. *Improving college and university teaching, 21,* 222–225.

Rutter, M. (1983). School effects on pupil progress: Research findings and policy implications. In L. S. Shulman & G. Sykes (Eds.), *Handbook of Teaching and Policy* (pp. 3–41). New York: Longman.

Salmon-Cox, L. (1980). *Teachers and tests: What's really happening?* Paper presented at Annual Meeting of the American Educational Research Association.

Sanders, J. C. R. (1999). *The impact of teacher effect on student math competency achievement,* EdD dissertation, University of Tennessee, Knoxville.

Sanders, W. L., & Rivers, J. C. (1996, November). *Cumulative and residual effects of teachers on future student academic achievement.* Research Progress Report, University of Tennessee Value-Added Research and Assessment Center.

Schab, F. (1978, January). Who wants minimal competencies? *Phi Delta Kappan, 59,* 350–352.

Schafer, W. D., Hultgren, F. H., Hawley, W. D., Abrams, A. L., Seubert, C. C., & Mazzoni, S. (1997). *Study of Higher-Success and Lower-Success Elementary Schools.* School Improvement Program, University of Maryland.

Schlawin, S. A. (1981, December). *The New York State testing program in writing: Its influence on instruction.* Paper presented at the International Conference on Language Problems and Public Policy. Cancun, Mexico.

Schleisman, J. (1999, October). *An in-depth investigation of one school district's responses to an externally-mandated, high-stakes testing program in Minnesota.* Paper presented at the Annual Meeting of the University Council for Educational Administration, Minneapolis, MN. (ERIC: ED440465)

Schmoker, M. (1996). *Results: The key to continuous school improvement.* Alexandria, VA: Association for Supervision and Curriculum Development (ASCD).

Schoenecker, C. (1996, May). *Developmental education outcomes at Minnesota community colleges.* Paper presented at the 36th annual forum of the Association for Institutional Research, Albuquerque, NM.

Serow, R. C. et al. (1982, Winter). Performance gains in a competency test program. *Educational Evaluation and Policy Analysis, 4*(4), 535–542.

Shab, F. (1978, January). Who wants what minimal competencies? *Phi Delta Kappan, 59,* 350–352.

Shanker, A. (1994, May 18.). *Making standards count: The case for student incentives.* Remarks by AFT President Albert Shanker at the Brookings Institution, Washington, DC.

Shohamy, E. (1993). *The power of tests: The impact of language tests on teaching and learning.* NFLC Occasional Paper. Washington, DC: National Foreign Language Center.

Singh, J. S., Marimutha, T., & Mukjerjee, H. (1990). Learning motivation and work: A Malaysian perspective. In P. Broadfoot, R. Murphy, & H. Torrance (Eds.), *Changing educational assessment: International perspectives and trends* (pp. 177–198). London: Routledge.

Singh, J., & McMillan, J. H. (2002, April). *Staff development practices in schools demonstrating significant Improvement on high-stakes tests.* Paper presented at the Annual Meeting of the American Educational Research Association, New Orleans, LA.

Skinner, B. F. (1954). The science of learning and the art of teaching. *Harvard Educational Review, 24*(3), 86–97.

Solberg, W. (1977, May 23–28). School leaving examinations: Why or why not?: The case for school leaving examinations: The Netherlands. In F. M. Ottobre (Ed.), *Criteria for awarding school leaving certificates: An international discussion. Based on the proceedings of the 1977 Conference of the International Association for Educational Assessment held at the Kenyatta Conference Center,* (pp. 37–46). Nairobi.

Solmon, L. C., & Fagnano, C. L. (1990, Summer). Speculations on the benefits of large-scale teacher assessment programs: How 78 million dollars can be considered a mere pittance. *Journal of Education Finance, 16,* 21–36.

Somanathan, R. (1996). *School systems, educational attainment, and wages.* PhD dissertation, Boston University.

Somerset, A. (1968). *Examination reform: The Kenya experience.* Report No. EDT64. Washington, DC: The World Bank.

Somerset, A. (1996). Examinations and educational quality. In A. Little & A. Wolf (Eds.), *Assessment in transition: Learning, monitoring, and selection in international perspective.* Oxford: Pergamon-Elsevier.

South Carolina Department of Education, Division of Public Accountability. (1990, September). The exit exam. *Perspectives on South Carolina Educational Reform, 1*(1)

Southern Regional Education Board. (1998). *High Schools That Work: Case Studies.* Available at www.sreb.org

Southern Regional Education Board. (1993). *Outstanding practices for raising the achievement of career-bound high school students.* Atlanta, GA.

Southern Regional Education Board, Bradby, D., & Dykman, A. (2002). *Effects of high schools that work practices on student achievement.* Atlanta: GA.

Staats, A. (1973). Behavior analysis and token reinforcement in educational behavior modification and curriculum research. In C. E. Thoreson (Ed.), *72nd yearbook of the NSSE, behavior modification in education.* Chicago, University of Chicago Press.

Stager, S. F., & Green, K. E. (1984). *Wyoming teachers' use of tests and attitudes toward classroom and standardized tests.* University of Wyoming, Dept. of Educational Foundations.

Stake, R., & Theobald, P. (1991). Teachers' views of testing's impact on classrooms. In R. G. O'Sullivan & R. E. Stake (Eds.), *Advances in program evaluation: Effects of mandated assessment on teaching* (pp. 41–74). JAI Press.

Standards Work, Inc. (2003, February). *Study of the effectiveness of the Virginia Standards of Learning (SOL) Reforms.*

Stanley, J. C. (1976 , November). Identifying and nurturing the intellectually gifted. *Phi Delta Kappan, 58*(3), 234–237.

Stark, J. S., Shaw, K. M., & Lowther, M. A. (1989). *Student goals for college and courses.* ASHE-ERIC Higher Education Report No. 6. Washington, DC: School of Education and Human Development, George Washington University.

Steedman, H. (1992). *Mathematics in vocational youth training for the building trades in Britain, France and Germany.* Discussion Paper No. 9. London: National Institute for Economic and Social Research.

Stevens, F. I. (1984, December). *The effects of testing on teaching and curriculum in a large urban school district.* ERIC/TM Report 86, ERIC Clearinghouse on Tests, Measurement, and Evaluation.

Stevenson, H. W., Chen, C., & Uttal, D. H. (1989). *Beliefs and achievement: A study of Black, White and Hispanic children.* Unpublished manuscript.

Stevenson, H. W., Lee, S. et al. (1997). *International comparisons of entrance and exit examinations: Japan, United Kingdom, France, and Germany.* U.S. Department of Education, Office of Educational Research and Improvement.

Strauss, R. P., & Sawyer, E. A. (1986). Some new evidence on teacher and student competencies. *Economics of Education Review,* p. 41.

Strozeski, M. (2000, April). *High stakes, high standards, massive testing, and improved student success.* Paper presented at the annual meeting of the National Council on Measurement in Education. New Orleans, LA.

Stuit, D. B. (Ed.). (1947). *Personnel research and test development in the Bureau of Naval Personnel.* Princeton, NJ: Princeton University Press.

Swanson, D. H., & Denton, J. J. (1976). *A comparison of remediation systems affecting achievement and retention in mastery learning.* ERIC ED 131037.

Task Force on Educational Assessment Programs. (1979). *Competency testing in Florida: Report to the Florida cabinet, Part 1.* Tallahassee, FL.

Tanner, D. E. (199, December 5). The competency test's impact on teachers' abilities. *Urban Review, 27*(4), 347–351.

Taylor, A., Valentine, B., & Jones, M. (1985, December). *What research says about effective schools.* National Education Association.

Taylor, B., Pearson, P. D., Clark, K. F., & Walpole, S. (1999). *Beating the odds in teaching all children to read.* Report No. 2-006. Ann Arbor, MI: Center for the Improvement of Early Reading.

Terman, L. M. (1947). Genetic studies of genius, Vol. 4. In L. M. Terman & M. H. Oden (Eds.), *The gifted child grows up.* Stanford, CA: Stanford University Press.

Terman, L. M. (1954). The discovery and encouragement of exceptional talent. *American Psychologist, 9,* 221–230.

Thomas, J. W. (1992, December). Expectations and effort: Course demands, students' study practices, and academic achievement. In T. M. Tomlinson (Ed.), *Hard work and high expectations: Motivating students to learn.*

Thompson, B. (2002, November). High stakes testing and student learning: A response to Amrein and Berliner. *EducationNews.org, Commentaries and Reports.*

Thompson, T. D. (1990). *When mastery testing pays off: The cost benefits and psychometric properties of mastery tests as determined from item response theory.* PhD dissertation, University of Oklahoma.

Tobias, B. (2000, April). *The systematic impact of standards and assessments on instruction and school management.* Paper presented at the annual meeting of the National Council on Measurement in Education. New Orleans, LA.

Toenjes, L. A., Dworkin, A. G., Lorence, J., & Hill, A. N. (2000, August). *The lone star gamble: high stakes testing, accountability, and student achievement in Texas and Houston.* Department of Sociology, University of Houston.

Toppino, T. C., & Luipersbeck, S. M. (1993, July / August). Generality of the negative suggestion effect in objective tests. *Journal of Educational Research, 86*(6), 357–362.

Trelfa, D. (1998, June). The development and implementation of education standards in Japan, chapter 2. In U.S. department of education, office of educational research and improvement, national institute on student achievement, curriculum, and assessment. *The Educational System in Japan: Case Study Findings.*

Tuckman, B. W. (1994, April 4–8). Comparing Incentive motivation to metacognitive strategy in its effect on achievement. Paper presented at the Annual Meeting of the American Educational Research Association. New Orleans, LA. ERIC ED368790

Tuckman, B. W., & Trimble, S. (1997, August). *Using tests as a performance incentive to motivate eighth-graders to study.* Paper presented at the Annual Meeting of the American Psychological Association, Chicago. ERIC: ED418785

Turney, A. H. (1931). The effect of frequent short objective tests upon the achievement of college students in educational psychology. *School and Society, 33,* 760–762.

Tyler, R. W. (1941, November). *The influence of tests on teaching.* Paper presented at the Invitational Conference on Testing Problems, Tenth Educational Conference, Committee on Measurement and Guidance, American Council on Education.

Tyler, R. W. (1949). *Basic principles of curriculum and instruction.* Chicago: University of Chicago Press.

Tyler, R. W. (1959). Effect on teachers and students. In A. Anastasi (Ed.), *Testing problems in perspective: Twenty-fifth anniversary volume of Topical readings from the Invitational Conference on Testing Problems.* American Council on Education.

U.S. Department of Education. (1987). *What works: Research about teaching and learning* (p. 54). Washington.

U.S. General Accounting Office. (1993a, April). *Educational testing: The Canadian experience with standards, examinations, and assessments.* GAO/PEMD-93-11. Washington, DC.

U.S. General Accounting Office. (1993b, January). *Student testing: Current extent and expenditures, with cost estimates for a national examination.* GAO/PEMD-93-8. Washington, DC.

van Dam, P. R. L. (2000). The effects of testing on primary education in the Netherlands: The pupil monitoring system. In *The effects and related problems of large scale testing in educational assessment.* Foreign Language Teaching and Research, IAEA.

Venesky, R. L., & Winfield, L. F. (1979, August). *Schools that succeed beyond expectations in teaching.* University of Delaware Studies on Education. Technical Report, No. 1.

Wall, D., & Alderson, J. C. (1993). Examining washback: The Sri Lankan impact study. *Language Testing, 10,* 41–69.

Walstad, W. B. (1984, May–June). Analyzing minimal competency test performance. *Journal of Educational Research, 77*(5), 261–266.

Ward, J. G. (1980). *Teachers and testing: A survey of knowledge and attitudes.* American Federation of Teachers.

Waters, T., Burger, D., & Burger, S. (1995, March). Moving up before moving on. *Educational Leadership, 52*(6), 35–40.

Webb, K. A. (1996). *The benefits of standardized and nationally applicable criterion-referenced job skills assessments in proprietary postsecondary schools.* PhD dissertation, The Union Institute.

Webster, W. J., Mendro, R. L., Orsack, T., Weerasinghe, D., & Bembry, K. (1997, September). *The Dallas value-added accountability system* (pp. 81–99), and *Little practical difference and pie in the sky* (pp. 120–131). In J. Millman (Ed.), *Grading Teachers, Grading Schools: Is Student Achievement a Valid Evaluation Measure?* Thousand Oaks, CA: Corwin Press.

Weinman, J. J. (1976). *Declining test scores: A state study.* Bureau of Research and Assessment, Massachusetts Department of Education.

Winfield, L. F. (1990, March). *School competency testing reforms and student achievement: Exploring a national perspective.* Research Report. Princeton, NJ: Educational Testing Service.

Wellisch, J. B., MacQueen, A. H., Carriere, R. A., & Duck, G. A. (1978, July). School management and organization in successful schools. *Sociology of Education, 51,* 211–226.

Wenglinsky, H. (2001, September). *Teacher classroom practices and student performance: How schools can make a difference.* Educational Testing Service, Research Report RR-01-19.

Wentling, T. L. (1973). Mastery versus nonmastery instruction with varying test item feedback treatments. *Journal of Educational Psychology, 65,* 50–58.

Westbrook, B. W. (1967). The effect of test reporting on self-estimates of scholastic ability and on level of occupational aspiration. *Journal of Educational Research, 60,* 387–389.

Weston, P. (Ed.). (1991, September). Assessment and motivation: Some issues from England and Wales. In *Assessment of pupil achievement: Motivation and school success: report of the educational research workshop held in Liège [Belgium] 12-15.* Council of Europe. Amsterdam: Swets & Zeitlinger.

Whetton, C. (1992). *Advice to U.S. systems contemplating performance assessment.* Paper presented at the 1992 Annual Meeting of the American Educational Research Association, San Francisco.

Whiteley, J. W. (1980). *Effects on student achievement of a coordinated district-wide system for developing criterion-referenced objectives and tests: A formative evaluation study.* EdD dissertation, University of San Francisco.

Wildemuth, B. M. (1977). *Minimal competency testing: Issues and procedures, an annotated bibliography.* ERIC ED150188.

Wiliam, D., & Black, P. (1996, December). Meanings and consequences: A basis for distinguishing formative and summative functions of assessment? *British Educational Research Journal, 22*(5), 537–548.

Willingham, W. W., & Morris, M. (1986). *Four years later: A Longitudinal study of advanced placement students in college.* (College Board Report 86-2). New York: College Entrance Examination Board.

Willingham, W. W., Lewis, C., Morgan, R., & Ramist, L. (1990). Implications of using freshman GPA as the criterion for the predictive validity of the SAT. *Predicting college grades: An analysis of institutional trends over two decades.* Princeton, NJ: Educational Testing Service.

Wilson, B. I., & Dickson Corbett, H. (1990). Statewide testing and local improvement: An oxymoron? In J. Murphy (Ed.), *The educational reform movement of the 1980s: Perspectives and cases.* Berkeley, CA: McCutcheon.

Winfield, L. F. (1987, March). *The relationship between minimum competency testing programs and students' reading proficiency: Implications from the 1983–1984 national assessment of educational progress of reading and writing.* Research Report, Educational Testing Service.

Winfield, L. F. (1990). School competency testing reforms and student achievement: Exploring a national perspective. *Education Evaluation and Policy Analysis, 12*(2), 157–173.

Woessman, L. (2000, December). *Schooling resources, educational institutions, and student performance: The international evidence.* Kiel Institute of World Economics. Kiel Working Paper No. 983.

Wolf, A., & Rapiau, M. T. (1993). The academic achievement of craft apprentices in France and England: Contrasting systems and common dilemmas. *Comparative Education, 29*(1).

Wolf, L. F., & Smith, J. K. (1995). The consequence of consequence: Motivation, anxiety, and test performance. *Applied Measurement in Education, 8*(3), 227–242.

Wood, R. G. (1953). A twenty-year pilot study of what has become of Ohio's superior high school graduates. In the *Tenth Yearbook of the National Council on Measurements in Education.*

Wrightstone, J. W. (1963). The relation of testing programs to teaching and learning. In N. B. Henry & H. G. Richey (Eds.), *Sixty-second yearbook of the National Society for the Study of Education, Part II: The impact and improvement of school testing programs.* Chicago: University of Chicago Press.

Yeh, J. P. (1978). *Test use in schools.* Washington, DC: National Institute of Education.

Yeh, J., Herman, J., & Rudner, L. M. (1983). A survey of the use of various achievement tests. In L. W. Rudner (Ed.), *Testing in our schools: Proceedings of the NIE Invitational Conference on Test Use.* Washington, DC: National Institute of Education, June 2, 1980.

Yussufu, A., & Angaka, J. A. (2000). National examinations and their effects on curriculum development and implementation in Kenya. In *The effects and related problems of large scale testing in educational assessment.* Foreign Language Teaching and Research, IAEA.

Zigarelli, M. A. (1996). An empirical test of conclusions from effective schools research. *Journal of Educational Research, 90*(2), 103–110.

Author Index

A

Aaron, 144, *146*
Abbott, 75, 86, *87*
Aber, 71, *87*
Allalouf, 162, *172*
Amrein, 29–31, 43, *50*
Anastasi, 116, *120*, 154, *157*, 195, *201*
Anderson, 97, *109*
Angel, 163, *172*
Angoff, *185*, 190, *201*
Apgar, 48
Archer, 249, *252*
Astuto, 73, 86, *87*
Averch, 73, *87*

B

Banerji, 40, 50
Bangert-Drowns, 72, 74, 86, *87*, 167, *172*
Barrett, 76
Battiste, 63, *88*
Beaudry, 40, *51*
Ben-Shakhar, 162, *172*
Berk, 190, *201*
Berliner, 29–31, 43, *50*
Bhola, 94, *109*
Bishop, 30, *51*, 71, 77–79, *87*
Bloom, 76

Bonnur, 167, *173*
Boudreau, 71, *87*
Bourque, xviii
Bowers, 20, 22
Bowman, 30, *51*
Bracey, 25, 27, *51*
Braun, 30, *51*, 80, *87*
Brennan, 94, *109*
Brody, 208, *218*
Brooks, 24, *51*
Brown, D., 168, *172*
Bruce, 105, *109*
Buckendahl, xvi, 94, 182, *185*
Butcher, 197, *201*

C

Callenbach, 167, *172*
Cameron, 65, *87*
Camilli, 42, 45, 46, *51*
Campanile, 168, *172*
Campbell, 209, *219*
Cannell, 164, *173*
Carlin, 218, 222
Carnoy, 30, *51*, 80
Carroll, 73, *87*
Carter, 41, *51*
Casella, *219*, 222
Chenoweth, 28, *51*

Cizek, xv, 26, 32, 42, 45, *51, 52,* 103, *109,*
  166, *173,* 183, *185*
Clark, 73, 86, *87*
Cleary, 189, 195, *201*
Cohen, 241, *253*
Cole, 57, 71, *87,* 189, *201, 203*
Cook, 94, *109*
Corbett, 18
Cotton, 73, 86, *88*
Cracium, 246, *252*
Crocker, xvi, 168, 171, *173*
Cronbach, 77, 187, *201*
Crooks, 73–76, *88*
Cunningham, xvi, 139, *146*

D

Damico, 188, *202*
Darlington, 189, *201*
Dawes, 188, *201*
Delisi, 159, 166, 168, *174*
Denny, 153, *158*
Dickens, 50, *51*
Divine, 105, *109*
Dobbs, 249, *252*
Doerr, 187, *202*
Doherty, 163, 165, *173*
Donaldson, 73, *87*
Dorn, 29, *51*
Dornbush, 72, 76, *89*
Driesler, 29, *51*
Dunn, 194, *201*
Duran, 191, *202*

E

Eckstein, 69
Edmonds, 73, *88*
Eignor, 94, *109*
Elam, 5–7, 10, *22*
Elliot, 41, *53*
Ellwein, 41, *52*
Engel, 37, *53*
Eyde, 191, *201*

F

Falstrom, 76, 86, *87*
Farkus, 4, *22*
Finn, 39, *51*
Flanagan, 79, *88,* 230, *252*
Flaugher, 189, *201*
Fontana, 68, *88*

Forte Fast, 102, *109*
Fredericksen, 67, 79, *88*
Fremer, vii
Friedman, 75, 86, *88*

G

Gallup, 6, *22*
Gardner, 189, *201*
Garner, 188, *203*
Gates, 72, 75, 86, *88*
Gay, 105, *109*
Geisinger, xvii, 189, 191, 192, 195, 197,
  199, 200, *201*
Gifford, 188, *202*
Gladwell, 206, *219*
Golan, 170, *173*
Goldberg, 38, *51*
Gooding, 56, 71, *90*
Goodman, xv, 107, *109*
Gorth, 64, *88*
Gould, 187, *202*
Graue, 164, *173*
Green, 133, 134, *146,* 182, *185*
Greene, 39, *52*
Grissmer, 79, *88,* 230, *252*
Gronlund, 116, *121*
Gruber, 241, *253*
Gullickson, 41, *52*
Guskey, 36, *52,* 72, 75, 86, *88*

H

Haas, 171, *173*
Haertel, 215, *218*
Haladyna, 171, *173*
Hamayan, 188, *202*
Hambleton, xv, 105–107, *109, 110,* 183,
  185
Hamilton, 166, *173,* 230, *252*
Haney, 187, *202,* 230, *252*
Hanson, 187, *202*
Hanushek, 30, *53*
Harper, 63, *88*
Harris, 12, *22*
Hartigan, 188, *202*
Hawisher, 63, *88*
Hayward, 44, *52*
Henke, 241, *253*
Henry, 77
Herman, 170, *173*
Hill, 206, *219,* 223
Hilliard, 27, *52*

Hillocks, 159, *173*
Hills, 37, *52*
Hiskay, 194, *202*
Hoff, 252
Hoffman, 187, *202*
Holland, 190, 193, *202*
Hombo, 168, *173*
Hoxby, 100, *109*
Huff, 94, *100*
Huffington, 2, *22*
Hunt, xvi
Hunter, J. E., 56, 71, *88, 90*
Hunter, R. F., 56, 71, *88*

I

Impara, 38, *52*, 105, *109*, 176, 181, 182, *185*

J

Jackson, 63, *88*
Jacobson, 79, *88*
Jaeger, 133, *146*, 183, *185*
Jenifer, 189, *202*
Jenkins, 79, *89*, 105, *109*
Jennings, 164, *173*
Johnson, 79, *89*
Jones, 71, 86, *88, 90*
Jungeblut, 105, *109*

K

Kamin, 188, 196, *202*
Kaminski, 170, *173*
Kane, M., 117, *120*
Kane, T., 206, 218, *219*
Kannapel, 28, *52*
Kawata, 79, *88*, 230, *252*
Keys, 77
Kiesling, 73, *87*
Kirkland, 63, 73, 74, 76, 77, *88*
Kirkpatrick, 77
Kirsch, L., 105, *109*
Kirsch, M., 56, 71, *90*
Klein, 230, *252*
Kohn, 27, 28, *52*, 159, *173*, 187, *202*
Kolen, 94, *109*
Kolstad, 105, *109*
Koretz, 166, *173*
Kulik, C. L., 72, 74, 75, 86, *87, 88*, 167, *172*
Kulik, J. A., 72, 74, 75, 86, *87, 88*, 167, *172*

L

Latham, 72, *89*
Lattimore, 28, *52*, 159, *173*
Lehman, *219*, 222
Lemann, 162, *173*, 187, *202*
Lewis, C., 56, 71, *185*
Lewis, D. M., *90*, 133, 134, *146*, 182
Linn, 116, *121*, 162, 164, *173*
Liverman, 105, *109*
Locke, 72, *89*
Loeb, 30, *51*, 80
Lohman, 195, *203*
Lotto, 73, 86, *87*
Louis, *218*, 222
Lugg, 42, *51*
Lukhele, 135, 137, 140, 141, *146*
Lyons, 187, *202*

M

Mabry, 138, *146*
Mackenzie, 73, *89*
Madaus, 28, *52*, 159, *173*, 187, *202*
Manno, 39, *51*
Manuel, 57, *89*
McCaffrey, 166, *173*, 230, *252*
McGrath, 241, *253*
McFarland, 100, *110*
McKenzie, 56, *90*
McPhail, 160, 168, *173*
Meara, 105, *110*
Mehrens, 26, 45, 50, *52*, 157, *158*, 166, 168, 170, *173*
Meisels, 28, *52*
Messick, 117, *121*, 153, *158*
Miller, 228, *252*
Millman, 162, 167, *173*
Mills, 183, *185*
Milton, 63, *89*
Miron, 39, *52*
Mitzel, 182, *185*
Morgan, 56, 71, *89, 90*
Morris, *219*, 222
Muldrow, 56, *90*
Mullis, 79, *89*
Murnane, 73, *89*

N

Nairn, 188, *202*
Natriello, 72, 76, *89*
Nelson, 39, *52*

Noah, 69
Noe, 56, 71, *90*
Nolan, 171, *173*
Novick, 189, *202*

O

O'Connor, 188, *202*
Ohanian, 27, *52*
Olmsted, 71, *89*
Olson, 233, 246, *253*
O'Neil, 94, *110*
Orlich, 30, *52*
Owen, 187, *202*

P

Paige, 250
Pancheri, 197, *201*
Patz, 182, *185*
Pauk, 162, 168, *173*
Pennock-Roman, 196, *202*
Perkins, 64, *88*
Peterson, 189, *202*
Phelps, viii, xiv–xv, 3, 22, 29, 41, *52, 53,*
       62, 79, 89, 97–100, *110*
Phillips, 151, 154, *158*
Pierce, 65, *87*
Pincus, 73, *87*
Pitoniak, 142–144, *146,* 152, *158*
Plake, xvii, 38, *52,* 176, 181–183, *185*
Popham, 157, *158,* 159, 164, 168, 170, 171,
       173
Powers, 162, 173
Pressey, 71, *89*
Purkey, 73, 86, *89*

R

Ramist, 56, 71, *89, 90*
Raymond, 30, *53*
Rebarber, 100, *110*
Reckase, 237, *253*
Reeves, 171, *174*
Richard, 250, *253*
Robelen, 231, 250, *253*
Rock, 162, *173*
Roderick, 37, *53*
Rodriguez, 136, *146*
Rogosa, xvii, 206, 207, 214–215, 217–218,
       219, 220, 223
Rose, 6, 11, 22
Rosenshine, 30, *53,* 73, 80, *89*
Rosswork, 76
Roswell, 38, *51*

Rottenberg, 28, *53,* 159, 170, *174*
Royer, 142–144, *146,* 152, *158*
Ryan, 168, *173*

S

Sacks, 159, *173,* 187, *202*
Salvia, 195, *202*
Samuda, 188, *202*
Sanders, 164, *173*
Sandoval, 191, *202*
Sarnacki, 167, *173*
Scheuneman, 190, *203*
Schmeiser, 162, *173,* 189, *203*
Schmidt, 56, 71, *88, 90*
Schmitt, 56, 71, *90*
Schneiders, 20, *22*
Schrag, 32, *53*
Scruggs, 167, *173*
Seastrom, 241, *253*
Seebach, 31, *53*
Shaw, 30, *53*
Shepard, 117, *121,* 164, *174*
Shoben, 149, *158*
Silber, 118
Sireci, xv–xvi, 94, *110,* 117, *121*
Skinner, 163, 165, *173*
Slater, 105, *109*
Smisko, 153, *158*
Smith, 80
Smith, J. K., 159, 166, 168, *174*
Smith, L. F., 159, 166, 168, *174*
Smith, M. L., 28, *53,* 159, 170, *174*
Smith, M. S., 73, 80, 86, *89*
Smith, R. W., 182, *185*
Staats, 73, *90*
Staiger, 218, *219*
Stake, 60
Stanley, 71, *90*
Starch, 41, *53*
Stecher, 166, *174,* 230, *252*
Sternberg, 144, *146*
Stiggins, 38, *53*
Stoddard, 57
Stuit, 77
Swerling, 144, *146*

T

Taylor, 86, *90*
Terman, 71, *90*
Theobald, 60
Thissen, 135, 137, 140, 141, *146*
Thompson, B., 30, *53,* 80, *90*

Thompson, S., 27, *53*
Thorndike, 195, *203*
Thurlow, 37, *53*
Tinkleman, 163, *174*
Tittle, 190, *203*
Trimble, 133, 134, *146*
Tuckman, 65, *90*
Tufte, 106, *110*
Turney, 77
Twing, 153, *158*

U

Urbina, 195, *201*

V

Valentine, 86, *90*
Vanourek, 39, *51*
Viator, 19, 20, *22*

W

Wainer, 105, 106, *110*, 135, 137, 140, 141, *146*, 190, 193, *202*

Webb, 94, *110*, 153, *158*
Wedman, 71, *90*
Weintraub, 30, 31, *53*
Wenglinsky, 80, *90*
West, 19, *22*
Westbrook, 76
White, 167, *173*
Wigdor, 188, *203*
Wildemuth, 63, *90*
Williams, 188, *203*
Williamson, 79, *88*, 230, *252*
Willingham, 56, 57, 71, *87*, *90*, 192, 199, *203*
Wilson, B. L., 18
Wilson, L. W., 166, 168, *174*
Winfield, 67, 79, *90*
Winter, 29, *54*
Woessman, 79, *90*
Wong, 229, *253*

Y

Ysseldyke, 37, *53*, 195, *202*

Subject Index

A

Academic Performance Index (API), xvii, 205–225
Accommodations, 37, 141–144, 190–200, 232
Accountability Systems and Reporting State Collaborative on Assessment and Student Standards, 107
Achieve, 29
ACT, 29, 100, 162, 189, 190, 193
Adequate Yearly Progress (AYP), 231, 233–235, 242–249
Adjustable Mortgage Approach, 233
Advanced Placement (AP) Exams, 39, 43, 135–138, 162, 163
Adverse Impact, 149–150
Age Discrimination in Employment Act (ADEA), 149
Albert Shanker Institute, 15
America 2000, 228
American Achievement Tests, 8, 228
American Association of School Administrators (AASA), 18, 19
American Educational Research Association (AERA), xvi, 40, 119, 120, 126, 147–150, 156, 170, 171, 192
American Federation of Teachers (AFT), 17
American National Standards Institute (ANSI), 147
American Psychological Association (APA), 119, 126, 147–150, 156, 170, 171, 192
American Test Publishers (ATP), 147
Americans with Disabilities Act (ADA) of 1990, 149, 191–195, 198–200
Analytical Judgment Method, 183
Anderson v. Banks, 151
Angoff Method, 133–134, 180–183
Annual Testing, 232, 233
Apgar Scoring, 48
Applied Measurement in Education, 41
Arizona, 30
Army *Alpha*, 196
Army *Beta*, 196
Association of American Publishers (AAP), 16
Association for Supervision and Curriculum Development (ASCD), 19
Atlantic Monthly, 32

B

Back Translation, 197–200
Backlash, 13–16, 27, 29
Bayes Theorem, 209–225
Bookmark Method, 103, 133, 134, 181, 182

337

Boston College, 17–20
Boston Herald, 44
Brookhart v. Illinois State Board of Education, 151
Buros Center, 120, 147
Bush, George H. W., xviii, 8, 228
Bush, George W., 9, 13, 227, 229, 230
Business Roundtable, 15, 29, 250

C

California, xvii, 30, 205–218
California Governor's Performance Awards (GPA), 207–215
Canada, 82, 83, 92
CBS, 15
Center for Educational Assessment (University of Massachusetts), 102
Center on Education Policy, 249
Cheating, 25, 31, 164, 170
Civil Rights Act of 1964, xvi, 149–152
Clinton, Bill, xviii, 8, 228–229
CNN, 18
Code of Fair Testing Practices in Education, 190
College Entrance Examination Board, 56, 57, 71, 189, 192–193
Consortium on Chicago School Research, 37
Criterion-Referenced, 93, 114–116, 125–127, 161, 164
CTB, 135, 190
Curricular Alignment, 42, 92–95, 150–153, 164–166, 232, 238–240, 248
Cutscore (*see* Passing Score)

D

Debra P. vs. Turlington, xvi, 41, 150–152
Disability Rights Advocates, 192
Dropouts, 25, 44, 108
Due Process, 150–152

E

Educate America Act, 37
Education Commission of the States, 245–246
Education Week, 18, 93–96, 99, 228, 231, 246
Educational Measurement: Issues and Practice, 28
Educational Resource Information Clearinghouse (ERIC), 63

Educational Testing Service (ETS), 22, 55, 67, 127, 135, 162, 163, 188, 189, 192
Elementary and Secondary Education Act (ESEA), 163, 164, 227–231, 249
English As a Second Language (ESL) (*see* Ethnic Minorities)
English Language Learners (ELL) (*see* Ethnic Minorities)
Equal Employment Opportunity Commission (EEOC), 149
Equating, 94
Ethnic Minorities, xvii, 139, 141–144, 148–150, 152, 190–198, 210–211, 213–218, 234
Evaluating Professional Development, 36

F

False Negatives, 213–218
False Positives, 213–218
Florida, 33, 40, 150–152
Florida Statutes, 33
Forte Fast, 107

G

Gallup, 4–6, 15, 17, 18, 20
GI Forum v. Texas Education Agency, xvi, 152–154
Goals 2000, 37
Graduate Record Examination (GRE), 114, 135, 162, 192, 200
Gwinnett County (GA) Public Schools, 49

H

Hazelwood School District v. the United States, 149
High School and Beyond (HSB), 66, 79

I

IAEP, 78
IDEA, 141–144
IEA-Reading, 78
Improving America's Schools Act, 36, 37
Integrated Judgment Method, 183
Integer Incrementation, 215–218
International Baccalaureate (IB), 39, 43
International Standards Organization (ISO), 147
International Test Commission (ITC), 147
INTASC, 124

Iowa Test of Basic Skills, 135
Items, 156, 157
    Bias, 100–102, 148, 190–194
    Constructed-Response, 93, 135–141,
        160, 179–183, 188
    Difficulty, 134, 140, 141, 190
    Multiple-Choice, 135–141, 160,
        178–180, 188

J

J. D. Franz Research, 16
Johnson, Lyndon B., 227–228

K

Kentucky, 28

L

Lake Wobegon Effect, 164
Language Minorities (*see* Ethnic Minorities)
Law School Admission Test (LSAT), 114
Limited-English Proficient (LEP) (*see* Ethnic Minorities)
Louis Harris, 12, 13, 19
Lower-Order Thinking, 30, 41, 114, 124
Luntz/Laszlo, 18

M

Maine, 40
Mantel-Haenszel Procedure, 102
Margin of Error, xvii, 205–215
Market Opinion Research, 11
Maryland, 108
Maryland School Performance Assessment Program (MSPAP), 38
Mass Insight Education, 44, 96
Massachusetts, 30, 44, 93, 95, 97
Massachusetts Comprehensive Assessment System (MCAS), 44, 45,
        96, 111–112
Massachusetts Department of Education, 93, 98
Mastery Learning, 71, 72, 75, 76, 86, 116, 171
Measurement-Driven Instruction, 165, 166

N

Nation at Risk, A, 8, 86, 229

National Assessment of Educational Progress (NAEP), 29, 66, 78–80, 100,
        105, 135, 145, 231–233, 236–245
National Assessment Governing Board (NAGB), 236
National Center for Education Statistics (NCES), 241
National Commission on Excellence in Education, 229
National Commission on Testing and Public Policy (NCTPP), 96, 97
National Council on Education Standards and Testing (NCEST), 228
National Council on Measurement in Education (NCME), 119, 126,
        147–150, 156, 170, 171, 192
National Council of Teachers of Mathematics (NCTM), 129
National Education Association (NEA), 16, 29
National Educational Longitudinal Study (NELS), 66, 79
National Goals Panel, 228–229
National Governors Association (NGA), 228, 250
National Occupational Certification Association (NOCA), 147
National Research Council (NRC), 86, 93, 188
National Science Foundation (NSF), 17, 19, 20
NCATE, 124
NCTAF, 124
Nebraska Test of Learning Aptitude, 194
New Jersey, 36
New Jersey Administrative Code, 36, 37
New Jersey Department of Education, 63
New Standards Project, 164
New York, 93, 104, 163
New York State Education Department, 93
New York State Regents Scholarship Examination, 163
New York Times, 29
No Child Left Behind (NCLB) Act, xvii,
        xviii, 9, 12–15, 26, 36, 37, 40, 91,
        93, 99, 100, 107, 123, 127, 131,
        144, 148, 153, 165, 206, 227–251
Norm-Referenced, 114–116, 125–127,
        130–132, 161, 164, 177, 194–195,
        247
North Carolina, xvii, 32, 38, 93
North Carolina Department of Public Instruction, 93

Northwest Regional Laboratory for Education Research, 73, 86

O

Ohio, 163
Opportunity-to-Learn, 124, 150–152
Orange County Register, 205–225

P

Paige, Rod, 250
Paraprofessionals, 235
Partial Incrementation, 215–218
Passing Score, xvi, xvii, 30–34, 102–104, 118, 119, 124, 130–135, 143, 156, 165, 175–185, 232
PBS, 118
Peabody Picture Vocabulary Test, 194
Pennsylvania Code, 33
Percentage-Point Differential, 9–16, 81–83
Peter D. Hart, 17
Phi Delta Kappa, 4–6, 15, 17, 18, 20, 21, 27
Polling the Nations, 7
PRAXIS, 127
Professional Development, 35–37, 171, 240–242
Project Head Start, 194
Psychological Corporation, 190
Public Agenda, 4, 16, 18, 85
Public Opinion Polls, xiv, 1–22

R

Rehabilitation Act of 1973, 191–192, 198–200
Reliability, xvi, 116–118, 137, 154, 195
Remediation, 96
Report Cards, State and District, 234, 235, 247
Richardson v. Lamar City Board of Education, 153
Riverside Corporation, 190
Rocky Mountain News, 31
Roper Center, 7

S

SAT, 43, 100, 117, 135, 161, 162, 187–190, 192, 195
Sacramento Bee, 30
Schools and Staffing Survey, 241
Schoolsite Employee Performance Bonus Program, 207

Science Research Associates, 190
Scope and Sequencing, 152
Scoring, 152–157
   Analytic, 137, 138, 182, 183
   Holistic, 137, 138, 182, 183
Selection (*see* Validity, Predictive)
Setting the Record Straight, 29
Society of Industrial-Organizational Psychologists (SIOP), 147
Southern Regional Education Board (SREB), 69
Standardized Tests, xvi, 113, 114
   Consequences of, xv, 11–15, 25–50, 62, 108, 150–152, 161, 187–188
   Costs, 96–100
   Extent of, 41, 96–98, 249–250
   High-Stakes xv, xvi, 11–15, 25–50, 62, 92–96, 108, 150–152, 161, 179, 184, 187, 188, 236
   IQ, 8, 188
   Minimum Competency. 8, 60, 63, 64
   "Teaching to," 28, 31, 94, 159–172
   Security, 98–99, 156
Standards, 32–34, 93
   Absolute, 127, 130–132
   Content, 32–34, 42, 92–94, 156, 165, 128–130, 232
   Performance (*see* Passing Score)
   Referenced, 125, 165
   Setting (*see* Passing Score)
Standards for Educational and Psychological Testing, xvi, 119, 120, 126, 147–157, 192
Standards of Learning (SOL), 43
Standards-based Education Reform (SBER), 124–145
Stanford Achievement Test (SAT9), 43, 135, 207
Stanley Kaplan, 161, 162
Steady Stair-Step Approach, 233
Sylvan Learning Centers, 19

T

Tarrance Group, 16
Task Force on Educational Assessment Programs, 68
Teacher Competency, 235, 242, 248
Terra Nova, 135
Test Corporation of America, 120
Test Preparation, xvi, 94, 95, 159–172
Test Scores
   Reporting, 38, 39, 94, 104–107, 119, 120, 144, 145, 147, 156, 193, 234, 235

Single, 31, 34, 95, 96
Volatility, xvii
Texas, 41, 152–154, 230
Texas Assessment of Academic Skills
(TAAS), 153, 230
Third International Mathematics and Science Study (TIMSS), 66, 78, 79
Title 1, 164, 227–251
Tyler v. Vickery, 153

U

USA Today, 18, 44
U.S. Constitution, 9, 55
14th Amendment, xvi, 150– 152
U.S. Education Department, 36, 127, 228, 231, 233, 238, 245, 246, 249–251
U.S. General Accounting Office, 96–100
U.S. Office of Technology Assessment, 97

V

Validity, xvi, 6, 116–118, 137–138, 160–162, 188, 189, 192
Consequential, 58
Construct, 142, 143
Content, 141, 170
Curricular, 150–153
Predictive, 56, 57, 71
Vanderbilt University, 194
Virginia, 43, 108
Virginian-Pilot, 43
Voluntary National Tests, 9, 229

W

Washington, 30, 163
Wisconsin, 32
Wisconsin Statutes, 32